Clinical Hematology: A Case-Based Approach

Clinical Hematology:
A Case-Based Approach

Edited by Malcolm Porter

hayle medical

New York

Hayle Medical,
750 Third Avenue, 9th Floor,
New York, NY 10017, USA

Visit us on the World Wide Web at:
www.haylemedical.com

ISBN: 978-1-63241-888-3

Cataloging-in-Publication Data

Clinical hematology : a case-based approach / edited by Malcolm Porter.
     p. cm.
Includes bibliographical references and index.
ISBN 978-1-63241-888-3
1. Hematology. 2. Hematology--Case studies. 3. Blood--Diseases.
4. Blood--Diseases--Treatment. I. Porter, Malcolm.
RC633 .C55 2020
616.15--dc23

Table of Contents

Preface

The purpose of the book is to provide a glimpse into the dynamics and to present opinions and studies of some of the scientists engaged in the development of new ideas in the field from very different standpoints. This book will prove useful to students and researchers owing to its high content quality.

The branch of medicine that is concerned with the cause, prognosis, prevention and treatment of disorders of the blood is known as hematology. The diseases affecting the production of blood and its components, such as hemoglobin, blood cells, bone marrow, blood proteins, spleen, blood vessels, etc. are also under the scope of hematology. This field largely focuses on the conditions of the bone marrow and the lymphatic organs, including platelet and blood count irregularities. Organs that are fed by blood cells, such as lymph nodes, thymus, spleen and lymphoid tissue are also studied under this field. Some hematological disorders are bleeding disorders and cancers, hemophilia and blood clots. Lymphoma and leukemia are hematological malignancies. Complete blood count is the most common hematological test. It is generally performed to detect anemia, blood cancers, infections, clotting anomalies and immune system disorders. Other hematological tests are blood enzyme test, blood chemistry test and blood tests for assessing risks of heart diseases. This book unfolds the innovative aspects of hematology which will be crucial for the progress of this field in the future. It will also provide interesting topics for research which interested readers can take up. The extensive content of this book provides the readers with a thorough understanding of the subject.

At the end, I would like to appreciate all the efforts made by the authors in completing their chapters professionally. I express my deepest gratitude to all of them for contributing to this book by sharing their valuable works. A special thanks to my family and friends for their constant support in this journey.

Editor

A Challenging Case of Kikuchi-Fujimoto Disease Associated with Systemic Lupus Erythematosus

Mihaela Găman [iD],[1,2] Ana-Maria Vlădăreanu,[1,2] Camelia Dobrea,[1] Minodora Onisâi [iD],[1,2] Cristina Marinescu [iD],[1,2] Irina Voican,[2] Daniela Vasile,[1,2] Horia Bumbea,[1,2] and Diana Cîşleanu[1,2]

[1]Carol Davila University of Medicine and Pharmacy, Bucharest, Romania
[2]Department of Hematology, University Emergency Hospital Bucharest, Bucharest, Romania

Correspondence should be addressed to Minodora Onisâi; minodorel@yahoo.com

Academic Editor: Kostas Konstantopoulos

Kikuchi–Fujimoto disease (KFD) or histiocytic necrotizing lymphadenitis is a rare disease that is frequently underdiagnosed due to clinical features that are similar to those of non-Hodgkin lymphomas, systemic lupus erythematosus (SLE), or infectious reactive lymphadenopathy. An excisional biopsy is required. We report a young Caucasian female diagnosed with KFD with skin lesions, complicating with SLE. The clinical course, laboratory, and CT findings are described, as are histopathologic features, for a better recognition of this rare disorder in clinical practice.

1. Introduction

Kikuchi–Fujimoto disease (KFD) is a self-limiting disease that is characterized by cervical adenopathies and fever [1, 2]. Although KFD is reported in various ethnic groups and geographical areas, young Asian females are frequently affected. The onset is acute or subacute, with painful cervical nodes and fever in previously young individuals who were previously healthy. Extranodal manifestations are rare [3]. The skin is commonly affected (16–40% of patients), with nonspecific lesions [4]. The diagnosis represents a challenge due to similar features to non-Hodgkin lymphoma (NHL), systemic lupus erythematosus (SLE), and reactive lymphadenopathy; however, examination by an experienced morphopathologist offers a correct diagnosis. KFD lymphadenitis presents coagulative necrosis and karyorrhectic debris [3].

Several reports have emphasized the importance of KFD and SLE association. KFD can precede or coexist with SLE [4]. Some authors recommend antinuclear antibody (ANA) screening at diagnosis and close follow-up, especially in patients with cutaneous lesions for the early detection of an autoimmune disease [5–8].

2. Case Report

A 26-year-old Caucasian female was admitted to the hospital with fever, chills, and malaise. The patient reported fever of up to 39°C for the past 4 weeks, intermittent arthralgia of bilateral proximal and distal interphalangeal joints of the hands. One year prior to this, she presented with a similar episode of fever and tender cervical lymph node. She underwent a biopsy with a diagnosis of reactive lymphadenitis. The symptoms resolved spontaneously. No tests to exclude an autoimmune disease were performed. Her medical history included insulin-dependent type 1 diabetes.

Clinical examination revealed a febrile patient with enlarged and tender bilateral cervical and axillary lymph nodes as well as hepatomegaly. Scattered erythematous macules were noted on the neck, trunk, and upper extremities.

Laboratory studies are presented in Table 1. She had a high erythrocyte sedimentation rate, moderate anemia, leukopenia with marked lymphopenia, negative inflammatory markers, increased hepatic enzymes, hypoalbuminemia, and albuminuria (1815 mg/24 h). Blood cultures were negative. Serologic tests for hepatitis B and C, HIV, Epstein–Barr virus, cytomegalovirus, and toxoplasmosis were negative. She had a positive ANA titer (1/3200) and positive double-strand DNA antibodies (2628 UI/mL), negative rheumatoid factor, C3 complement, and smooth muscle antibodies. Normocellular marrow with no tumor cells was found on bone marrow biopsy.

CT scan revealed generalized lymphadenopathy involving the submandibular, cervical, supraclavicular, and axillary areas, the mediastinum, and the intra-abdominal and inguinal regions ranging in size from 0.9 cm to 2.5 cm. CT also revealed hepatomegaly (right lobe 21 cm craniocaudal diameter) and pleural effusion (2.3 cm right side and 0.5 cm left side).

Excisional biopsy of axillary lymphadenopathy was diagnostic for KFD (Figure 1). There was an effaced architecture with foci of necrosis containing karyorrhectic debris, a polymorphic infiltration pattern with abundant histiocytes, large transformed lymphocytes with immunoblast morphology, and rare tangible macrophages. No polymorphonuclear leukocytes or plasma cells were identified. Immunohistochemical staining showed abundant CD3 dim positive immunoblastic activated cytotoxic T-cells that outnumbered CD20 immunoblastic B-cells, scattered CD56 NK cells, rare CD30 cells, and a large number of CD68/KP1 histiocytes. Pankeratin and ALK were negative.

Antipyretics and nonsteroidal anti-inflammatory drugs were started with slow clinical improvement. The patient was treated with prednisone 1 mg/kg/day × 2 weeks, which was then tapered. The arthralgias improved, fever did not reappear, and a gradual attenuation of skin lesions was noted. Soon after hospitalization in the Hematology Department, she was referred to the rheumatologist for evaluation and closer follow-up of her autoimmune disease.

3. Discussion

Kikuchi disease occurs in a wide age range of patients but usually affects young adults. The age of diagnosis in our patient was similar to that in other published series (median age of 20 to 30 years), including mostly Asian females with a male : female ratio of 1 : 2 [9–11]. Kikuchi disease may be underdiagnosed due to similarities with other disorders. Recent data reported increasing incidence outside of Asia for all races [12–14], yet very rare cases of KFD are reported in Caucasian population and the exact incidence is unknown.

Pathogenesis remains unclear. Various infections have been proposed, such as Epstein–Barr virus, human herpes virus, herpes simplex virus, hepatitis B, parvovirus B19, human T-lymphotrophic virus 1, Yersinia enterocolitica, and toxoplasma [4, 15]. This theory is based on the self-limited course, laboratory findings (atypical morphologic lymphocytes on peripheral blood smear, as well as elevated inflammatory cytokines interferon α, and interleukin 6), and histological features (CD8 + T-lymphocytes that induce cell apoptosis). These cells later undergo apoptosis themselves, resulting in a necrosis background [3, 16, 17]. However, the results are inconclusive, and it is not clear whether infections are responsible for pathogenesis. Other reports suggested an autoimmune origin because KFD has been reported to simultaneously occur or follow SLE. Our patient also associated with autoimmune

TABLE 1: Laboratory tests.

Parameter	Results	Normal range
ESR (mm/h)	68	<20
Hemoglobin (g/dl)	8.7	14–18
Hematocrit (%)	27.0	42–52
WBC (×10⁹/mmc)	2.2	4–10
Differential	80% neutrophils, 14% lymphocytes, 2% bands, 4% monocytes	
PLT (×10⁹/mmc)	238	150–450
CRP (mg/l)	3.88	<5
Procalcitonin (ng/mL)	<0.5	<0.5
AST (U/L)	89	2–40
ALT (U/L)	120	3–65
GGT (U/L)	190	5–85
LDH (U/L)	345	125–220
Albumin (g/dl)	1.9	3.4–5.2
Albuminuria (mg/dl)	72.6	0–3
Albuminuria/24 hours	1815 mg/24 h	

features—SLE criteria in addition to a 17-year-history of diabetes type 1. Other autoimmune diseases (Still's disease, Sjogren's syndrome, polymyositis, and rheumatoid arthritis) have rarely been reported to be associated with KFD [4, 18–20].

Lymphadenopathies are the most relevant manifestations. The cervical area is a frequently involved site with severe pain or tenderness. KFD usually presents as solitary or multiple enlarged cervical lymph nodes and rarely with generalized lymphadenopathies, such as in our case [21–23].

Fever is another manifestation, which is present in 30–50% of reported cases. Less common clinical findings include weight loss, malaise, chills, night sweats, or gastrointestinal symptoms [24].

Few reports noted hepatomegaly as presenting extranodular sites. Biopsies performed in published cases revealed that reactive changes and hepatic enzymes reverted to normal after a short period of time, as in our patient [11].

Nonspecific cutaneous manifestations (such as erythematous macules, papules, plaques, facial malar erythema, erosions, patches, and nodules) have been observed in up to 40% of cases [25]. In our case, skin lesions preceded the appearance of adenopathies and resolved 3-4 weeks after initiating treatment. Unfortunately, a skin biopsy was not performed. It would have been of great value to distinguish KFD from SLE skin lesions, and we strongly recommend it to be performed whenever possible. Histological findings such as perivascular and interstitial infiltration of CD68- and CD163-positive histiocytes, CD8-positive cytotoxic T-lymphocytes, nuclear debris, the absence of neutrophils, vacuolar degeneration, keratinocyte necrosis, and the presence of interface dermatitis have been described in KFD cutaneous lesions [26, 27]. The KFD cutaneous lesions could resemble clinically and morphologically with skin manifestations observed in SLE: the presence of interface dermatitis, dermal mucin deposition, and panniculitis. The

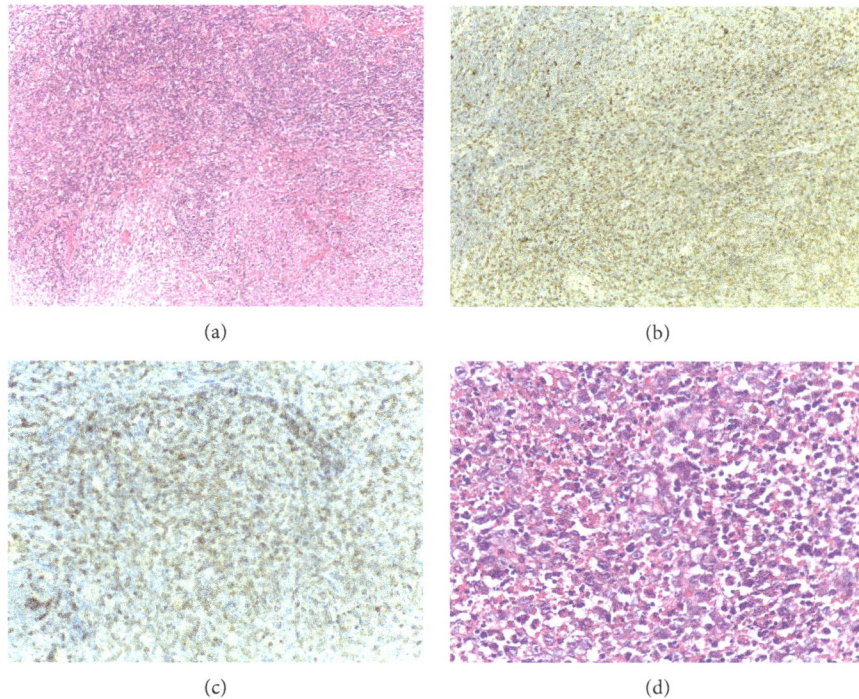

FIGURE 1: (a) H&E stained section (10x) of lymph node. Foci of necrosis containing abundant karyorrhectic debris. (b) Immunohistochemical stained section (10x). CD68-positive histiocytes. (c) Immunohistochemical stained section (10x). Abundant CD3 dim positive immunoblastic T-cells. (d) H&E stained section (40x) of lymph node. Infiltration pattern with abundant transformed lymphocytes with immunoblast morphology.

difference is in the absence of plasma cells that are commonly found in SLE [26].

Biological findings such as leukopenia, neutropenia, atypical lymphocytes on peripheral blood smear, thrombocytopenia, and anemia have been classically reported in KFD. It is notable that our patient displayed lymphopenia which is not commonly seen in KFD and has rather been reported when SLE associated with KFD [18, 28]. Reports also associate severe lymphopenia with more forms of KFD [28].

In addition to these, other biological abnormalities have also been reported: elevated inflammatory markers, elevated liver transaminases, increased LDH, ANA, and reduced C3 values [11, 29].

Our patient fulfilled SLE diagnosis criteria according to both ACR and SLICC classification [30], respectively (a total of 6 criteria): serositis (pleural effusion), arthritis (tenderness in bilateral proximal and distal interphalangeal joints of hands), proteinuria greater than 500 mg/24 hours (1815 mg), leukopenia (2200/mmc) with significant lymphopenia (approx. 300/mmc), double-stranded DNA, and ANA positivity (immunologic criteria). Sopeña et al. reported an incidence of 23% SLE cases in 20 patients with Kikuchi disease and autoimmune manifestations. The incidence was similar to those in previous literature [18]. According to Kucukardali et al., SLE-associated Kikuchi's disease is more common in Asian patients than in European patients. 28 patients were studied: 18 had simultaneous SLE and KFD, 6 presented with SLE after KFD diagnosis, and 4 were previously diagnosed with SLE [11]. The association between these two disorders is not completely understood. The clinical features are similar, and differentiation between them is based on lymph node histopathology [31]. The absence of hematoxylin bodies and neutrophils indicates KFD rather than SLE, and our patient showed definite features of Kikuchi's disease. Histopathologic features that support SLE include an increased number of plasma cells, hematoxyphilic bodies, DNA deposits in the vascular walls, neutrophilic infiltration, and varying degrees of coagulative necrosis with Azzopardi phenomenon [3]. Given the number of published clinical cases, the association between KFD and SLE cannot be random. Some authors have postulated that KFD is prodromal for SLE and recommend follow-up for KFD patients with cutaneous lesions for detecting an autoimmune disease. Others recommend ANA screening at the time of KFD diagnosis [7, 19, 27].

Differentiating KFD from other diseases such as lymphoma and reactive lymphadenopathies (e.g., sarcoidosis, tuberculosis, toxoplasmosis, and cat-scratch fever) is mandatory [22, 32]. Our patient was referred to the hematologist with the clinical suspicion of NHL, particularly angioimmunoblastic T-cell lymphoma, as it may associate with rash, arthralgias, and ANA positivity [33]. The differential diagnosis of the two most clinical relevant findings, fever and lymphadenopathy, is often challenging and requires an extensive work-up. This is emphasized in a group of 244 KFD patients published by Kucukardali et al. [11]. Our patient had a normal bone marrow examination and negative virology serological tests.

Even with adequate biopsy, appearances can be mistaken for NHL or reactive lymphadenopathies [22]. In our patient, an experienced morphopathologist confirmed KFD on the second biopsy. Coagulative necrosis with histiocytes proliferation and the absence of granulocytic infiltration is mandatory for diagnosis. Necrosis, karyorrhexis, and cellular debris are the hallmarks of the necrotizing type. Kuo proposed three histopathological stages: (a) a *proliferative stage* with histiocytes, plasmacytoid monocytes, lymphoid cells, karyorrhectic nuclear fragments, and eosinophilic apoptotic debris; (b) a *necrotizing stage* with coagulative necrosis; and (c) a *xanthomatous stage* with foamy histiocytes predominance [3]. In our case, the biopsy confirmed the necrotizing stage. A helpful histopathological feature is the absence of granulocytes in the necrotizing stage, which is used to distinguish KFD from SLE or reactive lymphadenopathy, especially given the coexistence of clinical or biological abnormalities that are similar to those of an autoimmune disease.

Recurrence is rarely reported (3–5%). Song et al. reported a higher incidence rate in ANA-positive cases and identified fever, fatigue, extranodal involvement, and positive fluorescence antinuclear antibody as predictive factors for relapse [34]. Our patient had presented a previous episode of fever and enlarged lymph nodes. However, the excisional biopsy did not suggest KFD and unfortunately was not available for reexamination. That is why we emphasize again the need for an expert morphopathologic evaluation in any case with features resembling KFD.

The *outcome* of these patients is generally favorable with a self-limited course. *Treatment* is symptomatic with NSAIDs and a short course of steroids. KFD coexisting with SLE can have a more aggressive course, and treatment is recommended to prevent relapse, as in our case. Rare cases with a fatal evolution have been reported; KFD was found to be complicated with hemophagocytic syndrome, heart failure, or recurrent aseptic meningitis that required intravenous immunoglobulin and corticosteroids [35–38].

4. Conclusions

Many of the symptoms, cutaneous manifestations, biological and histopathological features of KFD are similar to those of autoimmune diseases, particularly those of SLE, and differentiating between the two entities is challenging.

We present this case in order to highlight the rare clinical entity of Kikuchi's disease in Caucasian population, the need for an experienced pathologist and for long-term follow-up, especially for those cases with cutaneous manifestations, and high risk of associating autoimmune diseases such as SLE.

Consent

Informed consent from the patient was obtained prior to data collection.

Conflicts of Interest

The authors have no conflicts of interest.

References

[1] M. Kikuchi, "Lymphadenitis showing focal reticulum cell hyperplasia with nuclear debris and phagocytosis," *Acta Haematologica*, vol. 35, pp. 379-380, 1972.

[2] Y. Fujimoto, Y. Kozima, and K. Hamaguchi, "Cervical necrotizing lymphadenitis: a new clinicopathologic agent," *Nihon Naika Gakkai Zasshi*, vol. 20, pp. 920–927, 1972.

[3] T. Kuo, "Kikuchi's disease (histiocytic necrotizing lymphadenitis): a clinicopathologic study of 79 cases with an analysis of histologic subtypes, immunohistology, and DNA ploidy," *American Journal of Surgical Pathology*, vol. 19, no. 7, pp. 798–809, 1995.

[4] X. Bosch, A. Guilabert, R. Miquel, and E. Campo, "Enigmatic Kikuchi-Fujimoto disease: a comprehensive review," *American Journal of Clinical Pathology*, vol. 122, no. 1, pp. 141–152, 2004.

[5] C. Lopez, M. Oliver, R. Olavarria, M. Sarabia, and M. Chopite, "Kikuchi-Fujimoto necrotizing lymphadenitis associated with cutaneous lupus erythematosus: a case report," *American Journal of Dermatopathology*, vol. 22, no. 4, pp. 328–333, 2000.

[6] C. B. Hutchinson and E. Wang, "Kikuchi-Fujimoto disease," *Archives of Pathology and Laboratory Medicine*, vol. 134, no. 2, pp. 289–293, 2010.

[7] C. Martinez-Vazquez, G. Hughes, J. Bordon et al., "Histiocytic necrotizing lymphadenitis, Kikuchi-Fujimoto's disease, associated with systemic lupus erythematosus," *QJM*, vol. 90, no. 8, pp. 531–533, 1997.

[8] C. W. Davies and C. G. Wathen, "Kikuchi's disease and systemic lupus erythematosus," *Respiratory Medicine*, vol. 91, no. 2, pp. 117-118, 1997.

[9] H. C. Lin, C. Y. Su, C. C. Huang, C. F. Hwang, and C. Y. Chien, "Kikuchi's disease: a review and analysis of 61 cases," *Otolaryngology-Head and Neck Surgery*, vol. 128, no. 5, pp. 650–653, 2003.

[10] H. L. Yu, S. S. Lee, H. C. Tsai et al., "Clinical manifestations of Kikuchi's disease in southern Taiwan," *Journal of Microbiology, Immunology, and Infection*, vol. 38, no. 1, pp. 35–40, 2005.

[11] Y. Kucukardali, E. Solmazgul, E. Kunter, O. Oncul, S. Yildirim, and M. Kaplan, "Kikuchi-Fujimoto disease: analysis of 244 cases," *Clinical Rheumatology*, vol. 26, no. 1, pp. 50–54, 2007.

[12] D. J. Archibald, M. L. Carlson, and R. O. Gustafson, "Kikuchi-Fujimoto disease in a 30-year-old Caucasian female," *International Journal of Otolaryngology*, vol. 2009, Article ID 901537, 4 pages, 2009.

[13] S. Kaur, R. Mahajan, N. P. Jain, N. Sood, and S. Chhabra, "Kikuchi's disease-a rare cause of lymphadenopathy and fever," *Journal of the Association of Physicians of India*, vol. 62, no. 1, pp. 54–57, 2014.

[14] H. Duskin-Bitan, S. Kivity, D. Olchovsky, G. Schiby, D. Ezra, and M. Mouallem, "Kikuchi-Fujimoto disease," *Israel Medical Association Journal*, vol. 12, no. 10, pp. 617–621, 2010.

[15] C. F. Chiu, K. C. Chow, T. Y. Lin, M. H. Tsai, C. M. Shih, and L. M. Chen, "Virus infection in patients with histiocytic necrotizing lymphadenitis in Taiwan: detection of Epstein-Barr virus, type I humanT-cell lymphotropic virus, and parvovirus B19," *American Journal of Clinical Pathology*, vol. 113, no. 6, pp. 774–781, 2000.

[16] M. Kubota, R. Tsukamoto, K. Kurokawa, T. Imai, and K. Furusho, "Elevated serum interferon gamma and interleukin-6 in patients with necrotizing lymphadenitis (Kikuchi's disease)," *British Journal of Haematology*, vol. 95, no. 4, pp. 613–615, 1996.

[17] K. Kato, K. Ohshima, K. Anzai, J. Suzumiya, and M. Kikuchi, "Elevated serum-soluble fas ligand in histiocytic necrotizing lymphadenitis," *International Journal of Hematology*, vol. 73, no. 1, pp. 84–86, 2001.

[18] B. Sopeña, A. Rivera, C. Vázquez-Triñanes et al., "Autoimmune manifestations of Kikuchi disease," *Seminars in Arthritis and Rheumatism*, vol. 41, no. 6, pp. 900–906, 2012.

[19] S. C. Murthy, S. M. Dandin, A. S. Dandin, and M. Y. Patwardan, "Kikuchi's disease associated with systemic lupus erythematosus," *Indian Journal of Dermatology, Venereology and Leprology*, vol. 71, no. 5, pp. 338–341, 2005.

[20] A. Santana, B. Lessa, L. Galrão, I. Lima, and M. Santiago, "Kikuchi-Fujimoto's disease associated with systemic lupus erythematosus: case report and review of the literature," *Clinical Rheumatology*, vol. 24, no. 1, pp. 60–63, 2005.

[21] C. Rudniki, E. Kessler, M. Zarfati, H. Turani, Y. Bar-Ziv, and I. Zahavi, "Kikuchi's necrotizing lymphadenitis: a cause of fever of unknown origin and splenomegaly," *Acta Haematologica*, vol. 79, no. 2, pp. 99–102, 1988.

[22] R. F. Dorfman and G. J. Berry, "Kikuchi's histiocytic necrotizing lymphadenitis: an analysis of 108 cases with emphasis on differential diagnosis," *Seminars in Diagnostic Pathology*, vol. 5, no. 4, pp. 329–345, 1988.

[23] W. Y. Tsang, J. K. Chan, and C. S. Ng, "Kikuchi's lymphadenitis. A morphologic analysis of 75 cases with special reference to unusual features," *American Journal of Surgical Pathology*, vol. 18, no. 3, pp. 219–231, 1994.

[24] B. J. Baumgartner and E. R. Helling, "Kikuchi's disease: a case report and review of the literature," *Ear, Nose, and Throat Journal*, vol. 81, no. 5, pp. 331–335, 2002.

[25] T. T. Kuo, "Cutaneous manifestation of Kikuchi's histiocytic necrotizing lymphadenitis," *American Journal of Surgical Pathology*, vol. 14, no. 9, pp. 872–876, 1990.

[26] J. H. Kim, Y. B. Kim, S. I. In, Y. C. Kim, and J. H. Han, "The cutaneous lesions of Kikuchi's disease: a comprehensive analysis of 16 cases based on the clinicopathologic, immunohistochemical, and immunofluorescence studies with an emphasis on the differential diagnosis," *Human Pathology*, vol. 41, no. 9, pp. 1245–1254, 2010.

[27] A. R. Atwater, B. J. Longley, and W. D. Aughenbaugh, "Kikuchi's disease: case report and systematic review of cutaneous and histopathologic presentations," *Journal of the American Academy of Dermatology*, vol. 59, no. 1, pp. 130–136, 2008.

[28] G. Dumas, V. Prendki, J. Haroche et al., "Kikuchi-Fujimoto disease: retrospective study of 91 cases and review of the literature," *Medicine*, vol. 93, no. 24, pp. 372–382, 2014.

[29] B. Ruaro, A. Sulli, E. Alessandri, G. Fraternali-Orcioni, and M. Cutolo, "Kikuchi-Fujimoto's disease associated with systemic lupus erythematous: difficult case report and literature review," *Lupus*, vol. 23, no. 9, pp. 939–944, 2014.

[30] M. Petri, A. M. Orbai, G. S. Alarcón et al., "Derivation and validation of the Systemic Lupus International Collaborating Clinics classification criteria for systemic lupus erythematosus," *Arthritis and Rheumatism*, vol. 64, no. 8, pp. 2677–2686, 2012.

[31] G. A. Chamulak, R. K. Brynes, and B. N. Nathwani, "Kikuchi-Fujimoto disease mimicking malignant lymphoma," *American Journal of Surgical Pathology*, vol. 14, no. 6, pp. 514–523, 1990.

[32] J. Y. Song, H. J. Cheong, S. Y. Kee, J. Lee, J. W. Sohn, and M. J. Kim, "Disease spectrum of cervical lymphadenitis: analysis based on ultrasound-guided core-needle gun biopsy," *Journal of Infection*, vol. 55, no. 4, pp. 310–316, 2007.

[33] S. K. Kim, M. S. Kang, B. Y. Yoon et al., "Histiocytic necrotizing lymphadenitis in the context of systemic lupus erythematosus (SLE): is histiocytic necrotizing lymphadenitis in SLE associated with skin lesions?," *Lupus*, vol. 20, no. 8, pp. 809–819, 2011.

[34] J. Y. Song, J. Lee, D. W. Park et al., "Clinical outcome and predictive factors of recurrence among patients with Kikuchi's disease," *International Journal of Infectious Diseases*, vol. 13, no. 3, pp. 322–326, 2009.

[35] Y. M. Kim, Y. J. Lee, S. O. Nam, S. E. Park, J. Y. Kim, and E. Y. Lee, "Hemophagocytic syndrome associated with Kikuchi's disease," *Journal of Korean Medical Science*, vol. 18, no. 4, pp. 592–594, 2003.

[36] Y. Wano, K. Ebata, T. Masaki et al., "Histiocytic necrotizing lymphadenitis (Kikuchi-Fujimoto's disease) accompanied by hemophagocytosis and salivary gland swelling in a patient with systemic lupus erythematosus," *Rinsho Ketsueki*, vol. 41, pp. 54–60, 2000.

[37] U. Mahadeva, T. Allport, B. Bain, and W. K. Chan, "Haemophagocytic syndrome and histiocytic necrotising lymphadenitis (Kikuchi's disease)," *Journal of Clinical Pathology*, vol. 53, no. 8, pp. 636–638, 2000.

[38] T. Komagamine, T. Nagashima, M. Kojima et al., "Recurrent aseptic meningitis in association with Kikuchi-Fujimoto disease: case report and literature review," *BMC Neurology*, vol. 12, no. 1, p. 112, 2012.

Uncovering Clinical Features of De Novo Philadelphia Positive Myelodysplasia

Aristides Armas,[1] Chen Chen,[2,3] Martha Mims,[1,2,3,4] and Gustavo Rivero[1,2,3,4]

[1]Baylor St. Luke's Medical Center, Houston, TX 77030, USA
[2]Baylor College of Medicine, Section of Hematology and Oncology, 1 Baylor Plaza, Houston, TX 77030, USA
[3]Department of Pathology, Baylor College of Medicine, 1 Baylor Plaza, Houston, TX 77030, USA
[4]The Dan L. Duncan Comprehensive Cancer Center at Baylor College of Medicine, 1 Baylor Plaza, Houston, TX 77030, USA

Correspondence should be addressed to Gustavo Rivero; garivero@bcm.edu

Academic Editor: Akimichi Ohsaka

Myelodysplastic syndrome (MDS) is cytogenetically heterogeneous and retains variable risk for acute myeloid leukemia transformation. Though not yet fully understood, there is an association between genetic abnormalities and defects in gene expression. The functional role for infrequent cytogenetic alteration remains unclear. An uncommon chromosomic abnormality is the presence of the Philadelphia (Ph) chromosome. Here, we report a patient with Ph+ MDS treated with low dose Dasatinib who achieved hematologic response for 7 months. In addition, we also examined the English literature on all de novo Ph + MDS cases between 1996 and 2015 to gain insight into clinical features and outcome.

1. Case Description

A 74-year-old male was evaluated for refractory anemia. He had a history of gallbladder cancer treated with radiation (RT) in 2010. His Hb, mean corpuscular volume (MCV), and red cell distribution width (RDW) were 8.3 g/dL, 86.1 fL, and 19.8%. White blood cell count, absolute neutrophil count (ANC), and absolute monocyte count (AMC) were 5400/μL, 3800/μL, and 1080/uL. There was no evidence for basophilia or thrombocytosis. His reticulocyte count, erythropoietin (EPO), and vitamin D level were 0.8%, 25.8 MIU/ML (2.6–18.5), and 76 pg/mL. Ferritin level was 120 ng/mL. Physical exam demonstrated no hepatosplenomegaly. Peripheral blood smear showed normocytic, normochromic anemia with scattered target cells. White blood cells were unremarkable and platelets were adequate. His bone marrow was hypocellular with trilineage dysplasia. His erythroid cells showed nuclear irregularities, budding, and nuclear/cytoplasmic desynchronization (Figures 1(a) and 1(b)). Micromegakaryocytes were hypolobated (Figure 1(c)). Immunohistochemistry revealed no evidence of blasts or monocytosis. Bone marrow findings were consistent with refractory cytopenia with multilineage

dysplasia (MDS-MLD) [1]. Karyotype was 46, XY, t (9:22) [4], XY [16] (Figure 1(d)). MDS fluorescence in situ hybridization (FISH) including probes for 5q31, 7q31, 8 centromere, 11q23, and 20q12 was negative. Chromosome microarray analysis (CMA) showed no pathogenic copy number variation (CNV) or copy number neutral loss of heterozygosity (LOH). Next generation gene sequencing demonstrated no relevant leukemia mutations in *CSFR1, SF3B1, SRSF2, U2AF1, NRAS, KRAS, FLT3, JAK2, JAK3, DNMT3A, KIT, PHF6, PDGFRA, CDKN2A, IDH1, IDH2, TET2, EZH2, CEBPA, EP300, PTPN11, P53, CREBBP, IKZF1, IKZF3, NOTCH1, RUNX1, WT1*, and *NPM1*. Real time polymerase chain reaction (PCR) for BCR-ABL1 (Major p210 form) was 24.1180%, International Scale (IS). Estimated R-IPSS score was 3 (hemoglobin [8.3 g/dL] = 1; platelets [341000/μL] = 0; absolute neutrophil count [3800/μL] = 0; cytogenetic = 2; blast = [0%] = 0). Trilineage dysplasia, refractory anemia without basophilia, karyotypic, and molecular clonal evidence for Ph + disease prompted treatment with Dasatinib at 20 mg orally daily. A low dose was selected given potential risk for worsening cytopenias. His hemoglobin progressively increased by 3 g/dL after 12 weeks of treatment (Figure 1(e)). Response was

(a)

(b)

(c)

(d)

(e)

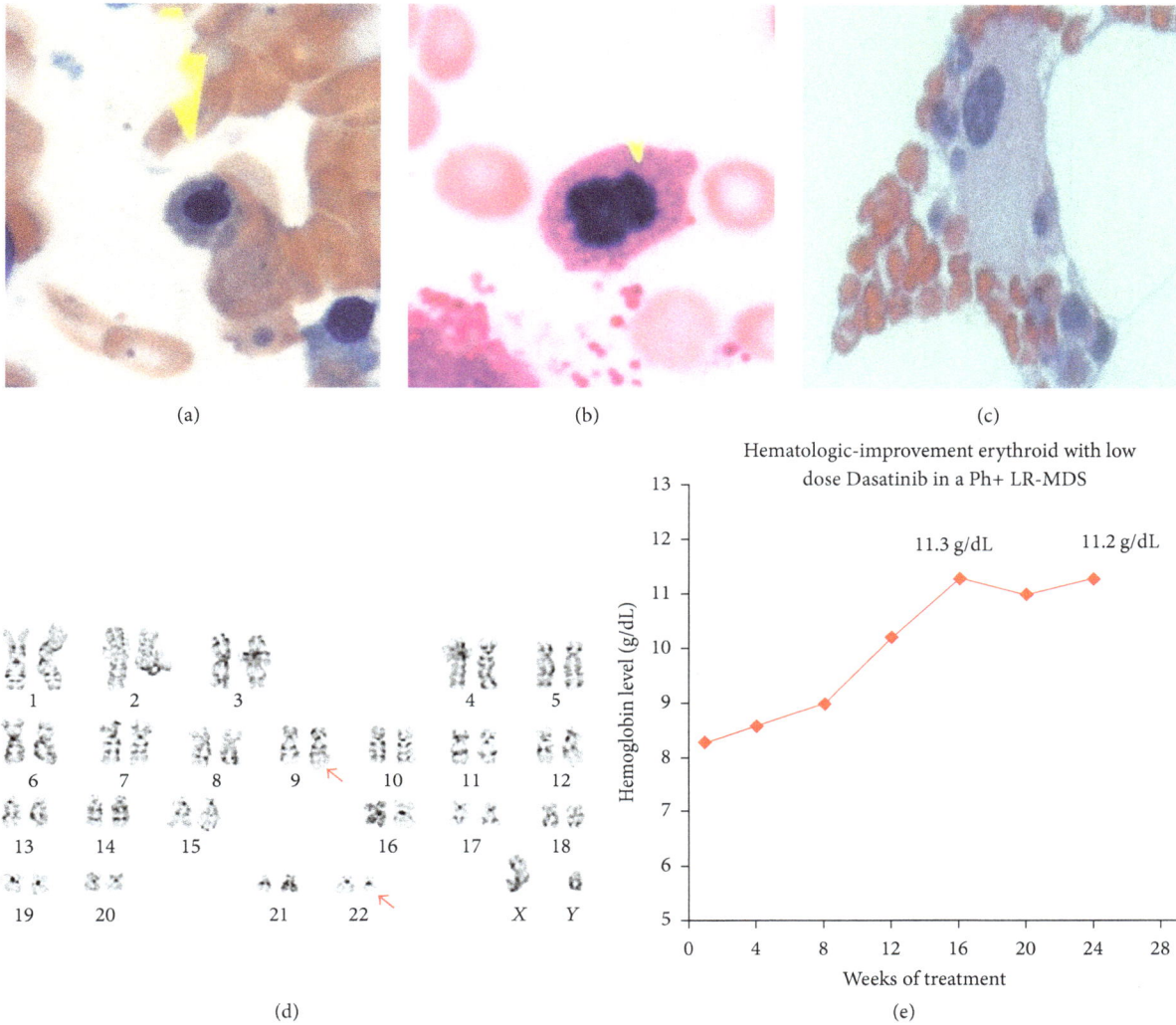

FIGURE 1: Bone marrow aspirate, biopsy, metaphases cytogenetic, and response to Dasatinib in a Ph+ LR-MDS patient. (a) Erythroid precursor with nuclear irregularity, budding, and nuclear/cytoplasm desynchronization. (b) Dysplastic erythroid precursors with karyorrhexis. (c) shows hypolobated dysplastic megakaryocytes. (d) Patient karyotype showing t (9; 22) translocation. (e) Progressive increase in hemoglobin level for a Ph + LR-MDS [RCMD] patient treated with low-dose Dasatinib. Progressive H-E was observed at 12 weeks. HI-E was sustained at 24 weeks of treatment.

maintained for a total of 24 weeks (Figure 1(e)). BCR-ABL1 transcripts were undetectable (0.0006%, IS) after 4 months of treatment. After 7 months of follow-up, patient opted for hospice care after developing pneumonia that led to respiratory failure.

2. Methods

In addition to our case, 9 patients diagnosed with de novo Ph+ MDS were identified from PubMed search [2–8]. De novo Ph+ MDS was defined as unequivocal morphologic evidence for myeloid dysplasia and initial karyotype examination positive for Ph abnormality. Given potential biologic confounders, treatment related MDS, CMML, and MDS/MPN Ph+ cases were excluded. In our 10 patients'

cohort, we investigated world health organization (WHO) 2008 classification, demographics, histopathologic bone marrow findings, and clinical outcome. Our primary aim was to identify relevant disease features that could facilitate disease management.

3. Cohort Analysis

Patient's characteristics and cytogenetic abnormalities are depicted in Table 1. Most of patients were males 6/10 (60%). Median age at diagnosis was 66 years (range, 49–74). According to WHO 2008, 3/7 (43%) and 2/7 (29%) patients were RAEB-2 and RCMD, respectively. RAEB-1 and RCUD (1 each) represented two additional patients with morphologic available data. Median hemoglobin, platelet, white, and blast

TABLE 1

Case	Age/sex	WBC*	Hemoglobin (g/dL)	Platelets (K/uL)	AMC** (uL)	Bone marrow blast (%)	WHO***	Cytogenetic	Treatment	Outcome±	Time to AML**** (months)	Ref.
1	49/F	6.5	8.2	425	585	0	MDS	46,XX,t(9;22)(q34;q11)	BSC^	AML	32	[2]
2	70/F	6.4	9.5	316	384	NA	MDS	46,XX[3]/46,XX,t(9q;22q)[12]	NA	Alive at 45 m		[3]
3	74/M (Case)	5.3	8.3	341	1080	0	RCMD+	44, XY, t (9;22) [4], 46,XY [16]	TKI	(alive) 7 months after diagnosis		
4	59/M	1.3	9.2	78	78	0	MDS	46,XY,t(9;22)(q34;q11)[20]	TKI+ + allo-stem cell transplant	(alive)	4ε	[4]
5	66/F	0.9	4.4	52	54	2	RCUD+++	46,XX,+8,t(9; 22;16)(q34;q11.2;q23)[4]/46,XX,idem,der(12)t(12;17)(p11.2;q11.2)[7]/46, XX [9].	Melphalan	(died) Developed skin Granulocytic sarcoma. (died)	9	[4]
6	67/M	2.7	10.4	52	81	4	RCMD	45, XY,+3,-5,-7,-20,+mar+mar/45,XY,+3,-4,-8,-9,-11,-18,-20,-21,-21,+mar,+mar,+mar,+mar,+mar,+breaks. FISH t(9;22)	TKI	1 year after diagnosis developed Fungal Pneumonia		[5]
7	62/M	1.8	11.9	3	NA	5	RAEBY-1	45,XY,-5,-7,+8, - 12, - 16,-22, + marE[?del(11)(q11)], + marC[?der(11)t(?;11;22)], + del(22)(q11)	BSC	(died)	2	[6]
8	67/F	3.4	11.5	111	NA	10	RAEB-2	46 XX, t(9;22)	TKI	(alive)	7	[7]
9	69/M	5.3	8.1	77	106	14	RAEB-2	45,XY,-5,-7,+8, - 12, - 16,-22, + marE[?del(11)(q11)], + marC[?der(11)t(?;11;22)], + del(22)(q11)	AraC+Mitho-xanthrone+Tenoposide	(died) Septicemia 5 months after diagnosis.		[8]
10	64/M	6.9	7.8	98	69	16	RAEB-2	46,XY[7]/47,XY,+8,t(9;22)(q34;q11)[6]	Hydroxyurea	(died)	9	[8]

*WBC = white blood cell count; AMC** = absolute monocyte count; WHO*** = World Health Organization; ±outcome reported at the time of publication; AML**** = acute myelogenous leukemia; ^BSC = best supportive care; ++TKI = tyrosine kinase inhibitor; εpatient was diagnosed in April 2001. He received Imatinib for 2 months until August 2001. Given AML transformation, BMT was performed and remained alive by the time of publication in June 2003; +RCMD = refractory cytopenia multilineage dysplasia; +++RCUD = refractory cytopenia multilineage dysplasia; YRAEB = refractory anemia excess of blast.

count were 8.75 g/dL, 88 K/uL, 4.35 K/uL, and 4%. Among 10 patients, Ph translocation, as a sole chromosomic abnormality, was detected in 5/10 (50%). Trisomy 8 occurred commonly as an additional karyotypic alteration in 4/10 (40%) of patients and was frequently associated with complex cytogenetic spanning monosomies 5 and 7. TKI treatment resulted in hematologic remission in 4 patients leading to a median response duration of 7 months. In 5 patients with available follow-up, median time to AML transformation was 7 months. Interestingly, in patients with de novo Ph+ MDS, a platelet count of more or less than 100 K/uL resulted in an overall survival (OS) of 32 versus 9 months.

4. Discussion

MDS is cytogenetically heterogeneous presenting with karyotypic abnormalities in about 50% of patients. Chromosomic gains and, most commonly, somatic loss of tumor suppressor genes (TSG) by structural and epiphenomenon's modifications result in impaired differentiation [9]. Translocation (9; 22) is frequently observed in chronic myelogenous leukemia (CML). The 2008 world health organization (WHO) and the 2016 revision for classification of myeloid neoplasm emphasizes that CML BCR-ABL1$^+$ phenotype must include significant myeloproliferation. A distinction for chronic myelomonocytic leukemia (CMML) is the prerequisite for persistent monocytosis in peripheral blood $\geq 1000^9$/L [1, 10]. Paradoxically, the translocation (9; 22) is rarely associated with dysplastic hematopoiesis suggesting that the abnormality may have antagonistic disease-initiating role. In this report, we describe a Ph+ MDS patient exhibiting refractory anemia and bone marrow trilineage dysplasia that attained HI-E after low dose Dasatinib. Lack of peripheral blood and bone marrow proliferation favored clonal disorder unrelated to myeloproliferative neoplasm. The presence of Ph+ metaphases and low-grade BCR-ABL transcripts suggest that his MDS was, at least in part, resultant from aberrant kinase overexpression. Given the rare nature of de novo Ph + MDS, we selected 9 additional cases to evaluate disease presentation and outcome. Previously, Keung et al. described three de novo Ph+ MDS cases and reviewed 18 additional patients [4]. However, contrasting with our de novo cohort, his study included Ph + treatment-related disease and CMML cases. In addition, about 48% of patients lacked Ph+ chromosomic abnormality and rather acquired the translocation sequentially at disease progression. It is possible that Keung et al. study design limits our ability to characterize disease initiating mechanisms and de novo disease outcome. We observed that 50% of patients present with t (9; 22) as a sole abnormality. However, typical MDS chromosomic abnormalities, such as +8, frequently coexist in complex Ph+ metaphases. The disease exhibits high-risk features characterized by complex karyotype and elevated proportion of blast and thrombocytopenia. Previous studies have demonstrated that thrombocytopenia adversely impacts MDS outcome [11]. Neukirchen et al. specifically highlights that patients presenting with platelet count lower than 100000/uL retained inferior outcome [12]. It is possible that Ph+ MDS exhibits similar prognostic variables as those observed in Ph negative MDS. A short median time to AML

transformation of 7 months suggests that Ph + MDS is a highly aggressive disease, especially if it is associated with complex karyotype and thrombocytopenia. In Keung et al. study [4], median time progression to AML was reported as 13 months. This most favorable prognosis may be biased by inclusion of indolent Ph+ myeloproliferative disorders.

Three Ph+ MDS patients developed isolated refractory anemia, normal platelets, low blast count, and more favorable outcome. This led us to hypothesize that their IE functionally originates from similar Ph negative low risk MDS mechanisms. Given potential BCR-ABL disease initiating role, TKI represents an attractive intervention. However, to date, the efficacy of this therapy on Ph+ MDS remains poorly characterized. In our cohort study, TKI treatment resulted in about 7 months' response in 4 patients. Similarly, TKI was feasible in our reported case demonstrating a correlation between HI-E and molecular remission. Interestingly, low dose of Dasatinib led to limited side effects. IE is associated with abnormal paracrine/autocrine pathways leading to hemopoietic failure; specifically elevated IL-1β, TNF-α, and INF-γ levels are central to low risk-MDS (LR-MDS) [13]. In recent years, the role of deregulated innate immunity has emerged as potential etiology for LR-MDS. Although our patient's HI-E could be attributed to Dasatinib induced BCR-ABL inhibition, it is possible that an "off-target" Dasatinib effect on deregulated cytokines facilitated IE improvement. In vitro studies have demonstrated that Dasatinib suppresses the production of IL-6 and TNFα and favors production of anti-inflammatory cytokines, such as IL-10 in primary macrophages [14]. In addition, Src-family kinases (SFK), a potential Dasatinib target, participates in toll-like receptor-2 (TLR-2) mediated NF-kB activation leading to elevated IL-6 and TNFα levels [15]. Recent reports link TLR-2 deregulation and MDS pathogenesis [16]. Dasatinib may potentially cooperate to normalize IL-6 and TNFα levels inappropriately elevated in LR-MDS.

There are limitations to our study. The retrospective nature of the study could have biased our survival estimation for patients with high and low risk features given inaccurate censoring at the time of publication. Concerning our case, the lack of posttreatment bone marrow evaluation limits our ability to assign a direct favorable TKI effect to improve dysplastic marrow features. However, low dose Dasatinib led to molecular remission and improved IE. This may suggest a favorable drug effect on Ph + MDS disease initiating mechanisms and chronic marrow inflammation. To date, our study is the first to investigate a cohort of newly diagnosed Ph + MDS. The disease potentially recapitulates low and high risk features observed in Ph negative disease. It is likely that high risk Ph+ MDS could exhibit short latency to AML necessitating early chemotherapy and even allo-stem-cell transplantation. Future directions should evaluate the role and potential mechanism of action of TKIs in Ph + MDS patients presenting with low risk features.

Competing Interests

All authors reported no competing interests.

Authors' Contributions

Dr. Armas, Mims, and Rivero contributed equally to manuscript writing. Dr. Chen provided hemopathologic description for the case. Dr. Rivero designed plan for investigation and report of the case.

References

[1] D. A. Arber, A. Orazi, R. Hasserjian et al., "The 2016 revision to the World Health Organization classification of myeloid neoplasms and acute leukemia," *Blood*, vol. 127, no. 20, pp. 2391–2405, 2016.

[2] D. G. Roth, C. M. Richman, and J. D. Rowley, "Chronic myelodysplastic syndrome (preleukemia) with the Philadelphia chromosome," *Blood*, vol. 56, no. 2, pp. 262–264, 1980.

[3] A. Berrebi, R. Bruck, M. Shtalrid, and J. Chemke, "Philadelphia chromosome in idiopathic acquired sideroblastic anemia," *Acta Haematologica*, vol. 72, no. 5, pp. 343–345, 1984.

[4] Y.-K. Keung, M. Beaty, B. L. Powell, I. Molnar, D. Buss, and M. Pettenati, "Philadelphia chromosome positive myelodysplastic syndrome and acute myeloid leukemia—retrospective study and review of literature," *Leukemia Research*, vol. 28, no. 6, pp. 579–586, 2004.

[5] S. Dutta, P. Kumari, N. Ks et al., "Philadelphia chromosome-positive myelodysplastic syndrome: is it a distinct entity?" *Acta Haematologica*, vol. 129, no. 4, pp. 215–217, 2013.

[6] J. H. Ohyashiki, K. Ohyashiki, H. Fujieda et al., "Myelodysplastic syndrome with Philadelphia-like chromosome without bcr rearrangement," *Cancer Genetics and Cytogenetics*, vol. 35, no. 2, pp. 151–158, 1988.

[7] M. W. Drummond, C. J. Lush, M. A. Vickers, F. M. Reid, J. Kaeda, and T. L. Holyoake, "Imatinib mesylate-induced molecular remission of Philadelphia chromosome-positive myelodysplastic syndrome," *Leukemia*, vol. 17, no. 2, pp. 463–465, 2003.

[8] J. F. Lesesve, X. Troussard, C. Bastard et al., "p190(bcr/abl) rearrangement in myelodysplastic syndromes: two reports and review of the literature," *British Journal of Haematology*, vol. 95, no. 2, pp. 372–375, 1996.

[9] G. Garcia-Manero, "Myelodysplastic syndromes: 2011 update on diagnosis, risk-stratification, and management," *American Journal of Hematology*, vol. 86, no. 6, pp. 490–498, 2011.

[10] J. W. Vardiman, J. Thiele, D. A. Arber et al., "The 2008 revision of the World Health Organization (WHO) classification of myeloid neoplasms and acute leukemia: rationale and important changes," *Blood*, vol. 114, no. 5, pp. 937–951, 2009.

[11] H. Kantarjian, F. Giles, A. List et al., "The incidence and impact of thrombocytopenia in myelodysplastic syndromes," *Cancer*, vol. 109, no. 9, pp. 1705–1714, 2007.

[12] J. Neukirchen, S. Blum, A. Kuendgen et al., "Platelet counts and haemorrhagic diathesis in patients with myelodysplastic syndromes," *European Journal of Haematology*, vol. 83, no. 5, pp. 477–482, 2009.

[13] S. M. Kornblau, D. McCue, N. Singh, W. Chen, Z. Estrov, and K. R. Coombes, "Recurrent expression signatures of cytokines and chemokines are present and are independently prognostic in acute myelogenous leukemia and myelodysplasia," *Blood*, vol. 116, no. 20, pp. 4251–4261, 2010.

[14] J. Ozanne, A. R. Prescott, and K. Clark, "The clinically approved drugs dasatinib and bosutinib induce anti-inflammatory macrophages by inhibiting the salt-inducible kinases," *Biochemical Journal*, vol. 465, pp. 271–279, 2015.

[15] J. Toubiana, A.-L. Rossi, N. Belaidouni et al., "Src-family-tyrosine kinase Lyn is critical for TLR2-mediated NF-κ activation through the PI 3-kinase signaling pathway," *Innate Immunity*, vol. 21, no. 7, pp. 685–697, 2015.

[16] Y. Wei, S. Dimicoli, C. Bueso-Ramos et al., "Toll-like receptor alterations in myelodysplastic syndrome," *Leukemia*, vol. 27, no. 9, pp. 1832–1840, 2013.

3

A Case Report of Nongerminal Center B-Cell Type Diffuse Large B-Cell Lymphoma Treated to Complete Response with Rituximab and Ibrutinib

Geoffrey Shouse [iD][1] **and Miemie Thinn**[2]

[1]*Division of Hematology and Oncology, Loma Linda University School of Medicine, Loma Linda, CA, USA*
[2]*Division of Hematology and Medical Oncology, Loma Linda Veterans Administration Medical Center, Loma Linda, CA, USA*

Correspondence should be addressed to Geoffrey Shouse; gshouse@llu.edu

Academic Editor: Kiyotaka Kawauchi

Diffuse large B-cell lymphoma (DLBCL) is a molecularly heterogeneous disease consisting of different subtypes with varying clinical behaviors. For example, the activated B-cell-like (ABC) type of DLBCL has lower cure rates with traditional chemotherapy regimens. The molecular pathway promoting tumorigenic growth of the ABC type includes a dependence on intracellular signaling by Bruton's agammaglobulinemia tyrosine kinase (BTK). This specific pathway has led to the investigation of the utility of ibrutinib in treatment of this type of lymphoma at relapse or in combination with standard chemotherapy. In elderly patients stricken with this disease, standard combination chemotherapy can pose significant toxicity. Some reduced intensity regimens have activity but significantly less favorable long-term outcomes and still pose significant toxicity to elderly patients. In the following case, we demonstrate induction of complete response in an elderly patient with significant comorbidities with nongerminal center B-cell type (NGCB) DLBCL treated with rituximab, ibrutinib, and prednisone. Toxicity included atrial fibrillation that ultimately led to heart failure as well as sepsis which ultimately led to the patient's demise. Despite this fact, the response to treatment appeared durable. This case illustrates the utility and limitations of molecularly targeted therapies to treat aggressive lymphoma in frail elderly patients.

1. Introduction

Diffuse large B-cell lymphoma (DLBCL) is a molecularly heterogeneous disease, with multiple subtypes that have variable clinical characteristics. Recent studies indicate that the molecular disruptions in various DLBCL subtypes may explain the observed differences in clinical behavior. For example, the two most common subgroups of DLBCL include the germinal center B-cell-like (GCB) and the non-GCB or activated B-cell-like (ABC) subtypes. The goal of many recent and ongoing studies has been to elucidate the underlying molecular mechanisms promoting cancer growth to identify pathways that can be potentially targeted with less toxic and more efficacious treatments, rather than toxic multiagent chemotherapy. One recent and significant targeted therapy that has revolutionized the treatment of CD20-positive lymphomas is the use of therapeutic anti-CD20 monoclonal antibodies, such as rituximab. The addition of rituximab to standard multiagent chemotherapy has improved survival across all DLBCL subtypes [1].

Despite significant gains in response rates, ABC DLBCL still has a lower rate of cure compared to the GCB type when using conventional R-CHOP chemotherapy [2]. The underlying molecular signaling pathways acting in the ABC subtype of DLBCL are thought to be responsible for this difference. The viability of the ABC subtype of DLBCL is sustained by signaling from the B-cell receptor (BCR) [3]. The BCR is critically important for normal B-cell development and is linked to the development of many of the B-cell malignancies including DLBCL. The BCR is a transmembrane immunoglobulin receptor associated with a heterodimer of CD79a and CD79b. Upon binding of the antigen, the BCR activates the tyrosine kinases LYN and SYK, which initiate a downstream signaling cascade activating intracellular messengers, ultimately leading to increased nuclear factor kappa b (NF-κB) activity, which promotes cell growth and inhibits apoptosis. In the ABC subtype of DLBCL, the NF-κB pathway is constitutively activated by mutations in the BCR and adaptor proteins, as well as the activity of MYD88. The critical link between BCR signaling and NF-κB activation is Bruton's agammaglobulinemia tyrosine kinase (BTK). Signaling from the BCR through LYN and SYK leads to activation of BTK which signals downstream to activate PI3K, phospholipase C2, and the mTOR pathway as well as the mitogen-activated protein kinase ERK, ultimately leading to upregulation and activation of the transcription factor NF-κB [4]. With the advent of the BTK inhibitor, ibrutinib, the potential for targeting this pathway in ABC DLBCL is attractive [5–7]. To date, early phase data indicate the potential for ibrutinib to induce a complete response (CR) in relapsed and refractory DLBCL as a single agent, with the ABC subtype preferentially responding. Studies combining ibrutinib with chemotherapy are ongoing; however, evaluation of a nonchemotherapy combination of both rituximab and ibrutinib has not been described to date [8, 9]. In the present case, we report an elderly patient with significant comorbidities, who was deemed not a candidate for standard therapy and was treated to CR with a combination of rituximab, ibrutinib, and prednisone.

2. Case Presentation

The patient was a 70-year-old Caucasian male with coronary artery disease, sick sinus syndrome with pacemaker dependence, chronic kidney disease, type 2 diabetes mellitus, dementia, and schizoaffective disorder, who was found to have spontaneous unilateral epistaxis and left-sided facial asymmetry. He lived at a board and care facility, and medical decisions were made in conjunction with the patient and his sister who was his power of attorney. Prior to these symptoms, the patient was Eastern Cooperative Oncology Group functional status (ECOG) of 2. Upon admission to the hospital, he was found to have a large nasal mass, palpable large left cervical lymphadenopathy. Timeline of events is outlined in Table 1.

CT imaging demonstrated a large infiltrative enhancing mass centered in the left side of the nasal cavity and left maxillary sinus as well as an enlarged left submandibular lymph node. Left submandibular lymph node fine-needle biopsy demonstrated sheets of lymphocytes with effacement of the normal lymph node architecture, with medium to large lymphocytes with nucleoli and vesicular chromatin. By immunohistochemistry, the atypical cells were Pax-5, CD20, MUM1, BCL2, and BCL6 positive and CD56, TdT, CD10, and cyclin D1 negative, with a Ki-67 of about 95%, consistent with diffuse large B-cell lymphoma, NGCB type (Figure 1). PET/CT was performed after the biopsy to complete staging, which demonstrated multifocal hypermetabolic tumor foci including bilateral nasopharynx, bilateral nasal cavity, left maxillary sinus with extension to the left parapharyngeal space, soft palate, lingual tonsil, palatine tonsil, left face, bilateral neck nodes including jugulodigastric, posterior cervical,

TABLE 1: Timeline of major events.

Date	Event
2/13/16	Patient admitted with large nasal mass found
2/13/16	CT demonstrated large infiltrative mass
2/13/16	Left mandibular lymph node fine needle biopsy demonstrating DLBCL NGCB type
3/10/16	Initial staging PET/CT
3/11/16	Cycle 1, day 1 of ibrutinib and rituximab
8/15/16	PET CT showing CR
10/6/16	Cycle 9 of ibrutinib and rituximab completed
10/6/16	First documentation of atrial fibrillation noted
10/17/16	Patient presented with heart failure and sepsis
10/24/16	Patient went to hospice

and the largest of which was a left submandibular node with central necrosis of 4 centimeters (Figure 2(a)). In addition, the liver and bone were diffusely increased in avidity suggestive of involvement by lymphoma (Figure 2(b)). The initial standardized uptake value (SUV) of the left submandibular node was 6.4, the liver was 3.2 SUV, and the bone marrow was 3.7 SUV. The patient and his sister refused biopsy of these sites to confirm the presence of disease pathologically. Based on these findings and a normal initial LDH level of 159 units per liter, he was considered stage IV, with International Prognostic Index (IPI) of 4 (high risk), as well as high risk for CNS involvement. After discussion with the patient and his sister, decision was made to pursue only "nonchemotherapy" treatments. As such, monoclonal antibodies, targeted therapies, and corticosteroids were all considered; however, intrathecal chemotherapy was declined.

The patient started treatment with ibrutinib, and the dose was escalated over several weeks to 420 mg daily by mouth. At the same time, 21-day cycles of rituximab 375 mg/m^2 IV on day 1 along with prednisone 1 mg/kg PO for days 1 through 5 were also initiated. Supportive care was initiated simultaneously with allopurinol for tumor lysis prophylaxis. In addition, since the patient was wheelchair bound and at risk for thromboembolism, he was started on prophylactic dose of enoxaparin at 40 mg subcutaneously daily. Baseline hepatitis B, C, and HIV testing was negative. The patient tolerated the treatment well with no hematologic toxicities, minimal tumor lysis, no effect on renal or liver function, and no significant infection. The patient had an excellent response to treatment, and after the first cycle of chemotherapy, his epistaxis had resolved and his pain and swelling had also subsided. After five cycles of treatment, the patient had repeat PET/CT imaging that demonstrated near-complete response (Figure 2(a)). The dominant submandibular lymph node decreased in size from more than 4 cm to less than 1.5 cm, there were only residual erosive changes in the maxilla with mild residual FDG avidity (SUV max 3.6), the FDG activity in the liver resolved to SUV 2.7, and however the bone marrow remained PET avid with SUV 3.8. After 4 additional cycles, the patient achieved a complete response on repeat PET imaging including resolution of the bone marrow avidity (Figure 2(a)). This response was durable, and even after cessation of therapy, he had no signs of recurrence.

After a total of 9 cycles of rituximab, prednisone, and ibrutinib, the patient had a complete response (Figure 2). At

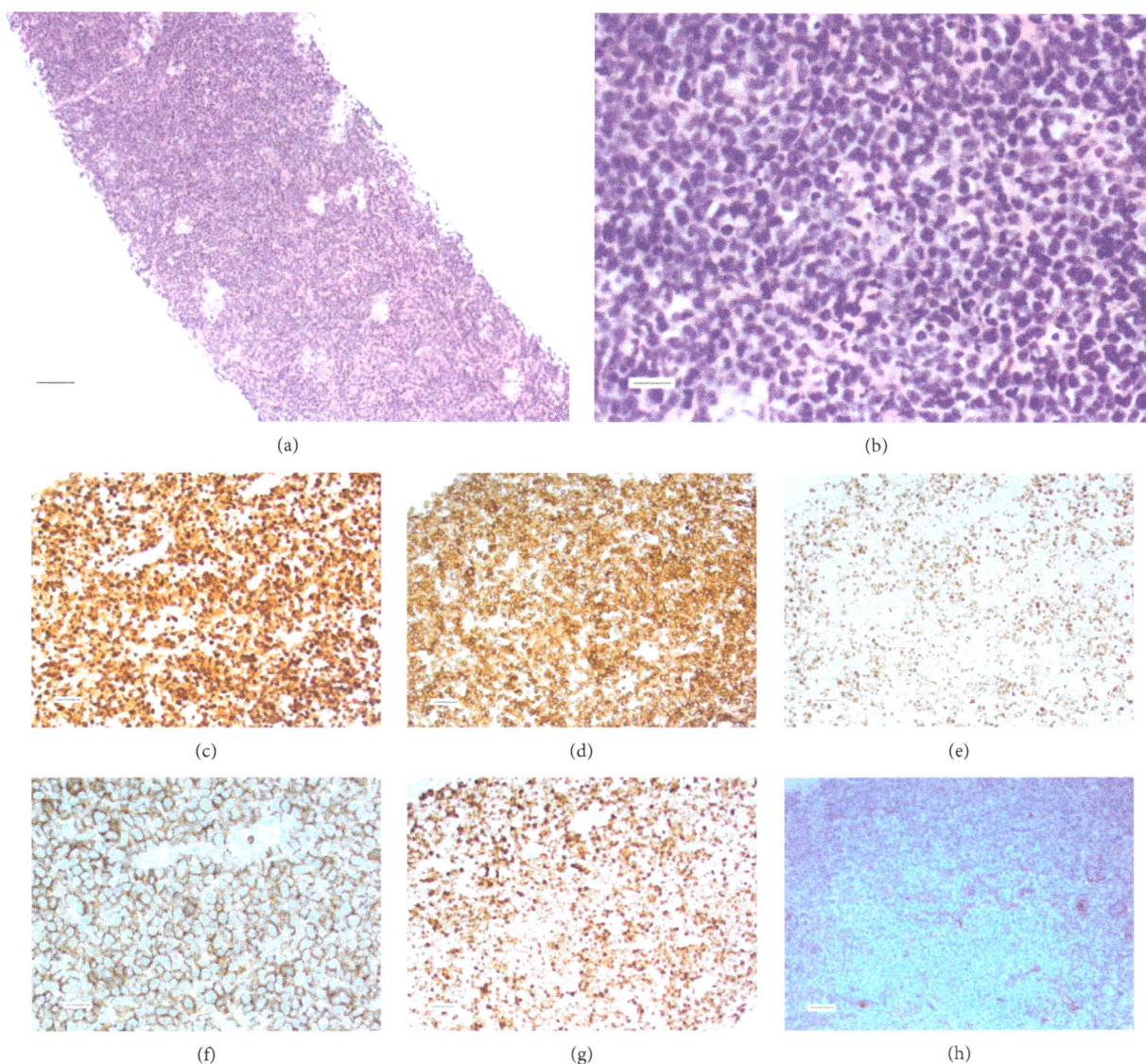

(a)

(b)

(c)

(d)

(e)

(f)

(g)

(h)

FIGURE 1: Pathology demonstrating staining consistent with ABC type DLBCL. Hematoxylin and eosin staining demonstrating large lymphocytes with active mitoses at both (a) 100x magnification with bar representing 100 microns and (b) 400x with bar representing 25 microns. (c) Ki-67 stain demonstrating high proliferative index. Various stains including positivity for (d) Bcl2, (e) Bcl6, and (f) CD20 magnified at 400x with bar representing 25 microns and (g) MUM1 as well as negativity for (h) CD10. All images are obtained at 200x magnification with bar representing 50 microns unless otherwise documented.

that time, however, ECG demonstrated that he was in atrial fibrillation with rapid ventricular response. He was referred to cardiology, and his dose of enoxaparin was increased to a therapeutic level at 1 mg/kg subcutaneously twice per day. He was started on beta blockade with control of his heart rate. At that point, the plan was to transition to rituximab maintenance every 2 months. Ibrutinib was continued as his atrial fibrillation seemed to be rate controlled. Repeat PET/CT showed the disease was still in remission one month later; however, prior to his first dose of maintenance rituximab, he presented to an outside hospital with fever, cough, shortness of breath, and atrial fibrillation with rapid ventricular response. He was diagnosed simultaneously with sepsis from pneumonia and respiratory failure from both

pneumonia and an acute exacerbation of heart failure. During the hospital course, the patient and his sister decided to stop all interventions and he was made comfort care. He died a few weeks later on hospice care. Despite being off of treatment for several weeks, however, there was no sign of recurrent disease at that time.

3. Discussion

In this study, we report a case of stage IV NGCB DLBCL in a patient with significant comorbidities who was treated to CR using 9 cycles of ibrutinib, rituximab, and prednisone. The patient had an excellent clinical response to treatment with resolution of epistaxis and decrease in pain and swelling

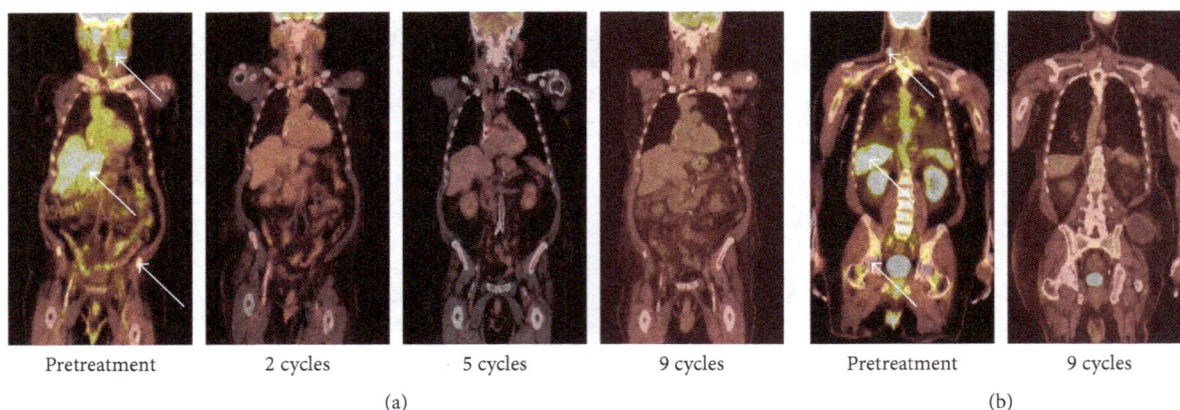

FIGURE 2: Staging imaging demonstrating response to treatment. (a) PET/CT imaging at initiation of treatment, after 2 cycles of treatment, 5 cycles of treatment, or 9 cycles of treatment as listed. (b) PET/CT imaging showing activity in the bone marrow and liver prior to treatment that was reduced to background levels after 9 cycles of treatment. White arrows indicate areas of active disease on the PET/CT.

of his face after the first cycle. His response was durable lasting almost a full year with no evidence of recurrence noted even when he was off therapy for several weeks. The patient initially tolerated the treatment very well with remarkable resolution of tumor burden and minimal effects on blood counts, renal function, liver function, and without significant bleeding, thrombosis, or infection. Of note, however, after achieving complete response, the patient developed atrial fibrillation, a known complication associated with ibrutinib therapy. In addition, at the same time he was noted to have acute onset of systolic heart failure with a drop in ejection fraction from 60% measured prior to treatment to 35%. Although the patient appeared to have the atrial fibrillation under control, after a nonneutropenia-associated infection led to sepsis, it was too overwhelming for his body to overcome. It was likely that ibrutinib was associated with both the atrial fibrillation and the sepsis, as ibrutinib blocks BTK signaling in normal B-cells which may predispose to infection-related complications. Ibrutinib had been stopped for several weeks due to the presumed cardiac toxicity, but despite this, the patient was still without evidence of lymphoma at the time of his death. No other significant dose-limiting toxicities were encountered during his treatment. Review of the literature demonstrates several case reports outlining chemotherapy regimens that have been effective at treating elderly patients, even though these lower toxicity regimens carry with them significant risk and toxic side effects [10–12]. In each of these reports, there were significant toxicities associated with treatment in order to achieve clinical response. Rituximab has been shown to add survival benefit to many CD20-positive B-cell malignancies [13]. Side effects and toxicities were generally mild and included infusion reactions and hypogammaglobulinemia in long-term use. Ibrutinib has demonstrated excellent responses in various hematologic malignancies including chronic lymphocytic leukemia and mantle cell lymphoma [14]. In general, ibrutinib was well tolerated with bleeding and atrial fibrillation being the most common significant side effects. Despite these, in general the medication was well tolerated even in elderly patients over the age of 70. Our case is unique in that our patient was not only elderly but had

borderline poor performance status and significant comorbidities. Our patient also had very high-risk disease, stage IV, with indication of both liver and bone marrow involvement based on PET/CT imaging. Finally, it was also unique in that classical cytotoxic chemotherapy was not administered at all. Of additional note, although the patient had significant risk for development of CNS disease, there was no clinical evidence of this occurring on exam or imaging. It is not clear whether this is due to effectiveness of ibrutinib at controlling CNS disease or some other unknown factors, although it was a very encouraging outcome, regardless.

In the field of cancer research and therapeutics, there is a steady movement toward the study, implementation, and use of targeted therapies to treat cancer. These therapies can be tailored to the particular molecular aberrations inherent to a specific subtype of cancer. The goal of these targeted therapies is to improve clinical outcomes, decrease toxicity, enhance response rates, and decrease relapse. In the case of DLBCL, recent studies indicate that the ABC subtype of lymphoma has an addiction to the driving signal from the BCR to NF-κB mediated by BTK. This yields this particular subtype of DLBCL to targeted therapy with ibrutinib. Although initial early phase studies have demonstrated good responses in relapsed and refractory DLBCL, there are limited data to indicate the efficacy of low-toxicity regimens such as that described in this case using rituximab, prednisone, and ibrutinib. The clinical response seen in this patient suggests that in elderly patients with significant comorbidities, complete responses can be achieved, leading to improvement in quality of life and likely duration of life as well. It is important to remember, however, that with new therapies come new important side effects and toxicities. In our case, the patient developed atrial fibrillation, a known toxicity associated with ibrutinib. He also developed uncompensated heart failure related to his atrial fibrillation as well as sepsis which was most likely related to ibrutinib use. It is therefore important to keep important toxicities of these medications in mind, especially in elderly patients with comorbidities. Additionally, it is important to be aware of the potential shortcomings of novel therapies. For ibrutinib in ABC DLBCL, there are known resistance mechanisms. It is important to be aware of these as they may potentially be associated with recurrent disease or disease that is primary refractory of ibrutinib therapy. One such pathway includes the PI3K-Akt-mTOR signaling cascade, either by over-expression of CD79B BCR subunit or mutations in the PLC gamma subunit [15, 16]. In vitro studies suggest these resistance mechanisms can be overcome by inhibition of the PI3K pathway and may represent a second potential target in A3C DLBCL [4]. It will be interesting to see the changes to treatment paradigms in the coming years as these new targeted agents are utilized to their full potential.

Consent

Consent to publish was obtained from the patient's next of kin, his wife.

Conflicts of Interest

The authors declare that they have no conflicts of interest.

Acknowledgments

The authors would like to acknowledge the rest of the Division of Hematology and Medical Oncology at the Veterans Administration Medical Center, Loma Linda, Loma Linda, CA, as well as the Veterans that the authors care for. Funding for this case report was provided by the Division of Hematology and Medical Oncology of the Loma Linda Veterans Administration Medical Center, Loma Linda, CA.

References

[1] J. Y. Hong, C. Suh, and W. S. Kim, "Evolution of frontline treatment of diffuse large B-cell lymphoma: a brief review and recent update," *F1000Research*, vol. 5, p. 1933, 2016.

[2] J. W. Friedberg, "Using the pathology report in initial treatment decisions for diffuse large B-cell lymphoma: time for a precision medicine approach," *Hematology*, vol. 2015, no. 1, pp. 618–624, 2015.

[3] K. A. Blum, "B-cell receptor pathway modulators in NHL," *Hematology*, vol. 2015, no. 1, pp. 82–91, 2015.

[4] S. A. Ezell, M. Mayo, T. Bihani et al., "Synergistic induction of apoptosis by combination of BTK and dual mTORC1/2 inhibitors in diffuse large B cell lymphoma," *Oncotarget*, vol. 5, no. 13, pp. 4990–5001, 2014.

[5] W. H. Wilson, R. M. Young, R. Schmitz et al., "Targeting B cell receptor signaling with ibrutinib in diffuse large B cell lymphoma," *Nature Medicine*, vol. 21, no. 8, pp. 922–926, 2015.

[6] N. S. Grover and S. I. Park, "Novel targeted agents in hodgkin and non-hodgkin lymphoma therapy," *Pharmaceuticals*, vol. 8, no. 4, pp. 607–636, 2015.

[7] A. Novero, P. M. Ravella, Y. Chen, G. Dous, and D. Liu, "Ibrutinib for B cell malignancies," *Experimental Hematology & Oncology*, vol. 3, no. 1, p. 4, 2014.

[8] A. Younes, C. Thieblemont, F. Morschhauser et al., "Combination of ibrutinib with rituximab, cyclophosphamide, doxorubicin, vincristine, and prednisone (R-CHOP) for treatment-naive patients with CD20-positive B-cell non-Hodgkin lymphoma: a non-randomised, phase 1b study," *Lancet Oncology*, vol. 15, no. 9, pp. 1019–1026, 2014.

[9] K. Maddocks, B. Christian, S. Jaglowski et al., "A phase 1/1b study of rituximab, bendamustine, and ibrutinib in patients with untreated and relapsed/refractory non-Hodgkin lymphoma," *Blood*, vol. 125, no. 2, pp. 242–248, 2015.

[10] Y. Y. Tien, B. K. Link, J. M. Brooks, K. Wright, and E. Chrischilles, "Treatment of diffuse large B-cell lymphoma in the elderly: regimens without anthracyclines are common and not futile," *Leukemia & Lymphoma*, vol. 56, no. 1, pp. 65–71, 2015.

[11] S. Luminari and M. Federico, "Case studies of elderly patients with non-Hodgkin's lymphoma," *Hematology Reports*, vol. 3, no. 3, p. e7, 2011.

[12] H. Gomez, L. Mas, L. Casanova et al., "Elderly patients with aggressive non-Hodgkin's lymphoma treated with CHOP chemotherapy plus granulocyte-macrophage colony-stimulating factor: identification of two age subgroups with differing hematologic toxicity," *Journal of Clinical Oncology*, vol. 16, no. 7, pp. 2352–2358, 1998.

[13] G. Salles, M. Barrett, R. Foa et al., "Rituximab in B-cell hematologic malignancies: a review of 20 years of clinical experience," *Advances in Therapy*, vol. 34, no. 10, pp. 2232–2273, 2017.

[14] C. S. Lee, M. A. Rattu, and S. S. Kim, "A review of a novel, Bruton's tyrosine kinase inhibitor, ibrutinib," *Journal of Oncology Pharmacy Practice*, vol. 22, no. 1, pp. 92–104, 2016.

[15] J. H. Kim, W. S. Kim, K. Ryu, S. J. Kim, and C. Park, "CD79B limits response of diffuse large B cell lymphoma to ibrutinib," *Leukemia & Lymphoma*, vol. 57, no. 6, pp. 1413–1422, 2016.

[16] J. A. Woyach, R. R. Furman, T. M. Liu et al., "Resistance mechanisms for the Bruton's tyrosine kinase inhibitor ibrutinib," *New England Journal of Medicine*, vol. 370, no. 24, pp. 2286–2294, 2014.

4

Amebic Encephalitis in a Patient with Chronic Lymphocytic Leukemia on Ibrutinib Therapy

Ensi Voshtina (iD),[1] Huiya Huang,[2] Renju Raj,[3] and Ehab Atallah[3]

[1]Department of Medicine, Medical College of Wisconsin, Milwaukee, WI, USA
[2]Department of Pathology, Medical College of Wisconsin, Milwaukee, WI, USA
[3]Department of Hematology and Oncology, Medical College of Wisconsin, Milwaukee, WI, USA

Correspondence should be addressed to Ensi Voshtina; evoshtina@mcw.edu

Academic Editor: Kiyotaka Kawauchi

Chronic lymphocytic leukemia (CLL) is the most common type of leukemia in Western countries. A common first-line therapy offered to qualifying patients includes ibrutinib, an oral covalent inhibitor of Bruton's tyrosine kinase. Treatment of CLL with ibrutinib therapy is generally well tolerated; however, serious opportunistic infections are being reported in patients treated with ibrutinib. In this report, we present a patient with CLL on ibrutinib therapy who developed rapidly declining neurological status concerning for the central nervous system (CNS) process related to his immunocompromised status. Despite multiple testing modalities, no evidence was found to explain the acute changes the patient was experiencing, and he had no improvement with common antimicrobial coverage. The patient ultimately expired, and autopsy of the brain revealed granulomatous amebic encephalitis due to opportunistic infection by *Acanthamoeba* species. As evidenced by this case, ibrutinib therapy, despite being generally well tolerated, has the potential to predispose patients to opportunistic infections like amebic encephalitis. Amebic encephalitis is a highly lethal CNS infection, and it is important for clinicians to recognize early on the potential for infection in patients on ibrutinib therapy presenting with CNS symptoms.

1. Introduction

Chronic lymphocytic leukemia (CLL) is the most common type of leukemia in western countries with an estimate of about 20,000 newly diagnosed cases [1]. Clinical course of CLL patients is highly variable and partly depends on the stage of the disease. Staging is commonly performed using the Rai staging or the Binet staging [2]. An impaired immune system predisposes CLL patients to frequent infections which is a common cause of death in these patients. Treatment for CLL is chosen based on cytogenetic abnormalities, age, and performance status of the patient. Currently, the first-line therapy offered to unfit elderly patients with multiple comorbidities as well as CLL patients with 17p deletion includes ibrutinib, an oral covalent inhibitor of Bruton's tyrosine kinase [2, 3]. Ibrutinib is generally well tolerated, and the rate of infections reported in clinical trials with ibrutinib was comparable to historical controls; however with long-term follow-up, serious infections are being reported in patients treated with ibrutinib [4–7].

The most common infection in patients with CLL undergoing immunosuppressive treatment has been associated with bacteria and frequently involves the respiratory and urinary tracts [8]. Amebic encephalitis is an extremely rare and highly lethal central nervous system (CNS) infection, with mortality rate above 90% [9]. The initial symptoms can be indistinguishable from bacterial meningitis or mimic a brain abscess, bringing challenge to early diagnosis. We report a patient with CLL who developed an opportunistic infection with amebic encephalitis while on ibrutinib therapy.

2. Case Presentation

The patient was a 72-year-old male who presented to the emergency department (ED) with complaints of headache and seizure-like activity with shaking of his bilateral upper extremities. His past medical history was significant for CLL with 13q deletion diagnosed 6 years prior to presentation. He was treated at that time with fludarabine and rituximab for 4 cycles; however, he was not able to complete a 5th cycle due to prolonged cytopenia. Two years later due to progression of disease, he was started on ibrutinib 420 mg daily and continued for 2 years. He developed severe neutropenia while on ibrutinib, and treatment was held for two months until resolution. He presented to the ED one month after resuming ibrutinib.

At presentation, the patient was alert with the only examination finding of episodic shaking movements. He was afebrile and had a leukocytosis of 15,200/μL with 66% lymphocytes. Initial workup included computed tomography (CT) of the head without contrast which showed no findings to explain presenting symptoms. Continuous electroencephalography (EEG) evaluation was negative for epileptiform activity. With persistent symptoms he was started on anticonvulsants with levetiracetam and phenytoin. A magnetic resonance imaging (MRI) of the brain with contrast was obtained, and it showed a nonspecific focal area of increased signal involving the right frontal cortex (Figure 1(a)). He was transferred to our institution for further workup and management.

On arrival, the patient was evaluated for progression of CLL by the chest, abdomen, and pelvis CT which was negative for any evidence of disease with no lymphadenopathy or splenomegaly. MRI of the spine was performed and was negative for any disease other than degenerative changes. Ophthalmological evaluation was unrevealing for any intraocular pathology. He was worked up for autoimmune processes with ANA, CRP, and ESR, all of which were insignificant. Infectious workup with blood culture, urine culture, quantiferon-TB, histoplasma, blastomyces, influenza, RPR screen, and HIV were negative. He had a lumbar puncture which showed cerebrospinal fluid (CSF) with elevated WBC 97/μL, polysegmented neutrophils (PMN) 2%, lymphocytes 82%, red blood cells (RBC) 4/μL, elevated protein 93 mg/dL, and normal glucose of 44 mg/dL. FilmArray meningitis and encephalitis panel was negative for all the following tested agents: *Escherichia coli*, *Haemophilus influenzae*, *Listeria monocytogenes*, *Neisseria meningitidis*, *Streptococcus* group B, *Streptococcus pneumoniae*, *Cytomegalovirus*, *Enterovirus*, *Herpes simplex* virus 1 and 2, *Human herpesvirus 6*, *Human parechovirus*, *Varicella zoster virus*, and *Cryptococcus neoformans*. Gram stain and culture also turned out to be negative. Cytologic analysis of CSF was negative for malignant cells or large cell transformation. CSF flow cytometry showed a minute population of 0.04% CD5+ B-CLL cells, which was not felt to be clinically significant and sufficient to explain the acute changes the patient was experiencing. Other CSF tests, which were negative, included angiotensin-1-converting enzyme, John Cunningham (JC) polyomavirus, cryptococcal antigen, fungal culture, and CSF toxoplasma serologies.

The patient became increasingly lethargic and started complaining of worsening headache. He also started having high fevers which persisted despite treatment with broad-spectrum antibiotics with vancomycin and

piperacillin/tazobactam and antivirals with acyclovir. His neurological status continued to decline and repeat MRI brain showed new and increase in size of previously known scattered hyperintensities with associated rim enhancement (Figure 1(c)). At this time, infectious etiology was favored, given the acuity of changes seen on imaging and patient status. The infectious coverage was expanded and included IV vancomycin, cefepime, and ampicillin for bacterial meningitis; IV amphotericin B for atypical fungal meningitis; and IV acyclovir was continued for viral encephalitis. The patient continued to decompensate clinically, and a repeat CT of the head showed hydrocephalus. An external ventricular drain was placed which did not improve his status. A leptomeningeal biopsy was not performed considering the difficult location and size of the lesions. As all workup continued to be unrevealing, progressive multifocal leukoencephalopathy (PML) was thought to be the most likely diagnosis to fit the patient's medical history and imaging and laboratory results; however, JC polyomavirus was tested negative on two separate CSF analyses, making this diagnosis unlikely. The patient ultimately expired within two weeks after he presented with the neurologic symptoms after support was withdrawn per family request, and an autopsy was performed.

Autopsy of the brain showed diffuse cerebral edema with right-sided predominance on gross findings. There were multiple areas of hemorrhagic necrosis including the bilateral frontal lobe, right parasagittal posterior frontal lobe, left temporal lobe, bilateral medial occipital lobe, and paraventricular areas. Microscopic findings revealed parenchymal necrosis with mixed inflammation, amebic trophozoites, and occasional cysts (Figures 2(a) and 2(b)). This mixed infiltrate was seen involving the meninges. The amebas were prominent around vessels, and occasional multinucleated giant cells were seen (Figures 2(c) and 2(d)). The autopsy brain was sent to the Centers for Disease Control and Prevention (CDC) and immunohistochemical stains were performed, which identified *Acanthamoeba* species with no evidence of *Naegleria fowleri*. His final diagnosis based on autopsy was necrotizing meningoencephalitis with morphologic and immunohistochemical evidence of *Acanthamoeba* species.

3. Discussion

A wide array of conditions can cause neurological symptoms in CLL patients. The incidence of leptomeningeal involvement of CLL is rare and has been reported at 0.8 to 2% based on autopsy case studies [10, 11]. Another concern is that CNS symptoms could represent a more malignant variant such as diffuse large B-cell lymphoma transformation as seen in Richter's syndrome (RS). Just as in CLL CNS involvement, only a few cases of isolated RS without systemic lymphoma have been reported [12]. Oftentimes, CLL cells tend to recruit to sites of inflammation in both infectious and inflammatory processes and to discern them as the etiology for the CNS manifestation can be clinically challenging [13]. A B-cell monoclonal lymphocytosis >5% by flow cytometry in the CSF was found to be associated with

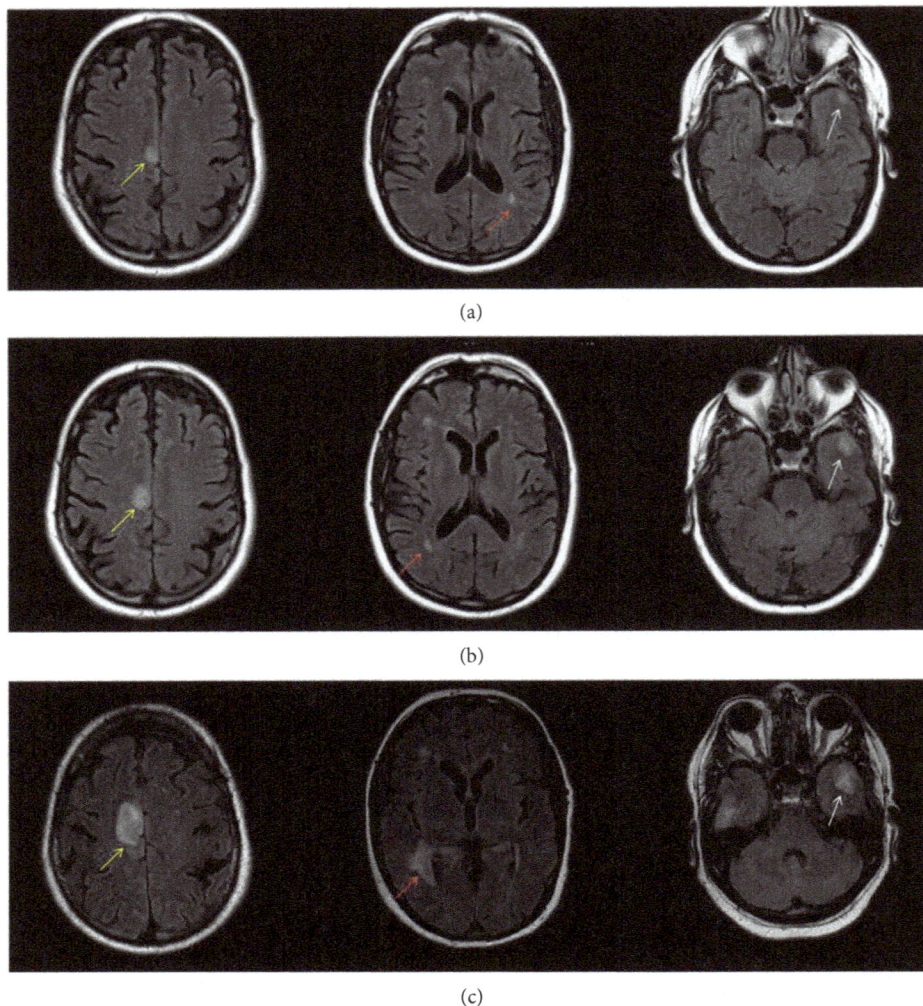

(a)

(b)

(c)

FIGURE 1: Axial T2-FLAIR MRI brain. (a) MRI at initial presentation shows the focal area of increased signal in the right frontal cortex (yellow arrow) along with areas of abnormal white matter signal abnormality in the left occipital lobe (red arrow) and the left temporal lobe (white arrow). (b) MRI obtained 2 days later with the increase in size of signal abnormality involving the right frontal cortex (yellow arrow) and multiple areas of signal abnormality in the right frontal, right occipital (red arrow), and left temporal lobes (white arrow). (c) Ten days from initial presentation, there were new and increase in previously known long TR hyperintensities involving the cortical (yellow arrow) and subcortical (red and white arrows) white matter. Given the short interval imaging findings, an infectious etiology was favored as the cause of the patient's symptoms.

clinically significant CNS involvement with CLL [14]. In our particular patient, because of the lack of pathological evidence of large cell transformation and the small amount of CLL cells seen in the CSF, CLL was not considered to be the etiology of neurological symptoms. Moreover, he was on ibrutinib which has been shown to cross the blood-brain barrier and have CNS penetration with other forms of non-Hodgkin's lymphoma [15]. Considering all of these factors, CNS involvement by CLL was not rendered as the clinical diagnosis.

The most commonly described neurologic complication in patients with CLL is opportunistic CNS infection [16]. One such infection-associated complication is PML, which is a demyelinating process in the CNS caused by JC virus infection. HIV infection accounts for 85% of PML cases. PML is also associated with hematologic malignancies such

as CLL, with a reported incidence rate of 11.1 per 100,000 person-years [17, 18]. Treatment with various chemotherapeutic agents has been linked to the development of PML [19–22]. There has been one case report of PML after treatment with ibrutinib therapy in a patient with CLL [23]. MRI often shows asymmetric lesions. Diagnosis via CSF analysis by PCR in immunosuppressed patients has been shown to have a sensitivity of 93% and specificity of 99% for detecting JC virus [24], though biopsy-proven disease remains to be the gold standard for diagnosis. In our case, however, both CSF analysis and autopsy results were negative for JC virus infection thus excluding PML.

Risk of infection and its complications in CLL patients have been associated with disease status and treatment-related immunosuppression [25, 26]. Ibrutinib therapy has been associated with a high rate of infection of 148.6/100

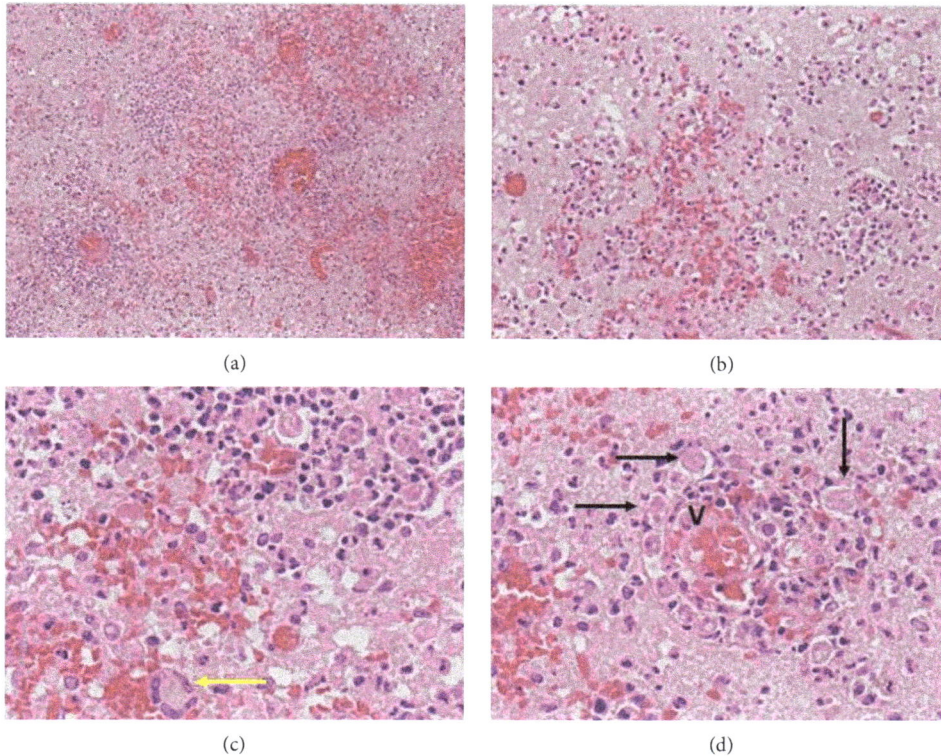

FIGURE 2: Microphotographs of autopsy brain sections. Hematoxylin and eosin stain. (a) A low-power view shows areas of parenchymal hemorrhage and necrosis with mixed inflammation, ×10 objective. (b) A higher power view demonstrates amebic trophozoites and occasional cysts, ×20 objective. (c) At high power, numerous amebic trophozoites can be seen intermixed with inflammatory cells and occasional multinucleated giant cells (yellow arrow), ×40 objective. (d) The amebae (black arrow) are prominent around vessels (V), ×40 objective.

person-year, especially in patients receiving treatment for relapsed or refractory CLL [5]. The majority of infections are bacterial, but there have also been case reports of rare opportunistic infections with military tuberculosis, invasive aspergillosis, cryptococcal meningoencephalitis, and disseminated fusarium infection [6, 27–31]. The most commonly seen atypical infection is found to be pneumocystis jiroveci pneumonia [7].

Amebic encephalitis is a rare CNS infection with high mortality rate caused by free-living amebae [9]. There are two entities of amebic encephalitis, primary amebic meningoencephalitis (PAM) and granulomatous amebic encephalitis (GAE). PAM caused by infection with *Naegleria fowleri* is a rapidly fatal hemorrhagic encephalitis typically occurring in immunocompetent children and young adults swimming in fresh water or inadequately chlorinated pools. GAE is less common and is due to opportunistic infection in immunosuppressed or debilitated hosts by *Acanthamoeba* species, most commonly found in lakes, tap water, and heating and air conditioning units, or *Balamuthia mandrillaris* [32]. Although *Acanthamoeba* encephalitis has also been reported in immunocompetent hosts [33], it is a mostly insidious and almost uniformly fatal encephalitic process [34], with acute and fulminant cases also reported [35, 36]. The patient usually presents with fever, nonspecific neurological symptoms, and enhancing edematous brain lesions found on MRI, but enhancement may or may not be seen despite the presence of an aggressive, necrotizing, parasitic infection [29]. The low incidence, nonspecific presentation, and imaging findings lead to difficulty in early diagnosis of the infection. Treatment regimens are mostly anecdotal and not well defined as most of the cases are diagnosed on autopsy. Our patient received amphotericin B and did not respond. Despite its rarity, clinicians should remain aware of this disease especially in immunocompromised patients. To our knowledge, this is the first case of amebic encephalitis in a patient receiving ibrutinib therapy for treatment of progressed CLL.

4. Conclusion

In this report, we present a patient with CLL on ibrutinib therapy who developed an opportunistic infection with amebic encephalitis. This is an extremely rare and highly lethal CNS infection that currently has no standard of treatment. It is important for clinicians to recognize the potential for infection in patients receiving ibrutinib therapy.

Conflicts of Interest

The authors have no conflicts of interest to report regarding the submission of this article.

References

[1] R. L. Siegel, K. D. Miller, and A. Jemal, "Cancer statistics," *CA: A Cancer Journal for Clinicians*, vol. 68, no. 1, pp. 7–30, 2018.

[2] M. Hallek, "Chronic lymphocytic leukemia: 2017 update on diagnosis, risk stratification, and treatment," *American Journal of Hematology*, vol. 92, no. 9, pp. 946–965, 2017.

[3] J. A. Burger, A. Tedeschi, P. M. Barr et al., "Ibrutinib as initial therapy for patients with chronic lymphocytic leukemia," *New England Journal of Medicine*, vol. 373, no. 25, pp. 2425–2437, 2015.

[4] S. O'Brien, R. R. Furman, S. E. Coutre et al., "Ibrutinib as initial therapy for elderly patients with chronic lymphocytic leukaemia or small lymphocytic lymphoma: an open-label, multicentre, phase 1b/2 trial," *The Lancet Oncology*, vol. 15, no. 1, pp. 48–58, 2014.

[5] A. M. Williams, A. M. Baran, P. J. Meacham et al., "Analysis of the risk of infection in patients with chronic lymphocytic leukemia in the era of novel therapies," *Leukemia and Lymphoma*, vol. 59, no. 3, pp. 625–632, 2018.

[6] D. Ghez, A. Calleja, C. Protin et al., "Early-onset invasive aspergillosis and other fungal infections in patients treated with ibrutinib," *Blood*, vol. 131, no. 17, pp. 1955–1959, 2018.

[7] I. E. Ahn, T. Jerussi, M. Farooqui, X. Tian, A. Wiestner, and J. Gea-Banacloche, "Atypical *Pneumocystis jirovecii* pneumonia in previously untreated patients with CLL on single-agent ibrutinib," *Blood*, vol. 128, no. 15, pp. 1940–1943, 2016.

[8] V. A. Morrison, K. R. Rai, B. L. Peterson et al., "Impact of therapy with chlorambucil, fludarabine, or fludarabine plus chlorambucil on infections in patients with chronic lymphocytic leukemia: Intergroup Study Cancer and Leukemia Group B 9011," *Journal of Clinical Oncology*, vol. 19, no. 16, pp. 3611–3621, 2001.

[9] A. Pana and S. S. Bhimji, *Amebic Meningoencephalitis*, StatPearls Publishing, Orlando, FL, USA, 2018, http://www.ncbi.nlm.nih.gov/pubmed/28613505.

[10] M. C. J. Hanse, M. B. Van't Veer, K. Van Lom, and M. J. Van Den Bent, "Incidence of central nervous system involvement in chronic lymphocytic leukemia and outcome to treatment," *Journal of Neurology*, vol. 255, no. 6, pp. 828–830, 2008.

[11] A. A. Moazzam, J. Drappatz, R. Y. Kim, and S. Kesari, "Chronic lymphocytic leukemia with central nervous system involvement: report of two cases with a comprehensive literature review," *Journal of Neuro-Oncology*, vol. 106, no. 1, pp. 185–200, 2012.

[12] A. Bagic, V. D. Lupu, C. M. Kessler, and C. Tornatore, "Isolated Richter's transformation of the brain," *Journal of Neuro-Oncology*, vol. 83, no. 3, pp. 325–328, 2007.

[13] G. S. Nowakowski, T. G. Call, W. G. Morice, P. J. Kurtin, R. J. Cook, and C. S. Zent, "Clinical significance of monoclonal B cells in cerebrospinal fluid," *Cytometry Part B: Clinical Cytometry*, vol. 63B, no. 1, pp. 23–27, 2005.

[14] P. Strati, J. H. Uhm, T. J. Kaufmann et al., "Prevalence and characteristics of central nervous system involvement by chronic lymphocytic leukemia," *Haematologica*, vol. 101, no. 4, pp. 458–465, 2016.

[15] S. Bernard, L. Goldwirt, S. Amorim et al., "Activity of ibrutinib in mantle cell lymphoma patients with central nervous system relapse," *Blood*, vol. 126, no. 14, pp. 1695–1698, 2015.

[16] J. H. Bower, J. E. Hammack, S. K. McDonnell, and A. Tefferi, "The neurologic complications of B-cell chronic lymphocytic leukemia," *Neurology*, vol. 48, no. 2, pp. 407–412, 1997.

[17] K. L. Amend, B. Turnbull, N. Foskett, P. Napalkov, T. Kurth, and J. Seeger, "Incidence of progressive multifocal leukoencephalopathy in patients without HIV," *Neurology*, vol. 75, no. 15, pp. 1326–1332, 2010.

[18] T. Weber, "Progressive multifocal leukoencephalopathy," *Neurologic Clinics*, vol. 26, no. 3, pp. 833–854, 2008.

[19] K. R. Carson, A. M. Evens, E. A. Richey et al., "Progressive multifocal leukoencephalopathy after rituximab therapy in HIV-negative patients: a report of 57 cases from the Research on Adverse Drug Events and Reports project," *Blood*, vol. 113, no. 20, pp. 4834–4840, 2009.

[20] S. L. Goldberg, A. L. Pecora, R. S. Alter et al., "Unusual viral infections (progressive multifocal leukoencephalopathy and cytomegalovirus disease) after high-dose chemotherapy with autologous blood stem cell rescue and peritransplantation rituximab," *Blood*, vol. 99, no. 4, pp. 1486–1488, 2002.

[21] J. García-Suárez, D. de Miguel, I. Krsnik, H. Bañas, I. Arribas, and C. Burgaleta, "Changes in the natural history of progressive multifocal leukoencephalopathy in HIV-negative lymphoproliferative disorders: impact of novel therapies," *American Journal of Hematology*, vol. 80, no. 4, pp. 271–281, 2005.

[22] H. Gonzalez, F. Bolgert, P. Camporo, and V. Leblond, "Progressive multifocal leukoencephalitis (PML) in three patients treated with standard-dose fludarabine (FAMP)," *Hematology and Cell Therapy*, vol. 41, no. 4, pp. 183–186, 1999.

[23] M. Lutz, A. B. Schulze, E. Rebber et al., "Progressive multifocal leukoencephalopathy after ibrutinib therapy for chronic lymphocytic leukemia," *Cancer Research and Treatment*, vol. 49, no. 2, pp. 548–552, 2017.

[24] I. J. Koralnik, D. Boden, V. X. Mai, C. I. Lord, and N. L. Letvin, "JC virus DNA load in patients with and without progressive multifocal leukoencephalopathy," *Neurology*, vol. 52, no. 2, pp. 253–260, 1999.

[25] M. Hensel, M. Kornacker, S. Yammeni, G. Egerer, and A. D. Ho, "Disease activity and pretreatment, rather than hypogammaglobulinaemia, are major risk factors for infectious complications in patients with chronic lymphocytic leukaemia," *British Journal of Haematology*, vol. 122, no. 4, pp. 600–606, 2003.

[26] C. A. Dasanu, "Intrinsic and treatment-related immune alterations in chronic lymphocytic leukaemia and their impact for clinical practice," *Expert Opinion on Pharmacotherapy*, vol. 9, no. 9, pp. 1481–1494, 2008.

[27] S.-Y. Wang, T. Ebert, N. Jaekel, S. Schubert, D. Niederwieser, and H. K. Al-Ali, "Miliary tuberculosis after initiation of ibrutinib in chronic lymphocytic leukemia," *Annals of Hematology*, vol. 94, no. 8, pp. 1419–1420, 2015.

[28] B. Arthurs, K. Wunderle, M. Hsu, and S. Kim, "Invasive aspergillosis related to ibrutinib therapy for chronic lymphocytic leukemia," *Respiratory Medicine Case Reports*, vol. 21, pp. 27–29, 2017.

[29] M. S. Lionakis, K. Dunleavy, M. Roschewski et al., "Inhibition of B cell receptor signaling by ibrutinib in primary CNS lymphoma," *Cancer Cell*, vol. 31, no. 6, pp. 833–843, 2017.

[30] T. S. Y. Chan, R. Au-Yeung, C.-S. Chim, S. C. Y. Wong, and Y.-L. Kwong, "Disseminated fusarium infection after ibrutinib therapy in chronic lymphocytic leukaemia," *Annals of Hematology*, vol. 96, no. 5, pp. 871–872, 2017.

[31] M. Baron, J. M. Zini, T. Challan Belval et al., "Fungal infections in patients treated with ibrutinib: two unusual cases of invasive aspergillosis and cryptococcal meningoencephalitis," *Leukemia and Lymphoma*, vol. 58, no. 12, pp. 2981–2982, 2017.

[32] J. J. Sell, F. W. Rupp, and W. W. Orrison, "Granulomatous amebic encephalitis caused by acanthamoeba," *Neuroradiology*, vol. 39, no. 6, pp. 434–436, 1997.

[33] J. Walochnik, A. Aichelburg, O. Assadian et al., "Granulomatous amoebic encephalitis caused by acanthamoeba amoebae of genotype T2 in a human immunodeficiency virus-negative patient," *Journal of Clinical Microbiology*, vol. 46, no. 1, pp. 338–340, 2008.

[34] V. Kaushal, D. K. Chhina, R. Kumar, H. S. Pannu, H. P. S. Dhooria, and R. S. Chhina, "*Acanthamoeba* encephalitis," *Indian Journal of Medical Microbiology*, vol. 26, no. 2, pp. 182–184, 2008.

[35] P. Lackner, R. Beer, G. Broessner et al., "Acute granulomatous acanthamoeba encephalitis in an immunocompetent patient," *Neurocritical Care*, vol. 12, no. 1, pp. 91–94, 2010.

[36] W. Meersseman, K. Lagrou, R. Sciot et al., "Rapidly fatal *Acanthamoeba* encephalitis and treatment of cryoglobulinemia," *Emerging Infectious Diseases*, vol. 13, no. 3, pp. 469–471, 2007.

5

An Atypical Presentation of Chronic Atrophic Gastritis: Hemolytic Anemia and Mesenteric Panniculitis

Zurab Azmaiparashvili, Vinicius M. Jorge, and Catiele Antunes

Albert Einstein Medical Center, Philadelphia, PA, USA

Correspondence should be addressed to Zurab Azmaiparashvili; azmaipaz@einstein.edu

Academic Editor: Kazunori Nakase

Microangiopathic hemolytic anemia (MAHA) requires an aggressive approach since primary thrombotic microangiopathy syndromes such as thrombotic thrombocytopenic purpura (TTP) can progress rapidly to a fatal outcome. Differential diagnosis can be challenging even for an experienced hematologist. We present a case of a 52-year-old male who presented with symptoms of mesenteric panniculitis and showed signs of MAHA. His condition was attributed to severe vitamin B12 deficiency secondary to chronic atrophic gastritis and initiation of appropriate therapy was met with complete resolution of symptoms and normalization of hematologic parameters.

1. Introduction

Thrombotic microangiopathies are a diverse group of disorders that may be congenital or acquired, present in childhood or in adults, and manifest an acute or a more gradual progressive course [1]. Clinically they are characterized by thrombocytopenia, microangiopathic hemolytic anemia (MAHA), and extremely elevated serum lactate dehydrogenase (LDH) levels with or without signs of end-organ damage [1, 2]. Differential diagnosis can be challenging as primary thrombotic microangiopathy syndromes such as thrombotic thrombocytopenic purpura (TTP) can progress rapidly to a fatal outcome without prompt initiation of effective therapy [3]. In this article, we discuss a case of severe vitamin B12 deficiency presenting as concurrent microangiopathic hemolytic anemia and mesenteric panniculitis.

2. Case Report

A 52-year-old Hispanic male with past medical history significant for essential hypertension, gastroesophageal reflux disease (GERD), and recently diagnosed anemia attributed to iron deficiency presented to the Emergency Department with three weeks' history of left flank pain. Pain was described as severe, sharp, and constant in nature, made worse with

prolonged fasting or following a meal. No recognizable alleviating factors were reported. Associated symptoms included nausea, vomiting of nonbloody, nonbilious secretions, and retrosternal burning. There was no hematemesis, melena, perrectal bleeding, or change in bowel habits. Patient also reported progressive weakness and fatigue for two weeks and weight loss of approximately ten pounds over the last two months. Patient was prescribed omeprazole and iron supplements for newly diagnosed anemia and abdominal pain by his primary care physician. He denied taking other prescription or over-the-counter medications, herbal supplements, or illicit drugs. Patient denied alcohol or tobacco use. There was no personal or family history of solid or hematologic malignancies or bleeding or thrombotic events.

Patient was afebrile on admission with normal hemodynamic parameters. Physical examination revealed conjunctival pallor and scleral icterus. Cardiovascular and pulmonary examination were within normal limits. Abdominal examination revealed mild to moderate left flank and epigastric tenderness with no rebound or involuntary guarding. There was no palpable hepatosplenomegaly or peripheral lymphadenopathy. The rest of the examination was largely unremarkable.

Complete blood count (CBC) on admission revealed hemoglobin 6.3 g/dL, hematocrit 17.9%, white blood cell

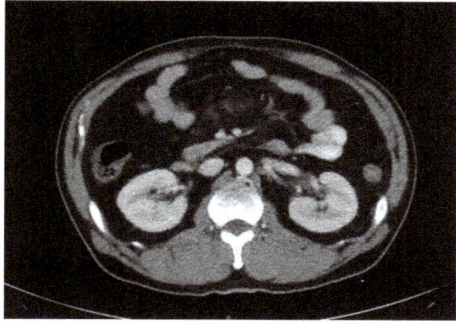

FIGURE 1: CT scan of the abdomen and pelvis showing inflammatory fat stranding in the small bowel mesentery (axial view).

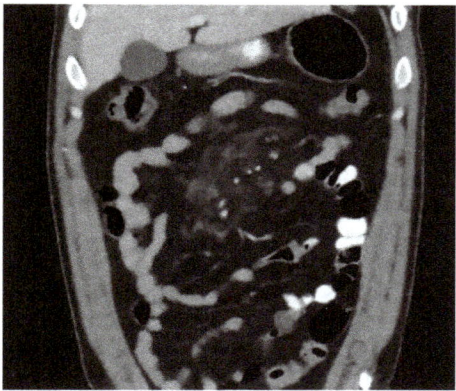

FIGURE 2: Redemonstration of inflammatory fat stranding in the small bowel mesentery (coronal view).

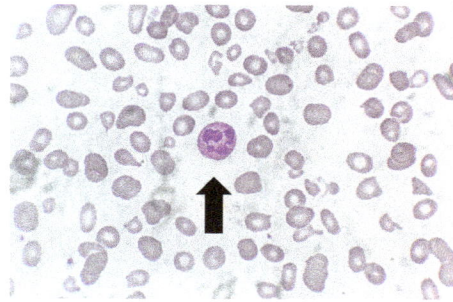

FIGURE 3: Peripheral blood smear showing poikilocytosis, schistocytosis, thrombocytopenia, and a hypersegmented neutrophil (arrow).

(WBC) count 4,100/μL, platelet count 88,000/μL, and reticulocyte count 0.86%. Mean corpuscular volume (MCV) was 96.2 fL and red blood cell distribution width (RDW) was 23.4%. Basic metabolic panel (BMP) showed normal serum electrolyte concentrations and normal renal function with creatinine 0.8 mg/dL and blood urea nitrogen (BUN) 14 mg/dL. Liver function tests (LFTs) on admission revealed elevated total bilirubin concentration of 4.5 mg/dL with direct fraction of 0.5 mg/dL and mildly elevated alanine aminotransferase (ALT) and aspartate aminotransferase (AST) levels of 67 IU/L and 165 IU/L, respectively. Coagulation profile showed international normalized ratio (INR) of 1.2 and partial thromboplastin time (PTT) of 25.4 seconds. Direct antiglobulin test and antibody screen were negative. Lactate dehydrogenase (LDH) was 6,235 IU/L while haptoglobin was <8.0 mg/dL.

Computed tomography (CT) scan of the abdomen and pelvis showed acute mesenteric inflammation involving central small bowel mesentery, compatible with the diagnosis of mesenteric panniculitis (see Figures 1 and 2).

Peripheral blood smear revealed an abundance of schistocytes and occasional hypersegmented neutrophils (see Figures 3 and 4). This, along with the initial laboratory findings, was concerning for an atypical presentation of thrombotic thrombocytopenic purpura (TTP).

At this point, the plan was to start urgent plasmapheresis. However, within the next hour, serum vitamin B12 level was reported at <109 pg/dL (normal range: 213–816 pg/dL) with serum homocysteine level of 86.8 μmol/L (normal range: 5.1–15.4 μmol/L). Plasmapheresis plans were stopped. Bone marrow smear and biopsy were performed confirming erythroid hyperplasia and megaloblastic anemia (see Figures 5 and 6). Cyanocobalamin repletion was promptly initiated.

Over the next 2 days, hemoglobin remained stable, reticulocyte count increased to 1.17%, and major improvement in the degree of hemolysis was noted. Furthermore, abdominal pain resolved and patient was tolerating regular diet. Gastroenterology team recommended upper endoscopy and considered mesenteric panniculitis reactive to underlying hematologic disorder. Late during the course of this admission, the sent-out laboratory tests showed methylmalonic acid level of 4080 nmol/L (normal range: 87–318 nmol/L), while the serologic tests for Intrinsic Factor Blocking Antibody and Anti-Gastric Parietal Cell Antibody were strongly positive. Together, these findings suggested autoimmune chronic atrophic gastritis as the underlying etiology of current presentation.

Esophagogastroduodenoscopy (EGD) was performed as outpatient showing two large, sessile polyps in the gastric body (see Figure 7) that were completely removed. The remainder of the EGD was within normal limits. Gastric polyp histologic examination was positive for well-differentiated neuroendocrine tumor and background changes of chronic atrophic gastritis.

Patient continues to receive cyanocobalamin replacement therapy as outpatient. Vitamin B12 replacement has been met with complete normalization of hematologic parameters and resolution of symptoms of mesenteric panniculitis.

This is the first case report of vitamin B12 deficiency secondary to chronic autoimmune gastritis, presenting with concurrent microangiopathic hemolytic anemia and mesenteric panniculitis.

3. Discussion

TTP has been classically diagnosed based on a pentad of MAHA, thrombocytopenia, neurologic abnormalities, renal dysfunction, and fever [3, 4]. However, with the introduction of plasmapheresis as the effective treatment modality,

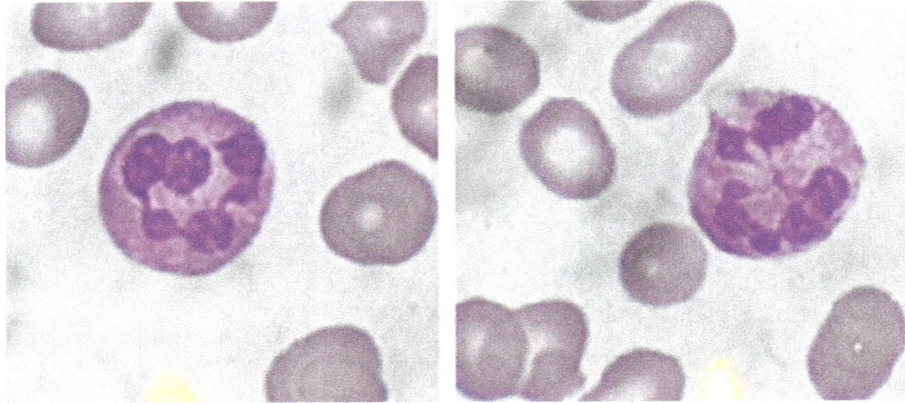

FIGURE 4: Magnified view of hypersegmented neutrophils.

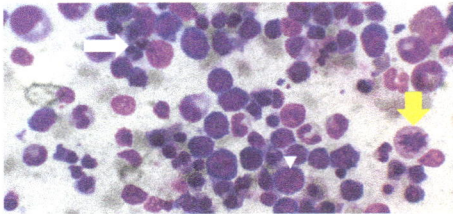

FIGURE 5: Bone marrow smear showing multinucleated red cell (white arrow), typical megaloblast (arrowhead), and mitotic phase cell (yellow arrow).

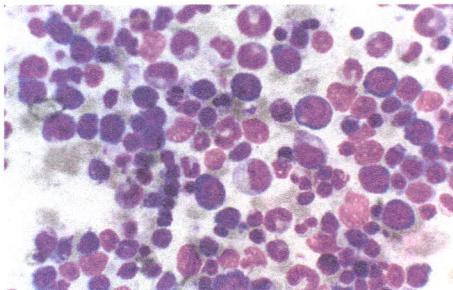

FIGURE 6: Bone marrow smear showing erythroid hyperplasia with dysplastic features and megaloblastic changes.

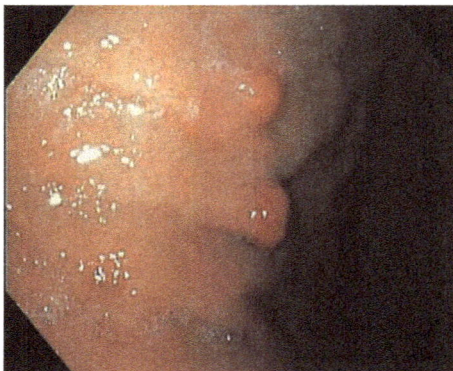

FIGURE 7: EGD showing two firm sessile polyps.

presumptive diagnosis is commonly made on the basis of MAHA and thrombocytopenia without an apparent cause [3, 5]. As a result, up to 10% of patients diagnosed with TTP and receiving plasmapheresis may be later found to have an alternate diagnosis [6], underlining the importance of continuous reevaluation.

The most common symptoms of TTP at presentation are generalized weakness, abdominal pain, nausea, and vomiting [3]. With suggestive clinical symptoms and characteristic laboratory findings, it is not surprising that our patient was presumptively diagnosed with TTP and planned for initiation of plasmapheresis. However, the possibility of vitamin B12 deficiency was also entertained in view of relatively mild thrombocytopenia, extremely elevated LDH level, and presence of hypersegmented neutrophils on blood smear.

Vitamin B12 deficiency causes dyssynchrony between nuclear and cytoplasmic maturation, resulting in ineffective erythropoiesis, intramedullary hemolysis, and characteristic features of megaloblastic anemia on blood smear: macrocytosis and hypersegmented neutrophils [7]. Other less common hematologic findings associated with vitamin B12 deficiency include thrombocytopenia, pancytopenia, and hemolytic anemia [8]. Furthermore, vitamin B12 deficiency has been implicated as a cause of thrombotic microangiopathy mimicking TTP [9–13]. The mechanism of thrombotic microangiopathy and resultant MAHA is not fully understood, but the presence of hyperhomocysteinemia has been suggested as the plausible link between vitamin B12 deficiency and endothelial dysfunction and microvascular thrombi formation [14, 15].

Mesenteric panniculitis is a relatively uncommon benign condition characterized by varying degrees of inflammation, fat necrosis, and fibrosis of the small bowel mesentery [16]. It may occur spontaneously or in association with other disorders, including abdominal trauma, hematologic and solid organ malignancies, and autoimmune conditions [16, 17]. The majority of cases are diagnosed incidentally during the work-up of an unrelated condition [17]. The most common symptoms in clinically apparent cases are abdominal pain, nausea and vomiting, change in bowel habits, and weight loss [18]. Confirmation of diagnosis generally requires histologic proof of mesenteric panniculitis; however, diagnosis is often suggested by typical radiologic findings [16, 17]. Treatment options are varied, nonstandardized, and typically reserved for symptomatic patients [16, 18]. A myriad of anti-inflammatory and hormonal therapies, including systemic corticosteroids and tamoxifen, alone or in combination, have been used with variable success. Most cases tend to resolve spontaneously with no intervention [16–18].

Mesenteric panniculitis has been reported in association with vitamin B12 deficiency and chronic atrophic gastritis [19]. The patient was treated with prolonged course of systemic corticosteroids with complete symptomatic and radiologic remission. We did not consider treatment of mesenteric panniculitis in our patient as the disease process was assumed to be secondary to concurrent hematologic abnormalities. To our knowledge, there have been no case reports of concurrent mesenteric panniculitis and thrombotic microangiopathy secondary to vitamin B12 deficiency.

Gastric carcinoid tumors, also called gastroenteropancreatic neuroendocrine tumors, comprise approximately 10% to 30% of all carcinoid tumors [20]. There are four different types of gastric carcinoid tumors with type 1 comprising the majority of cases [20, 21]. Type 1 carcinoid tumors are found in association with chronic atrophic gastritis and achlorhydria and are usually multiple, nodular, or polypoid in nature and less than 1 cm in size [20]. Endoscopic resection is the treatment of choice for type 1 gastric carcinoid tumors and they generally follow a benign course with >95% 5-year survival rate [20, 21].

4. Conclusion

Thrombotic microangiopathies are a diverse group of disorders that share microangiopathic hemolytic anemia and thrombocytopenia in common. Vitamin B12 deficiency may present in a similar fashion and pose a diagnostic and therapeutic challenge to the clinicians. We propose exploring further work-up for exclusion of vitamin B12 deficiency as the cause of thrombotic microangiopathy, especially for cases with extremely elevated LDH levels (>2500 IU/L), low reticulocyte counts, mild to moderate thrombocytopenia (>50,000/μL), and/or atypical findings on blood smear such as hypersegmented neutrophils.

Disclosure

The authors presented an earlier version of this article as an abstract at the ACP Internal Medicine Meeting 2017 in San Diego, CA.

Conflicts of Interest

The authors declare that there are no conflicts of interest regarding the publication of this paper.

References

[1] J. N. George and C. M. Nester, "Syndromes of thrombotic microangiopathy," *The New England Journal of Medicine*, vol. 371, no. 7, pp. 654–666, 2014.

[2] J. L. Moake, "Thrombotic microangiopathies," *The New England Journal of Medicine*, vol. 347, no. 8, pp. 589–600, 2002.

[3] J. N. George, "Thrombotic thrombocytopenic purpura," *The New England Journal of Medicine*, vol. 354, no. 18, pp. 1927–1935, 2006.

[4] E. L. Amorosi and J. E. Ultmann, "Thrombotic thrombocytopenic purpura: Report of 16 cases and review of the literature," *Medicine*, vol. 45, pp. 139–159, 1966.

[5] GA. Rock, KH. Shumak, NA. Buskard et al., "Comparison of plasma exchange with plasma infusion in the treatment of thrombotic thrombocytopenic purpura," *The New England Journal of Medicine*, vol. 325, pp. 393–397, 1991.

[6] J. N. George, S. K. Vesely, and D. R. Terrell, "The Oklahoma Thrombotic Thrombocytopenic Purpura-Hemolytic Uremic Syndrome (TTP-HUS) Registry: A Community Perspective of Patients with Clinically Diagnosed TTP-HUS," *Seminars in Hematology*, vol. 41, no. 1, pp. 60–67, 2004.

[7] S. P. Stabler, "Vitamin B$_{12}$ deficiency," *The New England Journal of Medicine*, vol. 368, no. 2, pp. 149–160, 2013.

[8] E. Andrès, S. Affenberger, J. Zimmer et al., "Current hematological findings in cobalamin deficiency. A study of 201 consecutive patients with documented cobalamin deficiency," *Clinical and Laboratory Haematology*, vol. 28, no. 1, pp. 50–56, 2006.

[9] A. K. Tadakamalla, S. K. Talluri, and S. Besur, "Pseudo-thrombotic thrombocytopenic purpura: a rare presentation of pernicious anemia," *North American Journal of Medical Sciences*, vol. 3, no. 10, pp. 472–474, 2011.

[10] K. Walter, J. Vaughn, and D. Martin, "Therapeutic dilemma in the management of a patient with the clinical picture of TTP and severe B12 deficiency," *BMC Hematol*, vol. 15, article 16, pp. 15-16, 2015.

[11] M. Malla and M. Seetharam, "To treat or not to treat: a rare case of pseudo-thrombotic thrombocytopenic purpura in a Jehovah's Witness," *Transfusion*, vol. 56, no. 1, pp. 160–163, 2016.

[12] T. S. Panchabhai, P. D. Patil, E. C. Riley et al., "When the picture is fragmented: Vitamin B12 deficiency masquerading as thrombotic thrombocytopenic purpura," *International Journal of Critical Illness and Injury Science*, vol. 6, no. 2, pp. 89–92, 2016.

[13] N. Noël, G. Maigné, G. Tertian et al., "Hemolysis and schistocytosis in the emergency department: consider pseudothrombotic microangiopathy related to vitamin B12 deficiency," *QJM*, vol. 106, no. 11, Article ID hct142, pp. 1017–1022, 2013.

[14] U. Acharya, J.-T. Gau, W. Horvath, P. Ventura, C.-T. Hsueh, and W. Carlsen, "Hemolysis and hyperhomocysteinemia caused by cobalamin deficiency: Three case reports and review of the literature," *Journal of Hematology and Oncology*, vol. 1, no. 1, article no. 26, 2008.

[15] E. Zittan, M. Preis, I. Asmir et al., "High frequency of vitamin B12 deficiency in asymptomatic individuals homozygous to MTHFR C677T mutation is associated with endothelial dysfunction and homocysteinemia," *American Journal of Physiology—Heart and Circulatory Physiology*, vol. 293, no. 1, pp. H860–H865, 2007.

[16] I. Issa and H. Baydoun, "Mesenteric panniculitis: various presentations and treatment regimens," *World Journal of Gastroenterology*, vol. 15, no. 30, pp. 3827–3830, 2009.

[17] M. Daskalogiannaki, A. Voloudaki, P. Prassopoulos et al., "CT evaluation of mesenteric panniculitis: prevalence and associated diseases," *American Journal of Roentgenology*, vol. 174, no. 2, pp. 427–431, 2000.

[18] K. Vlachos, F. Archontovasilis, E. Falidas, S. Mathioulakis, S. Konstandoudakis, and C. Villias, "Sclerosing Mesenteritis: Diverse clinical presentations and dissimilar treatment options. A case series and review of the literature," *International Archives of Medicine*, vol. 4, no. 1, article no. 17, 2011.

[19] R. Ribeiro, I. Bargiela, and C. Duarte, "A clinical case of mesenteric panniculitis associated with chronic gastritis and biliary lithiasis – diagnosis, treatment and morbidity," *Rev Clin Hosp Prof Dr Fernando Fonseca*, vol. 3, no. 1, pp. 27–29, 2015.

[20] J. W. Wardlaw and J. W. Wardlaw RSmith, "Gastric carcinoid tumors," *The Ochsner Journal*, vol. 8, pp. 191–196, 2008.

[21] K. Borch, B. Ahrén, H. Ahlman, S. Falkmer, G. Granérus, and L. Grimelius, "Gastric carcinoids: Biologic behavior and prognosis after differentiated treatment in relation to type," *Annals of Surgery*, vol. 242, no. 1, pp. 64–73, 2005.

6

Immune-Mediated Autonomic Neuropathies following Allogeneic Stem Cell Transplantation in Acute Myeloid Leukemia

Abhishek Mangaonkar,[1] **Hassan Al Khateeb,**[1] **Narjust Duma,**[1]
Erik K. St. Louis,[2] **Andrew McKeon,**[2] **Mrinal Patnaik,**[1] **William Hogan,**[1]
Mark Litzow,[1] **and Taxiarchis Kourelis**[1]

[1]*Division of Hematology, Department of Medicine, Mayo Clinic, Rochester, MN, USA*
[2]*Department of Neurology, Mayo Clinic, Rochester, MN, USA*

Correspondence should be addressed to Abhishek Mangaonkar; mangaonkar.abhishek@mayo.edu

Academic Editor: Masayuki Nagasawa

Background/Aims. Autonomic dysfunction (AD) after allogeneic stem cell transplant (SCT) is a rare occurrence and likely immune-mediated in etiology. There is limited literature on this topic and hence, we wish to briefly describe management of two cases at our institution and their outcomes. *Methods.* We retrospectively identified two patients with immune-mediated AD after SCT from our database. Immune-mediated AD was defined as AD secondary to an immune-mediated etiology without an alternative cause and responding to immunosuppression. *Results.* The first case is of a 32-year-old man with acute myeloid leukemia (AML) who underwent double umbilical cord allogeneic SCT. The second patient was a 51-year-old woman with secondary AML who underwent matched-related donor allogeneic SCT. Both underwent an extensive work-up for an underlying etiology prior to treatment with intravenous immunoglobulin (IVIG). *Conclusions.* AD after SCT is a rare yet significant clinical entity. A work-up of underlying etiology should be performed. IVIG is a treatment option for these patients.

1. Introduction

Immune-mediated neuropathies (IMN) after autologous and allogeneic stem cell transplant (SCT) are rare, with prevalence of 0.36 percent reported among 3305 SCT patients at the Mayo Clinic [1, 2], which is higher when compared to the general population and is suggestive of a causal association between SCT and IMN [3]. Cases of immune-mediated autonomic dysfunction (AD) following SCT have also been described [4]. Herein, we describe two cases of AD after SCT responding to immunosuppressive treatment and briefly discuss their clinical course and management. We retrospectively identified patients with immune-mediated AD after a SCT seen at the Mayo Clinic between January of 1998 and January of 2016. Immune-mediated AD was defined as AD presumed secondary to an immune-mediated etiology

without another plausible cause and a documented clinical response to immunosuppressive treatments.

2. Case 1

A 32-year-old man with a history of acute myelogenous leukemia (AML) secondary to myelodysplastic syndrome underwent double umbilical cord allogeneic SCT after fludarabine (Flu), cyclophosphamide (Cy), thiotepa, and total body irradiation (TBI) conditioning 6 months after his AML diagnosis. A few weeks after his SCT, he developed severe gastroparesis requiring the placement of a feeding tube. Following this event, his tacrolimus and prednisone doses were increased due to suspicion of graft versus host disease (GVHD) of the gastrointestinal tract. Random mucosal biopsies after an upper and lower gastrointestinal endoscopy were negative for GVHD and the patient continued to require a feeding tube for nutrition. Approximately 14 months after his transplant and while tapering of immunosuppressive agents, he developed severe symptomatic orthostatic hypotension requiring hospitalization for intravenous (IV) fluids. Adrenal insufficiency was thought unlikely due to an appropriately elevated cortisol level and a lack of response to stress dose steroids. An autonomic reflex screen demonstrated severe autonomic dysfunction. Patient underwent a tilt test for 1.5 minutes, following which there was severe progressive blood pressure drop with symptom of dizziness, weakness, and inadequate heart rate response. Beat-to-beat blood pressure responses to Valsalva maneuver showed absent late phase II and phase IV overshoot and prolonged blood pressure recovery time. The quantitative axon reflex sweat test responses were reduced at all sites except forearm. Severe orthostatic symptoms persisted despite maximal doses of midodrine and fludrocortisone and cerebrospinal fluid (CSF) analysis showed elevated protein of 109 mg/dl with normal cell count, glucose, and cytology. Serum autoimmune dysautonomia evaluation which consisted of antibodies to anti-neuronal nuclear antibodies (ANNA-1), striated muscle, acetylcholine receptor (AChR muscle binding and neuronal ganglionic), neuronal K+ channel, GAD-65, and N and P/Q type calcium channel, and ganglioside was negative. Serum and urine protein electrophoresis, HIV testing, and antinuclear antibodies were also negative. Since the development of his AD coincided with tapering of his immunosuppression, an autoimmune etiology was thought as the most likely underlying mechanism. A 5-day treatment course with intravenous immunoglobulin (IVIG) at a dose of 0.4 gm/kg daily resulted in significant improvement in orthostasis and gastroparesis. Posttreatment autonomic reflex screen was not performed due to significant clinical improvement. Soon thereafter, he was able to tolerate oral intake and his functional status significantly improved. A diagnosis of seronegative autoimmune autonomic ganglionopathy was made and he was discharged with maintenance twice weekly IVIG treatments. Orthostasis symptoms recurred following nonadherence, and resumption of IVIG led to rapid clinical improvement. At the time of last follow-up, the response has been sustained for four months.

3. Case 2

A 51-year-old woman with AML secondary to myelodysplastic syndrome with associated myelofibrosis underwent matched-related donor allogeneic SCT after Cy/TBI conditioning at first remission. She received cyclosporine and steroids for immunosuppression. Approximately 8 months after her SCT she developed orthostatic hypotension, confirmed by an autonomic reflex screen which showed significant adrenergic failure with mild cardiovagal and probable distal postganglionic sudomotor impairment. Heart rate responses to deep breathing and Valsalva maneuver were reduced. The quantitative sudomotor axon reflex tests were normal for all sites except marked reduction at foot. Nerve conduction studies (NCS) demonstrated reduced right ulnar and peroneal compound muscle action potential amplitudes, reduced right ulnar motor nerve conduction velocity,

prolonged right peroneal motor distal latency, and borderline reduced right sural sensory nerve conduction velocity. Prolonged bilateral blink responses were also noted. Needle examination revealed scattered fibrillation potentials in both proximal and distal muscles. Mildly enlarged motor unit potentials with reduced recruitment were noted in predominantly lower extremity muscles and thoracic paraspinal muscles. Overall, NCS findings were consistent with a diffuse neurogenic disorder with demyelinating features. Antibodies to ANNA-1, amphiphysin, Purkinje Cell (PCA-1), striated muscle, N and P/Q type calcium channels, acetylcholine receptor binding, neuronal K+ channel, GAD-65, P/Q type calcium channels, and ganglioside were all undetectable. Serum protein electrophoresis did not reveal monoclonal protein. An extensive infectious diseases work-up including HIV and hepatitis panel was also negative. CSF analysis showed an elevated protein at 93 mg/dl, with otherwise normal parameters. Fludrocortisone and compression stockings were initiated, and she was treated with a five-day course of IVIG at 0.4 gm/kg daily and then switched to daily plasmapheresis and prednisone at 1 mg/kg. Plasmapheresis was slowly tapered off to three and then 2 times per week as symptoms improved. Steroids were tapered over 2 weeks. She responded to this therapy within 2 weeks and eventually orthostatic symptoms resolved by the end of the hospitalization. A posttreatment autonomic reflex screen showed normal heart rate responses to deep breathing and Valsalva maneuver and normal quantitative sudomotor axon reflex tests at all sites except the foot. Her leukemia eventually relapsed after four months and she passed away subsequently from an unrelated cause. Table 1 summarizes the results of clinical, laboratory tests, treatment, and its response in the two cases.

4. Discussion

In this brief report, we demonstrate that autonomic IMNs may rarely develop late after an allogeneic SCT. They are associated with significant morbidity but fortunately tend to respond rapidly to treatments directed at the antibody immune response, such as IVIG and plasmapheresis.

Demyelinating neuropathies following SCT have been identified in 0.5% patients [4]. IMNs with isolated autonomic dysfunction are even rarer and limited to isolated case reports [1, 4, 5]. Nakane et al. found that all 5 patients undergoing a reduced intensity SCT developed a decrease in heart rate variability, indicative of autonomic dysfunction [6].

The possible underlying pathophysiologic mechanisms for IMNs following SCT are an immune reconstitution syndrome, GVHD, or a paraneoplastic phenomenon [1]. In both our cases, disease relapse was ruled out and response to immunosuppression was rapid and sustained, supportive of an immune-mediated mechanism. Furthermore, the absence of skin, GI, or liver involvement made GVHD appear less likely. However, neurologic manifestations of chronic GVHD can also present as IMNs [7]. Acute or chronic inflammatory demyelinating polyneuropathies are two examples of transplant-related IMNs impacting large fiber nerves [8]. These immune-mediated neurologic disorders seem more common in allogeneic SCT patients when compared to the

TABLE 1: Table summarizing results of clinical/laboratory testing, treatment response, and outcomes in the two cases.

Test	Case 1	Case 2
Autonomic reflex screen	(i) Moderate cardiovagal, widespread postganglionic sudomotor and severe adrenergic impairment on this study. (ii) Decreased heart rate responses to deep breathing and Valsalva maneuver. (iii) QSWEAT responses reduced at all sites except the forearm.	(i) Significant adrenergic failure with mild cardiovagal and probable distal postganglionic sudomotor impairment. (ii) Heart rate responses to deep breathing and Valsalva maneuver were reduced. (iii) The quantitative sudomotor axon reflex tests were normal for all sites except marked reduction at foot.
Antibody tests (all were undetectable) *Antibodies tested in addition for case 2	ANNA-1, striated muscle, acetylcholine receptor (AChR muscle binding and neuronal ganglionic), neuronal K+ channel, GAD-65, and N- and P/Q type calcium channel, ganglioside, amphiphysin*, Purkinje Cell (PCA-1)*.	
Treatment	IVIG 0.4 gm/kg for 5 days.	IVIG at 0.4 gm/kg for 5 days, daily plasmapheresis, prednisone at 1 mg/kg.
Response	Significant symptomatic improvement. Posttreatment autonomic reflex testing not performed.	Significant symptomatic improvement in two weeks. Posttreatment autonomic reflex screen showed normal heart rate responses to deep breathing and Valsalva maneuver and normal quantitative sudomotor axon reflex tests at all sites except the foot.

general population, which suggests a causal association [3]. Karam et al. demonstrated that such disorders are also seen following autologous SCT, suggesting that the underlying pathogenesis may be related to a nonspecific activation of the host's immune system rather than a graft versus host mechanism [1]. Further, the fact that both patients had an elevated CSF protein is supportive of an inflammatory process.

An inferred autoimmune etiopathologic mechanism is important to guide empiric therapy. In our two patients, favorable response to IVIG and plasmapheresis is specifically supportive of an antibody-mediated mechanism. Long term outcomes were favorable for both patients consistent with previous reports, although clinical improvement can be incomplete with persistent residual deficits [9, 10].

Limitations of our study include its retrospective nature, limited number of patients, and the short follow-up. However, we corroborate prior results that IMN following SCT is rare and a thorough work-up for relapsed disease and other causes of AD (chemotherapy, infectious, paraneoplastic, and endocrinologic etiologies) is critical prior to initiating empiric therapy for a presumed autoimmune cause. Furthermore, we probably underestimated the incidence of immune-mediated autonomic neuropathy due to lack of uniform diagnostic criteria and some patients may have limited autonomic disorders, such as isolated gastrointestinal dysmotility that may be poorly recognized. Our limited experience suggests that an empiric short-term trial of IVIG or plasma exchange is reasonable, with continued maintenance treatment for patients who exhibit a therapeutic response. Additional therapies directed at reducing antibodies against self-antigens such as rituximab and plasmapheresis may be reasonable options for long term management of these patients. Steroids may also be beneficial, at least in the short-term. Further analysis of a larger patient cohort will be necessary to confirm the association of IMN with SCT and potentially identify clinical factors that may predict IMN occurrence, prognosis, and best therapeutic approaches.

Conflicts of Interest

The authors declare no conflicts of interest or funding sources.

References

[1] C. Karam, M. L. Mauermann, P. B. Johnston, R. Lahoria, J. K. Engelstad, and P. J. B. Dyck, "Immune-mediated neuropathies following stem cell transplantation," *Journal of Neurology, Neurosurgery and Psychiatry*, vol. 85, no. 6, pp. 638–642, 2014.

[2] J.-M. Kang, Y.-J. Kim, J. Y. Kim et al., "Neurologic complications after allogeneic hematopoietic stem cell transplantation in children: analysis of prognostic factors," *Biology of Blood and Marrow Transplantation*, vol. 21, no. 6, pp. 1091–1098, 2015.

[3] H. C. Lehmann, G. M. Z. Horste, H.-P. Hartung, and B. C. Kieseier, "Pathogenesis and treatment of immune-mediated neuropathies," *Therapeutic Advances in Neurological Disorders*, vol. 2, no. 4, pp. 261–281, 2009.

[4] A. M. Delios, M. Rosenblum, A. A. Jakubowski, and L. M. Deangelis, "Central and peripheral nervous system immune mediated demyelinating disease after allogeneic hemopoietic stem cell transplantation for hematologic disease," *Journal of Neuro-Oncology*, vol. 110, no. 2, pp. 251–256, 2012.

[5] M. A. Roskrow, S. M. Kelsey, M. McCarthy, A. C. Newland, and J. P. Monson, "Selective automatic neuropathy as a novel complication of BMT," *Bone Marrow Transplantation*, vol. 10, no. 5, pp. 469-470, 1992.

[6] T. Nakane, H. Nakamae, T. Muro et al., "Cardiac and autonomic nerve function after reduced-intensity stem cell transplantation for hematologic malignancy in patients with pre-transplant cardiac dysfunction," *Annals of Hematology*, vol. 88, no. 9, pp. 871–879, 2009.

[7] O. Grauer, D. Wolff, H. Bertz et al., "Neurological manifestations of chronic graft-versus-host disease after allogeneic haematopoietic stem cell transplantation: report from the consensus conference on clinical practice in chronic graft-versus-host disease," *Brain*, vol. 133, no. 10, pp. 2852–2865, 2010.

7

Listeria monocytogenes Infection in Hairy Cell Leukemia

James C. Barton Ⓘ[1,2,3] **and Hayward S. Edmunds Jr.**[4]

[1]*Department of Medicine, University of Alabama at Birmingham, Birmingham, AL, USA*
[2]*Southern Iron Disorders Center, Birmingham, AL, USA*
[3]*Department of Medicine, Brookwood Medical Center, Birmingham, AL, USA*
[4]*Cunningham Pathology Associates, Birmingham, AL, USA*

Correspondence should be addressed to James C. Barton; ironmd@isp.com

Academic Editor: Akimichi Ohsaka

Listeria monocytogenes infections have been described in patients with diverse types of malignancy, especially leukemia. We report the case of a 65-year-old man with previously untreated hairy cell leukemia characterized by CD5 positivity and trisomy 12 (3% of blood lymphocytes) who developed bacteremia due to *L. monocytogenes* serotype 1/2b. We summarize clinical features and treatment of this patient and five previously reported patients with hairy cell leukemia who also had *L. monocytogenes* infections. All six patients were men. Their mean age at infection diagnosis was 70 y. Three men had undergone splenectomy 4–11 y before they developed *L. monocytogenes* infection. The central nervous system was the primary site of infection in four men. Bacteremia alone occurred in two other men. At diagnosis of infection, one man was receiving antileukemia chemotherapy and another man was receiving treatment for Kaposi's sarcoma. Two other patients had other comorbid conditions. All six men recovered from their infections.

1. Introduction

Hairy cell leukemia (HCL) is characterized by small mature B-lymphocytes with distinctive morphology and surface protein expression, hemocytopenias (especially neutropenia and monocytopenia), marrow fibrosis, splenomegaly, and an indolent clinical course [1]. The median age of patients with HCL is between 50 and 55 y [1]. Approximately 80% of persons with HCL are men [1]. Some persons with HCL develop autoimmune conditions unrelated to the severity of HCL [1, 2]. Cladribine therapy induces durable hematologic remissions in a high proportion of previously untreated patients [3].

We report the case of a man with previously untreated HCL who developed *Listeria monocytogenes* bacteremia. We summarize clinical features and treatment of this patient and five previously reported patients with HCL who were also diagnosed to have *L. monocytogenes* infections and discuss manifestations, management, and outcomes of *L. monocytogenes* infections in persons with HCL.

2. Case Report

A 64-year-old white man presented with a 10-month history of fatigue, lymphocytosis, microcytosis (elevated RDW), and subnormal platelet counts. He had bipolar disorder. Five months before presentation, he was treated as an outpatient for pneumonia not otherwise specified. Daily medications were duloxetine, lamotrigine, olanzapine, acetaminophen, fish oil, and melatonin. He tended horses and handled their silage daily. Physical examination revealed mild pallor. Lymph nodes, liver, and spleen were not enlarged.

Complete blood count revealed hemoglobin 110 g/L, erythrocytes 4.79×10^{12}/L, mean corpuscular volume 73 fL, red blood cell distribution width 17.2%, leukocytes 15.6×10^9/L, neutrophils 4.4×10^9/L, lymphocytes 10.5×10^9/L, monocytes 0.5×10^9/L, and platelets 125×10^9/L. Serum iron level was 5.7 μmol/L, transferrin saturation was 7%, and serum ferritin was 23 pmol/L. Comprehensive chemistry profile values were within respective reference limits. Total

TABLE 1: Immunophenotypes of clonal blood B-lymphocytes in a man with hairy cell leukemia[1].

Surface antigen	Month 1 (diagnosis of leukemia)	Month 16 (*Listeria* bacteremia)	Month 18 (initial cladribine therapy)	Month 24 (after initial cladribine therapy)	Month 28[2]
CD5	+	+	+	+	+
CD10	nd	−	nd	−	nd
CD11c	+	nd	+ Bright	+ Bright	+ Bright
CD19	+	+	+	+ Bright	nd
CD20	+ Bright	+ Bright	+ Bright	+ Bright	nd
CD22	+	+	+ Bright	+ Bright	nd
CD23	−	−	+ Dim	−	nd
CD25	+	nd	+	+	+
CD45	+	+	+	+	nd
CD103	+	nd	+	+	+
FMC-7	+	+	+	+	nd
HLA-DR	+	nd	+	+	nd
Lambda	+	+ Bright	+	+	nd

[1]Immunophenotypes were determined using flow cytometry; nd = not done; [2]complete blood count: hemoglobin 120 g/L, erythrocytes 4.05×10^{12}/L, mean corpuscular volume 97 fL, leukocytes 3.7×10^9/L, neutrophils 2.5×10^9/L, lymphocytes 0.9×10^9/L, and platelets 88×10^9/L. 0.9% of blood lymphocytes had a hairy cell leukemia immunophenotype.

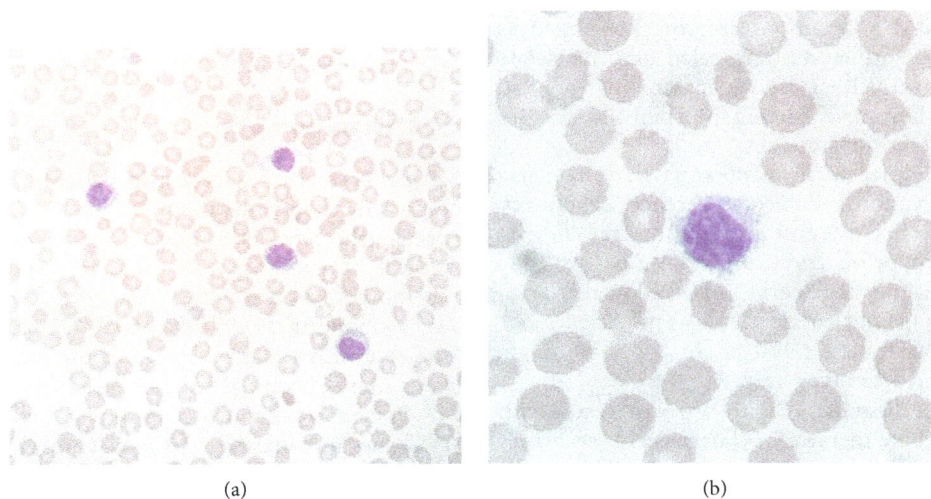

(a)   (b)

FIGURE 1: Photomicrographs of blood leukemic B-lymphocytes in a man with untreated hairy cell leukemia. (a) Original magnification 400x. (b) Original magnification 1000x.

immunoglobulin (Ig) G was 9.76 g/L. IgG subclass values were within respective reference limits. A HCL immunophenotype was detected in 68% of blood lymphocytes by flow cytometry (Table 1). Morphology of his leukemic blood lymphocytes is displayed in Figures 1 and 2. Fluorescent in situ hybridization revealed trisomy 12 in 3% of blood lymphocytes (reference < 1.3%). t(11;14) was not detected. He declined to undergo bone marrow evaluation or CT scanning.

Fecal occult blood testing was positive, although upper gastrointestinal tract endoscopy and colonoscopy did not reveal a site of blood loss. He was treated with four 500 mg infusions of iron as iron dextran. His fatigue resolved and his hemoglobin, erythrocytes, and mean corpuscular volume increased to 133 g/L, 485×10^{12}/L, and 88 fL, respectively. Transferrin saturation and serum ferritin increased to 16% and 357 pmol/L, respectively.

Fifteen months after diagnosis, his physical examination revealed mild pallor. Hemoglobin was 102 g/L, neutrophil count was 6.2×10^9/L, midrange cells were 5.8×10^9/L, lymphocyte count was 36.9×10^9/L, and platelet count was 72×10^9/L. There was no evidence of recurrent iron deficiency.

At age 65 y, 16 months after diagnosis, he was admitted to hospital because he had temperature 103.1° and chills. Hemoglobin was 99 g/L, erythrocytes were 3.10×10^{12}/L, mean corpuscular volume was 101 fL, leukocytes were 59.9×10^9/L, neutrophils were 3.0×10^9/L, lymphocytes were 56.9×10^9/L (88% with HCL immunophenotypes), and platelets were 83×10^9/L. The immunophenotype of his monoclonal blood lymphocytes was unchanged since diagnosis (Table 1). There was no apparent source of infection. He was treated initially with oral acetaminophen and

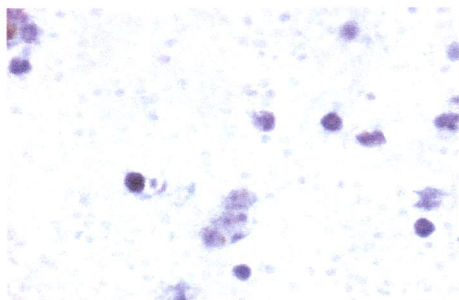

FIGURE 2: Photomicrograph of blood leukemic B-lymphocytes in a man with treated hairy cell leukemia stained to demonstrate tartrate-resistant acid phosphatase. Rare lymphoid cells are weakly to moderately positive (Genoptix, Carlsbad, CA) (original magnification 400x).

intravenous fluids. On the second hospital day, he was treated empirically with oral levofloxacin 750 mg daily and became afebrile. He was discharged on the fourth hospital day to continue taking levofloxacin 750 mg daily (7 days total). He recovered fully. After discharge, it was reported that aerobic and anaerobic blood cultures drawn at hospital admission revealed a Gram-positive rod interpreted as *Corynebacterium* sp. Further study revealed that the isolate was *L. monocytogenes*. Neither the patient nor his wife had consumed uncooked or unpasteurized food items sometimes associated with *Listeria* transmission.

Subtyping of the present *L. monocytogenes* isolate was performed at the National Enteric Reference Laboratory (Centers for Disease Control and Prevention, Atlanta, GA) using growth phenotype on Trypticase™ Soy Agar with 5% Sheep Blood (BD Diagnostics, Sparks, MD) and nucleic acid-based analyses (average nucleotide identity and AccuProbe® culture identification testing (Hologic Inc., Marlborough, MA)). Testing detected serotype 1/2b.

In month 18 after diagnosis (Table 1), he was treated with subcutaneous cladribine therapy [1, 4] because his recurrent anemia was best explained by decreased erythropoiesis due to marrow progression of HCL [1]. In month 23 (4 months after last cladribine injection), his hemoglobin was 118 g/L, erythrocytes were 4.09×10^{12}/L, mean corpuscular volume was 97 fL, leukocytes were 3.6×10^9/L, neutrophils were 2.5×10^9/L, lymphocytes were 0.8×10^9/L, and platelets were 113×10^9/L. Three percent of blood lymphocytes had a HCL immunophenotype (Table 1).

Mutation analysis to detect *BRAF* p.V600E (c.1799T > A) was performed for the first time in month 28 after diagnosis and 10 months after cladribine therapy (Table 1) by Genoptix (Carlsbad, CA) using the Cobas® 4800 V600 Mutation Test (Roche Molecular Systems, Inc., Branchburg, NJ). *BRAF* p.V600E was not detected.

3. Literature Search

We performed a computerized search of the National Library of Medicine and other sources to identify reports of patients with HCL who developed *L. monocytogenes* infections. We enhanced the computerized search by reviewing details of

individual patients in selected case series of *L. monocytogenes* infections.

4. Six Patients with Hairy Cell Leukemia and *L. monocytogenes* Infections

We identified previous reports of *L. monocytogenes* infections in five patients with HCL, although their HCL immunophenotypes were not reported [5–9] (Table 2). Including the present patient, all six were men. Mean age of the six men at infection diagnosis was 70 y (standard deviation 13 y). Three men had undergone splenectomy 4–11 y before they developed *L. monocytogenes* infection. The central nervous system was the primary site of infection in four men. Bacteremia alone occurred in two other men. Possible sources of *L. monocytogenes* were reported in two men. At diagnosis of infection, one man was receiving antileukemia chemotherapy and another man was receiving treatment for Kaposi's sarcoma. Two other patients also had other comorbid conditions. Antibiotic therapy was reported in five men, four of whom were treated with ampicillin in combination with other agents. All six men recovered from their infections (Table 2). *L. monocytogenes* serotyping and detailed flow cytometry and fluorescent in situ hybridization analyses were not described in the previous five reports [5–9].

5. Discussion

L. monocytogenes infection in patients with HCL has been reported infrequently [5–9]. The mean age and sex of the five previously reported cases and the present patient were typical of patients with HCL [1]. Splenectomy, current chemotherapy, and other comorbid conditions were common among these six patients. Four men had infections of the central nervous system, and the other two had bacteremia alone. Each patient recovered from his infection.

Persons with normal immunity who ingest *L. monocytogenes* in contaminated food typically have no manifestations or self-limited fever and diarrhea [10]. Those with persistent fever and positive stool cultures may benefit from antibiotic treatment [10]. Persons who have compromised defenses against *L. monocytogenes* include pregnant women; neonates; those with malignancy, diabetes mellitus, or chronic renal disease; those with acquired immunodeficiency syndrome; those who take glucocorticosteroid medications; and those > 50 years of age [10, 10–14]. Presenting symptoms of listeriosis in these persons include fever, myalgias, headache, confusion, loss of balance, and seizures. Most persons with compromised defenses who develop listeriosis require hospitalization, antibiotic therapy, and supportive care [10]. Serious complications include miscarriage and premature delivery; infection of neonates; and bacteremia, meningitis, and death [10–14].

Bacteremia without an evident focus is the most common manifestation of *L. monocytogenes* infections in compromised hosts [12]. In a 2004 review of 118 patients with malignancy and *L. monocytogenes* infections, the most common site of infection was also blood alone (53%) [13], consistent with the present case. Fifty-three percent of the 118 patients had

TABLE 2: *Listeria monocytogenes* infections in 6 patients with hairy cell leukemia[1].

Patient number	Age (y), sex	Previous leukemia management	Infection[2]	Comorbid condition(s)	Antibiotic(s)[3]	Reference
1	70, M	ns	Meningoencephalitis	ns	Ampicillin + trimethoprim/ sulfamethoxazole	[5]
2	62, M	Splenectomy 11 y before	Meningitis	Asthma treated with prednisone 5 mg daily	Ampicillin + gentamycin	[6]
3	73, M	Splenectomy 6 y before	Meningitis	Acquired immunodeficiency syndrome; thrombocytopenia; Kaposi's sarcoma treated with vinblastine, electron beam	Ampicillin + gentamycin	[7]
4	53, M	Splenectomy 4 y before	Cutaneous lesions, bacteremia, cerebritis	Seropositive for hepatitis B	Ampicillin + gentamycin; corticosteroids	[8]
5	93, M	ns	Bacteremia	Antileukemia chemotherapy	ns	[9]
6	66, M	No therapy	Bacteremia	None	Levofloxacin	Present report

[1]Age at diagnosis of *L. monocytogenes* infection; ns = not stated; [2]possible sources of infection were reported as soft cheese and meat/poultry cold cuts in patient number 2 and horses and silage in the present case; [3]predominant antibiotic therapy during acute infection. In patient number 2, infection progressed on initial ciprofloxacin therapy. Before *L. monocytogenes* was identified in cultures, some patients received other antibiotics that were subsequently discontinued, as appropriate. Some patients received protracted antibiotic therapy after resolution of the acute phase of infection. Each of these six men survived his respective infection.

leukemia (chronic lymphocytic leukemia, 21%; acute lymphoblastic leukemia and variants, 15%; acute myelogenous leukemia, 7%; chronic myelogenous leukemia, 6%; HCL, 3% [7, 8, 15]; and other leukemia, 2%) [13]. There were strong associations of *L. monocytogenes* infection with recent corticosteroid therapy (50%), recent chemotherapy (43%), or previous stem cell transplantation (17%). Mortality among patients with *L. monocytogenes* bacteremia alone was 18% [13].

BRAF p.V600E was detected at diagnosis in each of 48 patients with HCL reported by Tiacci et al. [16]. *BRAF* p.V600E was not detected in the present patient ten months after cladribine therapy. At that time, flow cytometry detected a hairy cell immunophenotype in only 0.9% of blood lymphocytes. The limit of detection of the assay used is 5% mutant alleles in a background of 95% wild-type alleles [17]. Thus, one cannot conclude that HCL in the present patient is not associated with *BRAF* p.V600E.

Features of the present case that distinguish it from variant HCL include lack of prominent nucleoli (Figure 1); positivity for CD11c, CD25, and CD103 (Table 1); and excellent response to cladribine [18]. Leukocyte counts were reported in 47 of 48 patients with HCL and *BRAF* p.V600E, among whom 12 (25.5%) had leukocyte counts at diagnosis $> 11.0 \times 10^9$/L (range 11.4–55.0 $\times 10^9$/L) [16]. Thus, we do not interpret leukocytes 15.6 $\times 10^9$/L (lymphocytes 10.5 $\times 10^9$/L) at diagnosis of the present patient as evidence that he has variant HCL.

Leukemic lymphocytes in the present patient were positive for CD5. Although CD5 positivity is not typical of HCL [19], this phenotype has been described in a small proportion of HCL cases [20]. Whether CD5 positivity represents a distinctive subtype of lymphoid malignancy is unknown [20]. Trisomy 12 occurred in three percent of blood lymphocytes in the present case. Trisomy 12 is not typical of HCL [3, 21] but has been described in a small

proportion of patients [22, 23]. In such cases, the proportion of cells that display trisomy 12 is small [22, 23], like the present case. Except the appearance of dim CD23 positivity in leukemic lymphocytes in month 18, the leukemia cell immunophenotype in the present patient did not change.

Limitations of the present study include the possibility that we overlooked other reports of *L. monocytogenes* infections in patients with HCL in our manual literature review. Cases of other patients with HCL who developed *L. monocytogenes* infections may be unreported. Foodborne *L. monocytogenes* sometimes causes epidemic acute, febrile gastroenteritis that lasts two days [24]. Some patients with HCL and *L. monocytogenes* gastroenteritis may have been mistakenly diagnosed to have non-*Listeria* gastroenteritis.

Authors' Contributions

James C. Barton conceived the study, treated the patient, tabulated data, and drafted the manuscript. Hayward S. Edmunds performed flow cytometry, interpreted hematologic data, performed photomicrography, and contributed to the manuscript.

Conflicts of Interest

The authors have no conflicts of interest to report.

Acknowledgments

This work was supported in part by Southern Iron Disorders Center. The National Enteric Reference Laboratory (Centers for Disease Control and Prevention, Atlanta, GA) identified the serotype of the present *L. monocytogenes* isolate.

References

[1] J. B. Johnston and M. R. Grever, "Hairy cell leukemia," in *Wintrobe's Clinical Hematology, Chapter 91*, J. P. Greer, D. A. Arber, B. Glader et al., Eds., Wolters Kluwer/Lippincott Williams & Wilkins, Philadelphia, PA, USA, 2014.

[2] E. H. Kraut, "Clinical manifestations and infectious complications of hairy-cell leukaemia," *Best Practice & Research: Clinical Haematology*, vol. 16, no. 1, pp. 33–40, 2003.

[3] M. R. Grever, O. Abdel-Wahab, L. A. Andritsos et al., "Consensus guidelines for the diagnosis and management of patients with classic hairy cell leukemia," *Blood*, vol. 129, no. 5, pp. 553–560, 2017.

[4] F. Lauria, E. Cencini, and F. Forconi, "Alternative methods of cladribine administration," *Leukemia & Lymphoma*, vol. 52, no. 2, pp. 34–37, 2011.

[5] M. Merle-Melet, L. Dossou-Gbete, P. Maurer et al., "Is amoxicillin-cotrimoxazole the most appropriate antibiotic regimen for listeria meningoencephalitis? Review of 22 cases and the literature," *Journal of Infection*, vol. 33, no. 2, pp. 79–85, 1996.

[6] N. M. Grumbach, E. Mylonakis, and E. J. Wing, "Development of listerial meningitis during ciprofloxacin treatment," *Clinical Infectious Diseases*, vol. 29, no. 5, pp. 1340-1341, 1999.

[7] W. Hocking, G. Lazar, M. Goldsmith, and S. Foreman, "Kaposi's sarcoma associated with hairy cell leukemia, immune thrombocytopenia, and opportunistic infection," *Cancer*, vol. 54, no. 1, pp. 110–113, 1984.

[8] R. A. Salata, R. E. King, F. Gose, and R. D. Pearson, "*Listeria monocytogenes* cerebritis, bacteremia, and cutaneous lesions complicating hairy cell leukemia," *American Journal of Medicine*, vol. 81, no. 6, pp. 1068–1072, 1986.

[9] L. A. Cone, M. S. Somero, F. J. Qureshi et al., "Unusual infections due to *Listeria monocytogenes* in the Southern California Desert," *International Journal of Infectious Diseases*, vol. 12, no. 6, pp. 578–581, 2008.

[10] B. Lorber, "Listeria monocytogenes," in *Mandell, Douglas, and Bennett's Principles and Practice of Infectious Diseases, Chapter 207*, G. L. Mandell, J. E. Bennett, and R. Dolin, Eds., Saunders, London, UK, 2014.

[11] R. Bortolussi, C. Krishnan, D. Armstrong, and P. Tovichayathamrong, "Prognosis for survival in neonatal meningitis: clinical and pathologic review of 52 cases," *Canadian Medical Association Journal*, vol. 118, no. 2, pp. 165–168, 1978.

[12] B. G. Gellin, C. V. Broome, W. F. Bibb, R. E. Weaver, S. Gaventa, and L. Mascola, "The epidemiology of listeriosis in the United States–1986. Listeriosis Study Group," *American Journal of Epidemiology*, vol. 133, no. 4, pp. 392–401, 1991.

[13] A. Ramsakal, H. Nadiminti, T. Field et al., "*Listeria* infections in cancer patients," *Infections in Medicine*, vol. 21, no. 7, 2004.

[14] Centers for Disease Control and Prevention, "*Listeria* (listeriosis)," June 2017, https://www.cdc.gov/listeria/index.html.

[15] J. M. Guerin, P. Meyer, and Y. Habib, "*Listeria monocytogenes* infection and hairy cell leukemia," *American Journal of Medicine*, vol. 83, no. 1, p. 188, 1987.

[16] E. Tiacci, V. Trifonov, G. Schiavoni et al., "*BRAF* mutations in hairy-cell leukemia," *New England Journal of Medicine*, vol. 364, no. 24, pp. 2305–2315, 2011.

[17] Package Insert, *Cobas® 4800 V600 Mutation Test*, Roche Molecular Systems, Inc., Branchburg, NJ, USA, 2011.

[18] T. Robak, E. Matutes, D. Catovsky, P. L. Zinzani, and C. Buske, "Hairy cell leukaemia: ESMO Clinical Practice Guidelines for diagnosis, treatment and follow-up," *Annals of Oncology*, vol. 26, no. 5, pp. v100–v107, 2015.

[19] M. Stetler-Stevenson and P. R. Tembhare, "Diagnosis of hairy cell leukemia by flow cytometry," *Leukemia & Lymphoma*, vol. 52, no. 2, pp. 11–13, 2011.

[20] D. Jain, P. Dorwal, S. Gajendra, A. Pande, S. Mehra, and R. Sachdev, "CD5 positive hairy cell leukemia: a rare case report with brief review of literature," *Cytometry Part B: Clinical Cytometry*, vol. 90, no. 5, pp. 467–472, 2016.

[21] F. Sole, S. Woessner, L. Florensa et al., "Cytogenetic findings in five patients with hairy cell leukemia," *Cancer Genetics and Cytogenetics*, vol. 110, no. 1, pp. 41–43, 1999.

[22] K. Vallianatou, V. Brito-Babapulle, E. Matutes, S. Atkinson, and D. Catovsky, "p53 gene deletion and trisomy 12 in hairy cell leukemia and its variant," *Leukemia Research*, vol. 23, no. 11, pp. 1041–1045, 1999.

[23] A. Cuneo, R. Bigoni, M. Balboni et al., "Trisomy 12 in chronic lymphocytic leukemia and hairy cell leukemia: a cytogenetic and interphase cytogenetic study," *Leukemia & Lymphoma*, vol. 15, no. 1-2, pp. 167–172, 1994.

[24] S. T. Ooi and B. Lorber, "Gastroenteritis due to *Listeria monocytogenes*," *Clinical Infectious Diseases*, vol. 40, no. 9, pp. 1327–1332, 2005.

8

Aggressive Systemic Mastocytosis in Association with Pure Red Cell Aplasia

Dhauna Karam (ID),[1,2] **Sean Swiatkowski,**[1,2] **Mamata Ravipati,**[1,2] **and Bharat Agrawal**[1,2]

[1]*Rosalind Franklin University, 3333 Green Bay Road, North Chicago, IL 60064, USA*
[2]*Captain James A. Lovell Federal Health Care Center, 3001 Green Bay Road, North Chicago, IL 60064, USA*

Correspondence should be addressed to Dhauna Karam; dhauna.karam@gmail.com

Academic Editor: Håkon Reikvam

Aggressive systemic mastocytosis (ASM) is characterized by mast cell accumulation in systemic organs. Though ASM may be associated with other hematological disorders, the association with pure red cell aplasia (PRCA) is rare and has not been reported. Pure red cell aplasia (PRCA) is a syndrome, characterized by normochromic normocytic anemia, reticulocytopenia, and severe erythroid hypoplasia. The myeloid and megakaryocytic cell lines usually remain normal. Here, we report an unusual case of ASM, presenting in association with PRCA and the management challenges.

1. Introduction

Aggressive systemic mastocytosis is a rare disorder characterized by abnormal accumulation of mast cells in bone marrow and internal organs (liver, spleen, lymph nodes, and gastrointestinal tract) [1]. Mastocytosis was initially classified as one of the subtypes of "myeloproliferative neoplasms (MPN)." In the 2016 revision of the World Health Organization (WHO) classification of tumors of the hematopoietic and lymphoid tissues, mastocytosis was classified as a separate entity [2, 3]. Chemical mediators such as tumor necrosis factor produced by mast cells can suppress erythropoiesis, and some mast cell diseases can cause hypoplastic anemia, though the pathogenesis is not clear. Our case report highlights an unusual and rare presentation of ASM with PRCA. Such an association has not been reported in the literature, except in one case report where mast cell activation disorder and PRCA occurred together [4].

2. Case Presentation

2.1. Patient's Symptoms/History. A 64-year-old white male, with past medical history of depression, presented with progressive weakness, unintentional weight loss, and exercise intolerance since past 1 month. He was a very healthy and active person; he enjoyed biking and rollerblading. The above symptoms were very unusual for him. The patient reported intermittent episodes of epistaxis, 3-4 times a week since the past month, lasting for a few minutes. He also endorsed 2-3 episodes of loose stools daily since the past month. Of note, the patient had history of exposure to Agent Orange between years 1969 and 1971; the first exposure was forty-five years earlier. Physical examination revealed stable vital signs with a palpable spleen of six finger-breadths below the left costal margin and mild hepatomegaly. Cardiopulmonary, lymphatic, and dermatologic examination, including Darrier's sign were all negative.

2.2. Diagnosis. On admission, the patient was found to have a hemoglobin count of 5.1 g/dl, which was a significant drop from the patient's baseline hemoglobin of 13-14 g/dl. Other basic laboratory studies are presented in Table 1. Urine analysis, stool for blood test, serum haptoglobulin, LDH, hepatitis B and C testing, PNH by flow cytometry, and hemochromatosis gene mutation were normal or negative. Serum tryptase level was elevated at 1110 ng/ml (normal < 11.4 ng/ml). Bone marrow biopsy and clot section performed as a part of anemia workup revealed hypercellularity with markedly increased maturing granulopoiesis

TABLE 1: Laboratory values.

Laboratory analysis	Patient's values on initial hospitalization	Patient's values on second hospitalization	Normal range
Hemoglobin	5.1 g/dl	7.4 g/dl	13–17
MCV	97 fl	90.4 fl	82–99
MCHC	31.5 g/dl	32.9 g/dl	31–37
WBC count	6 k/μL	5.1 k/μL	4–10
Platelet count	91 k/μL	90 k/μL	150–400
Absolute eosinophil count	2 k/μL	2 k/μL	
Neutrophil	30%	30.8%	40–80
Lymphocyte	24%	23.5%	15–45
Eosinophil	33.5%	33.3%	0–6
Basophil	0%	0%	0–2
Glucose	140 mg/dl	117 mg/dl	70–99
BUN	16 mg/dl	14 mg/dl	7–21
Creatinine	0.87 mg/dl	0.83 mg/dl	0.67–1.17
AST	16 U/L	96 U/L	10–37
ALT	22 U/L	55 U/L	10–65
Alkaline phosphatase	475 U/L	130 U/L	50–136
Total bilirubin	0.8 mg/dl	21.3 mg/dl (direct 16.7 mg/dl)	0–1
Stool occult blood	Negative		
Haptoglobulin	214 mg/dl		30–200
Reticulocyte %	0.6		0.5–2.5
LDH	147 U/L		84–246
PT	12.8 s	27 s	9–12
INR	1.2		0.9–1.1
aPTT	33.1 s	77 s	23–34
Iron	202 μg/dl		65–175
TIBC	203 μg/dl		250–450
Iron saturation	100%		10–50
Ferritin	949.9 ng/ml		26–388
Vitamin B12	1680 pg/ml		193–986
Folate	19.6 ng/ml		8.7–55.4
TSH	1.48 uIU/ml		0.358–3.74
Fibrinogen		410	
SPEP—protein	6.8 g/dl		6.4–8.2
Albumin	2.8 g/dl	1.3 g/dl	3.5–5.0
Alpha-1 globulin	0.5 g/dl		0.2–0.4
Alpha-2 globulin	1.0 g/dl		0.5–1.0
Beta globulin	0.7 g/dl		0.5–1.1
Gamma globulin	1.8 g/dl		0.6–1.5

with increased number of neutrophils and eosinophils. Erythropoiesis was markedly decreased with only very rare proerythroblasts present (Figure 1). Megakaryocytosis with dysmegakaryopoiesis was also appreciated. Several perivascular fibrotic areas containing mast cell aggregates were also identified (Figures 2 and 3). The mast cells were positive for mast cell tryptase and aberrant expression of CD2 and CD25 (Figures 4 and 5). c-KIT and D 816 V mutations were detected. The above findings were suggestive of ASM. FISH, cytogenetic, and flow cytometric analyses were unrevealing. Parvovirus immunostain was negative.

2.3. Treatment. After the diagnosis of ASM and PRCA, the patient left our hospital against medical advice. He became completely transfusion-dependent and was receiving weekly red cell transfusions from a nearby community hospital. He returned to our hospital after 5 weeks with worsening anemia, thrombocytopenia, liver function tests, and coagulopathy. The patient reported lack of transportation and

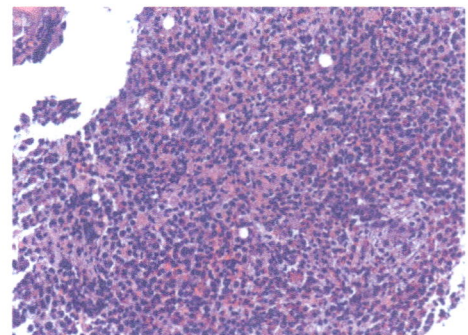

FIGURE 1: Area of hypercellular bone marrow with red cell aplasia.

social support to return to hospital for treatment. Peripheral smear revealed normochromic normocytic anemia with occasional ovalocyte, rare target cell, and dacrocyte. No nucleated red blood cell was identified. Granulocytes appeared mature without abnormal granulation or segmentation.

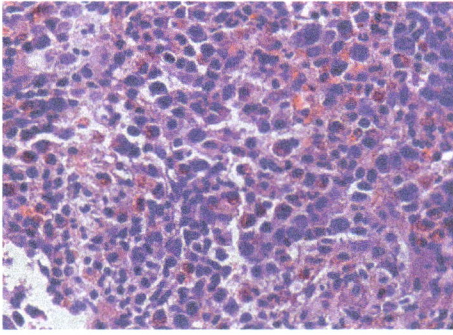

FIGURE 2: Bone marrow with hypercellularity and increased mast cells.

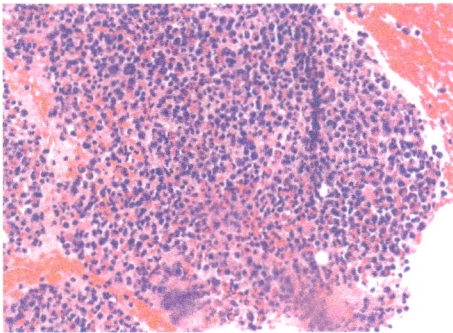

FIGURE 3: Clot section which shows hypercellularity and increased mast cells.

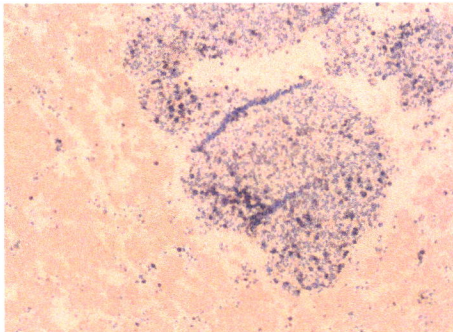

FIGURE 4: Clot stained with CD2 which is positive in mast cells.

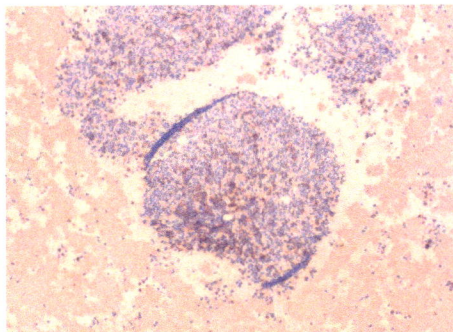

FIGURE 5: Clot stained with CD25 which is positive in mast cells.

Eosinophils were increased (30% with an absolute number of 1400/mcL) without abnormal features. Monocytes were increased to 12.9% without absolute monocytosis. Imaging studies (ultrasound and CT scan of abdomen) revealed hepatomegaly (liver 19.7 cm in length) and splenomegaly (spleen 19.1 cm in length) with multiple retroperitoneal lymph nodes.

With the patient's prior history of depression and ongoing thrombocytopenia, interferon alfa and 2-chlorodeoxyadenosine were not recommended for treatment of ASM. New avenues of treatments were discussed. Since the mast cells were CD30+, brentuximab vedotin was administered at a dose of 1.8 mg/kg. After therapy, patient developed worsening neutropenia, despite filgrastim and worsening anemia, and thrombocytopenia. The patient also developed Gram-negative bacteremia secondary to a urinary tract infection and became hypotensive and hypoxemic with lactic acidosis. The patient died 2 weeks later in the intensive care unit. Our patient lived for a short time after diagnosis of ASM; hence, there was not enough time for many sequential therapies. He did receive high-dose steroids before and concurrently with brentuximab therapy.

2.4. Outcome. The patient deceased within 2 months of initial diagnosis.

3. Discussion

Aggressive systemic mastocytosis is an uncommon disorder characterized by neoplastic mast cell accumulation in various organs. The skeletal system, bone marrow, gastrointestinal tract, and spleen are commonly involved. Mast cell infiltration of bone marrow leads to cytopenias, the so-called "C" findings [5, 6]. Systemic mastocytosis patients have poor prognosis because of multiorgan involvement and dysfunction [7].

Our patient presented with systemic symptoms and severe anemia, workup of which led to diagnosis of underlying systemic mastocytosis and pure red cell aplasia. The diagnosis of ASM was made by a constellation of clinical, cytogenetic, and molecular analyses [8]. Pure red cell aplasia was confirmed by normochromic anemia with very low reticulocyte percentage in presence of normal white cell and platelet counts, along with the finding of cellular marrow that revealed normal myelopoiesis, lymphopoiesis, and megakaryocytopoiesis, but very rare, if any erythroid precursors [9]. The association of mast cell disorder with pure red cell aplasia is rare and has been described only once in the literature [4].

Our patient had first exposure to Agent Orange 45 years earlier and then for the next three years. Agent Orange is a mixture of two chemicals that are phenoxy herbicides: 2,4 dichlorophenoxyacetic acid and 2,4,5 trichlorophenoxyacetic acid (2,4,5 T). The 2,4,5 T in Agent Orange was contaminated with small amount of dioxins. The main dioxin involved was 2,3,7,8-tetrachlorobenzo-p-dioxin or TCBD, which is one of the most toxic of dioxins and is classified as a human carcinogen by the U.S. Environmental

Protection Agency. In the Vietnam War, between 1962 and 1971, the US military sprayed these herbicides. The Centre for Disease Control and Prevention notes that, in particular, there are increased number of cases of acute/chronic leukemias, Hodgkin's and non-Hodgkin's lymphomas, head and neck cancers, prostate cancer, lung/colon cancers, and soft tissue sarcomas occurring in the exposed population. Other reports have included multiple myeloma, AL amyloidosis, and other benign hematologic changes like anemia, leukopenia, and thrombocytopenia. Role of Agent Orange exposure in cytopenia or systemic mastocytosis in our patient remains of concern but cannot be stated with certainty. The complete blood count 2 years before diagnosis of ASM was normal in our patient.

The etiology of anemia in our patient was probably multifactorial: anemia of chronic disease/malignancy, bone marrow mastocytosis, splenomegaly, and pure red cell aplasia. Myelodysplastic syndrome (MDS) and autoimmune hemolytic anemia contributing to the patient's anemia could not completely be excluded. Serum protein electrophoresis was negative for monoclonal gammopathy, and quantitative measurements of IgG, IgA, and IgM were normal. Direct antiglobulin test was not performed initially. Despite frequent red cell transfusions, no crossmatching difficulties were reported by the blood bank. But, 3 weeks prior to the patient's demise, the blood bank reported difficulty in crossmatching for compatible red cells. A direct antiglobulin test performed then detected an IgG-negative complement-mediated positive test. The serum erythropoietin level was elevated at 1234 IU/L. High-dose methylprednisone 80–100 mg IV was initiated over the next week. In view of the severe reticulocytopenia and rising liver enzymes, coagulopathy as a result of hepatic involvement of ASM, response to steroids could not be determined. The patient remained transfusion-dependent and developed progressively severe pancytopenia.

Similarly, the etiology of thrombocytopenia was also multifactorial: infiltrating mast cells in the bone marrow and splenic sequestration. Increased megakaryopoiesis as well as dysmegakaryopoiesis in bone marrow raise the possibility of immune thrombocytopenia and MDS, respectively. MDS mutational analysis and FISH was performed to evaluate for critical regions in myelodysplastic syndrome which included deletion of 5q31 and 7q31, enumeration of chromosome 8, and deletion of long arm of chromosome 20. The studies were negative for all four regions, and JAK 2 study was also negative. Hence, in absence of abnormal cytogenetics, FISH, and flow cytometric studies, the diagnosis of MDS could not be confirmed. Flow cytometry did not demonstrate any increase in the blasts or immature cells. Immunostain for CD34 was positive only in rare cells in the bone marrow. FISH analysis for t(9:22) BCR/ABL 1 translocation, PDGFRA (4q12), FGFR 1(t 8:11), and PDGRB (5q33) rearrangement was negative. Mutational analysis for MDS detected mutation of ASXL1 and EZH2 genes. These genes are not specific for MDS and have been reported in many myeloid disorders as well as in ASM with unfavourable prognosis [10, 11]. Mutations in IDH1, IDH2, KRAS, NRAS, and TET 2 were negative.

The favoured diagnosis of bone marrow was ASM. The interpretation was supported by the presence of "C" findings including cytopenia indicating bone marrow dysfunction, in association with elevated liver enzymes suggesting liver damage and splenomegaly probably associated with hypersplenism. The patient also had diarrhea on presentation. As an infiltrative process, a proliferation of mast cells in the intestinal submucosa causes malabsorption. Release of histamine, both locally and systemically, other peptides, proteases, and generation of excessive quantities of mediators, such as prostaglandin D2, leukotriene C4, and platelet-activating factor are likely to alter gastrointestinal function and motility.

The patient presented with rapidly accumulating, extremely high iron saturation, and raised ferritin level, with negative mutation in HFE gene, which included C282 Y and H63D. Of note, iron saturation and ferritin levels were normal 4 months before diagnosis of ASM. Other causes of iron overload included ineffective erythropoiesis seen in MDS/sideroblastic anemia, thalassemia, and congenital or acquired hemolytic anemia associated with multiple transfusions. These conditions were unlikely in our patient because of the short time course for iron accumulation. A number of acute and chronic liver diseases causing liver inflammation can release stored iron into circulation raising serum ferritin [12]. One such inflammatory condition is hemophagocytosis syndrome (HPS). It is an extremely lethal condition in which excessive activation of immunity leads to tissue destruction. This condition was unlikely in our patient as the ferritin levels are usually over 5000 ng/ml in hemophagocytosis syndrome, whereas it was below 1000 ng/ml in our patient. The other feature of HPS patients is the acuity of illness with multiorgan involvement. Though our patient had multiorgan involvement from ASM, the cardinal features of HPS such as fever or rheumatologic symptoms were lacking, making the diagnosis unlikely in our patient. Malignancy can also be associated with elevated ferritin as suggested by a clinical trial published in 2015 [13]. Our patient had both an underlying malignancy and liver injury, the latter most likely contributing to the increased ferritin levels.

Management of any form of mastocytosis involves 3 different strategies: (a) general measures to prevent anaphylaxis, (b) antihistamine (cetirizine, hydroxyzine, and doxepin) and antileukotriene therapy (montelukast and zileuton) to treat symptoms associated with mast cell mediator release, and (c) cytoreductive therapy for advanced disease [10, 14, 15]. Midostaurin is a KIT inhibitor, first-line agent used in advanced disease, regardless of KIT mutation status [16]. Our patient did not receive the drug as it was approved by FDA only recently (April 2017). Tyrosine kinase inhibitors (TKI) such as imatinib have been used in ASM patients who do not have D816V mutation [17]. Our patient did express the D816V mutation and hence did not qualify for TKI therapy. At that time, the available cytoreductive therapies were interferon alfa and 2-CDA (chlorodeoxyadenosine). These drugs tend to have significant side effects with response lasting for short duration. This has led to an increasing need for novel agents with longer response and fewer side effects. Another potential therapeutic target CD30 (Ki-1) antigen was identified in patients with advanced ASM, and brentuximab vedotin has been used as an alternative therapy. Our patient received the same [18, 19]. Though brentuximab vedotin has a better safety profile, our patient was unable to tolerate even a single dose.

Cladribine is indicated in patients with rapidly progressive mastocytosis for rapid debulking and those who failed to respond to midostaurin or TKI. Hydroxyurea is also used in ASM patients, especially those with leukocytosis and/or splenomegaly-associated myeloproliferative neoplasms [20, 21]. None of the above therapies could be initiated in our patient due to worsening general condition after brentuximab. Hematopoietic stem cell transplant is the only curative option, though it is typically performed in younger adults [22]. PRCA, with or without ASM, is generally managed with regular transfusions for anemia, followed by immunosuppressive or cytotoxic therapy [23].

Conflicts of Interest

The authors declare that they have no conflicts of interest.

References

[1] D. D. Metcalfe, "Classification and diagnosis of mastocytosis: current status," *Journal of Investigative Dermatology*, vol. 96, no. 3, pp. S2–S4, 1991.

[2] D. A. Arber, A. Orazi, R. Hasserjian et al., "Classification of mastocytosis: a consensus proposal," *Leukemia Research*, vol. 25, no. 7, pp. 603–625, 2001.

[3] J. W. Vardiman, "The 2016 revision to the World Health Organization (WHO) classification of myeloid neoplasms and acute leukemia," *Blood*, vol. 127, no. 20, pp. 2391–2405, 2016.

[4] L. B. Afrin, "Mast cell activation disorder masquerading as pure red cell aplasia," *International Journal of Hematology*, vol. 91, no. 5, pp. 907-908, 2010.

[5] P. Valent, C. Akin, W. R. Sperr et al., "Aggressive systemic mastocytosis and related mast cell disorders: current treatment options and proposed response criteria," *Leukemia Research*, vol. 27, no. 7, pp. 635–641, 2003.

[6] A. W. Hauswirth, I. Simonitsch-Klupp, M. Uffmann et al., "Response to therapy with interferon alpha-2b and prednisolone in aggressive systemic mastocytosis: report of five cases and review of the literature," *Leukemia Research*, vol. 28, no. 3, pp. 249–257, 2004.

[7] L. Afrin, "Presentation, diagnosis, and management of mast cell activation syndrome," in *Mast Cells: Phenotypic Features, Biological Functions, and Role in Immunity*, D. Murray, Ed., Nova Science Publishers, Happauge, NY, USA, 2013.

[8] L. B. Schwartz and A. M. Irani, "Serum tryptase and the laboratory diagnosis of systemic mastocytosis," *Hematology/Oncology Clinics of North America*, vol. 14, no. 3, pp. 641–657, 2000.

[9] K. Sawada, N. Fujishima, and M. Hirokawa, "Acquired pure red cell aplasia: updated review of treatment," *British Journal of Haematology*, vol. 142, no. 4, pp. 505–514, 2008.

[10] M. Jawhar, J. Schwaab, S. Schnittger et al., "Additional mutations in SRSF2, ASXL1 and/or RUNX1 identify a high-risk group of patients with KIT D816V+ advanced systemic mastocytosis," *Leukemia*, vol. 30, no. 1, p. 136, 2016.

[11] F. Traina, V. Visconte, A. M. Jankowska et al., "Single nucleotide polymorphism array lesions, TET2, DNMT3A, ASXL1 and CBL mutations are present in systemic mastocytosis," *PloS One*, vol. 7, no. 8, Article ID e43090, 2012.

[12] D. Karam, S. Swiatkowski, P. Purohit, and B. Agrawal, "High-dose steroids as a therapeutic option in the management of spur cell haemolytic anaemia," *BMJ Case Reports*, vol. 2018, 2018.

[13] A. M. Schram, F. Campigotto, A. Mullally et al., "Marked hyperferritinemia does not predict for HLH in the adult population," *Blood*, vol. 125, no. 10, pp. 1548–1552, 2015.

[14] J. Turk, J. A. Oates, and L. J. Roberts, "Intervention with epinephrine in hypotension associated with mastocytosis," *Journal of Allergy and Clinical Immunology*, vol. 71, no. 2, pp. 189–192, 1983.

[15] A. S. Worobec, "Treatment of systemic mast cell disorders," *Hematology/Oncology Clinics of North America*, vol. 14, no. 3, pp. 659–687, 2000.

[16] J. Gotlib, H. C. Kluin-Nelemans, T. I. George et al., "Efficacy and safety of midostaurin in advanced systemic mastocytosis," *New England Journal of Medicine*, vol. 374, no. 26, pp. 2530–2541, 2016.

[17] A. Vega-Ruiz, J. E. Cortes, M. Sever et al., "Phase II study of imatinib mesylate as therapy for patients with systemic mastocytosis," *Leukemia Research*, vol. 33, no. 11, pp. 1481–1484, 2009.

[18] A. Mehta, V. V. Reddy, and U. Borate, "Anti CD-30 antibody-drug conjugate brentuximab vedotin (ADCETRIS®) may be a promising treatment option for systemic mastocytosis (SM)," *Blood*, vol. 120, p. 2857, 2012.

[19] U. Borate, A. Mehta, V. Reddy, M. Tsai, N. Josephson, and I. Schnadig, "Treatment of CD30-positive systemic mastocytosis with brentuximab vedotin," *Leukemia Research*, vol. 44, pp. 25–31, 2016.

[20] K. H. Lim, A. Pardanani, J. H. Butterfield, C. Y. Li, and A. Tefferi, "Cytoreductive therapy in 108 adults with systemic mastocytosis: outcome analysis and response prediction during treatment with interferon-alpha, hydroxyurea, imatinib mesylate or 2-chlorodeoxyadenosine," *American Journal of Hematology*, vol. 84, no. 12, pp. 790–794, 2009.

[21] A. Tefferi, "Treatment of systemic mast cell disease: beyond interferon," *Leukemia Research*, vol. 28, no. 3, pp. 223-224, 2004.

[22] C. Ustun, A. Reiter, B. L. Scott et al., "Hematopoietic stem-cell transplantation for advanced systemic mastocytosis," *Journal of Clinical Oncology*, vol. 32, no. 29, pp. 3264–3274, 2014.

[23] K. Sawada, M. Hirokawa, and N. Fujishima, "Diagnosis and management of acquired pure red cell aplasia," *Hematology/Oncology Clinics of North America*, vol. 23, no. 2, pp. 249–259, 2009.

9

Drug-Induced Thrombotic Microangiopathy due to Cumulative Toxicity of Ixazomib

Suheil Albert Atallah-Yunes⑩ **and Myat Han Soe**⑩

Department of Medicine, Baystate–University of Massachusetts Medical School, Springfield, MA, USA

Correspondence should be addressed to Myat Han Soe; myathansoe@gmail.com

Academic Editor: Alessandro Gozzetti

Drug-induced thrombotic microangiopathies (DTMAs) are increasingly being recognized as an important category of thrombotic microangiopathies (TMAs). Cancer therapeutic agents including proteasome inhibitors (PIs) are among the most common medications reported to cause DTMA. PIs could cause DTMA either by an immune mechanism or dose-dependent/cumulative toxicity. Eleven cases of DTMA have been reported with bortezomib and carfilzomib. To the best of our knowledge, only one case of DTMA has been reported with ixazomib due to an immune-mediated mechanism. Here, we report the first case of ixazomib-induced DTMA due to cumulative toxicity rather than immune-mediated mechanism. In this article, we discuss the precipitating factors for cumulative toxicity of ixazomib, resulting in DTMA, diagnostic workup, and management of DTMA. We also discuss clinical reasoning based analysis of DTMA versus cancer-associated TMA as well as DTMA versus cyclic thrombocytopenia seen in PI use.

1. Introduction

Thrombotic microangiopathies are a group of disorders characterized by thrombocytopenia, microangiopathic hemolytic anemia, and ischemic end organ damage mostly involving the kidneys and brain caused by disseminated occlusive microvascular thrombosis [1]. TMA is well known to occur in the setting of thrombotic thrombocytopenic purpura (TTP) and hemolytic uremic syndrome (HUS). Other causes of TMA include atypical HUS, various malignancies, rheumatological diseases, and medications [1, 2]. TMA caused by malignancy has been mostly reported with adenocarcinomas metastasizing to bone marrow. Common solid tumors that have been linked to cancer-induced TMA include gastric, breast, lung, and prostate adenocarcinomas, with gastric adenocarcinoma being the most reported. It has also been reported with hematologic malignancies such as lymphoma and multiple myeloma [3]. TMA caused by drugs is called drug-induced TMA (DTMA) [4], and cancer therapeutic agents are among the most common medications reported to cause DTMA. Many cases of DTMA linked to bortezomib and carfilzomib have been reported [5].

Table 1 illustrates the most common cancer therapeutic agents known to cause DTMA, with the most common mechanism being either toxic or immune mediated or both [6–8].

Proteasomes are multicatalytic enzymatic complexes located in both nucleus and cytoplasm that aid in intracellular protein homeostasis by degradation and recycling of proteins [9]. They are an important target in the treatment of multiple myeloma as plasma cells producing paraproteins are highly dependent on these enzyme complexes for survival. PIs prevent degradation of proapoptotic factors and permit activation of programmed cell death in myeloma cells [10]. They also act by stabilization of nuclear factor kB (NF-kB) which ultimately decreases the proliferation of myeloma cells. Bortezomib and carfilzomib are the first and second generation PIs approved by FDA for treatment of multiple myeloma [11–14]. Side effects with these two PIs include gastrointestinal disturbances, peripheral neuropathy, and cyclic thrombocytopenia. The presence of a wide range of side effects and the emergence of chemoresistance required the introduction of newer generation of PIs with fewer side effects such as ixazomib.

TABLE 1: Common anticancer chemotherapeutic agents causing drug-induced thrombotic microangiopathy via immune-mediated mechanism or dose-dependent toxicity or both [4, 7].

Cancer therapeutic agent	Immune-mediated mechanism	Dose-dependent toxicity
Bevacizumab	—	X
Bortezomib	X	—
Carfilzomib	X	—
Ixazomib	X	—
Gemcitabine	X	X
Mitomycin	—	X
Oxaliplatin	X	—
Pentostatin	—	X
Sunitinib	—	X
Imatinib	X	—
Docetaxel	—	X

Ixazomib is the third generation proteasome inhibitor used in the treatment of refractory or relapsing multiple myeloma in combination with dexamethasone and lenalidomide. It has less side effects and several advantages over bortezomib and carfilzomib [15]. Studies show that ixazomib is associated with less frequent and less severe peripheral neuropathy [16, 17]. Another advantage is that ixazomib could be administered orally [18]. The most common side effects reported with ixazomib are gastrointestinal disturbances including nausea, vomiting, diarrhea, and constipation [15].

Thrombocytopenia is also another commonly reported adverse effect as PIs interfere directly with the budding of megakaryocytes rather than causing direct damage to the bone marrow [19]. Thrombocytopenia commonly seen with PIs is called cyclic thrombocytopenia in which the platelet count usually nadirs around day 11 of the cycle and then improves. The decrease in the platelet count is rarely severe, and the platelet count usually nadirs to a minimum of 60% of baseline [19]. The literature also provides a strong evidence of PIs causing TMA in which thrombocytopenia is more severe and accompanied by intravascular hemolytic anemia and renal dysfunction. Clinicians should be familiar with this thrombocytopenia pattern and severity in order to differentiate between benign cyclic thrombocytopenia and TMA in the setting of PI use. When proven to be TMA, another challenge is to differentiate whether TMA is caused by the PI or the multiple myeloma itself as both are managed differently. It is crucial to be familiar with this very rare side effect of ixazomib and other PIs causing TMA, as the principle treatment is to stop the implicated medication [2]. To the best of our knowledge, only one case of immune-mediated DTMA caused by ixazomib has been reported [6]. Here, we report the first case of ixazomib-induced DTMA due to cumulative toxicity rather than immune-mediated mechanism.

2. Case Description

A 71-year-old female with multiple myeloma status after 5 cycles of ixazomib, lenalidomide, and dexamethasone, chronic kidney disease stage III, previous stroke, hypertension, gout, and peripheral arterial disease presented to the hospital with generalized weakness, vomiting, and diarrhea as well as acute on chronic kidney injury in which serum creatinine and creatinine clearance (CrCl) were 3.3 mg/dl and 15 ml/min, respectively (baseline creatinine of 1.9 mg/dl with CrCl of 30 ml/min). Blood test showed thrombocytopenia with a platelet count of 84000/dl and anemia with hemoglobin of 12 g/dl. Regarding multiple myeloma, she was diagnosed with kappa light chain multiple myeloma with extensive lytic lesions in bones as well as renal dysfunction a few years ago. Diagnosis was made by bone marrow biopsy which demonstrated 80%–90% cellular marrow with 61% plasma cells. FISH study was abnormal for chromosome 1q, chromosome 13q, and 17p deletion. Based on patient's average CrCl of 30 ml/min, ixazomib was started at a dose of 3 mg on days 1, 8, and 15 of a 28-day treatment cycle along with lenalidomide and dexamethasone. After the second cycle of ixazomib, the patient had been having intermittent GI disturbances including diarrhea, and biweekly blood test revealed thrombocytopenia with a nadir of about 75000/dl (Figure 1), which were both attributed to ixazomib. Ixazomib was held on admission due to significant vomiting, abdominal pain, and diarrhea. Clostridium difficile toxin and stool culture were negative, ruling out infectious causes. One week after admission, the platelet count decreased dramatically to 9000/dl from 84000/dl on admission. The patient also developed intravascular hemolysis evident by an elevated LDH level (1366 units/L), decreased haptoglobin level (10 mg/dl), elevated total bilirubin (1.6 mg/dl), and indirect bilirubin (1.3 mg/dl). Peripheral blood smear also showed profound schistocytes. Coomb's test was negative, and DIC was ruled out as the fibrinogen level was normal (521 mg/dl). Acute thrombocytopenia, Coomb's negative hemolytic anemia with profound schistocytes, and acute renal injury raised the concern for TMA. Given the high morbidity of TMA, the patient received fresh frozen plasma and underwent plasmapheresis while further workup was in progress. Normal ADAMTS13 activity ruled out TTP. Normal complement levels and negative stool culture made atypical HUS and HUS less likely. Plasmapheresis was stopped after 5 days due to lack of clinical improvement and negative workup for TTP. Approximately three weeks after the onset of TMA, the platelet count started to improve spontaneously with supportive management. The gradual and spontaneous improvement in the platelet count pointed suspicion away from malignancy-induced TMA and favored DTMA caused by cumulative toxicity of ixazomib, likely precipitated by acute renal dysfunction and hypoproteinemia from malnutrition and chronic diarrhea related to ixazomib side effect. The presentation of this patient was consistent with ixazomib-induced DTMA from cumulative toxicity as the clinical picture of TMA improved after stopping ixazomib, independently of plasmapheresis. Also, the lack of recurrence of TMA after stopping ixazomib supported the diagnosis in our case.

3. Discussion

In the presence of possible offending medication, DTMA should be suspected in patients having acute onset

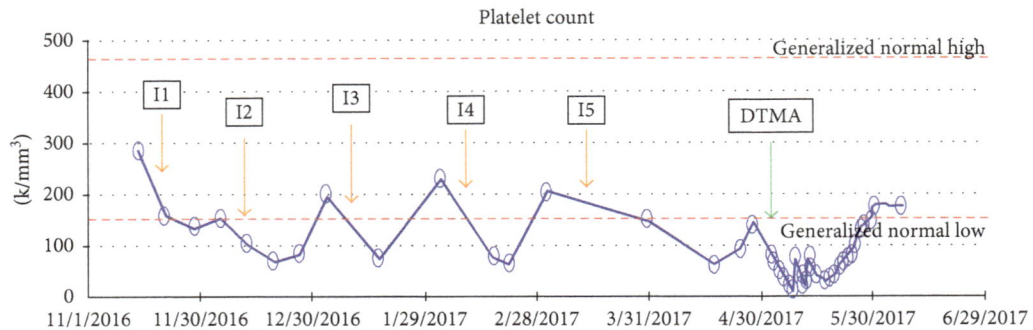

FIGURE 1: Cyclic thrombocytopenia in relation to cycles of ixazomib indicated by orange arrows (I1–I5) and the onset of DTMA indicated by green arrow.

thrombocytopenia, nonimmune intravascular hemolytic anemia with schistocytes and renal injury, with resolution of TMA after stopping the medication and ruling out other causes of TMA. Diagnosis of DTMA is supported if TMA reoccurs after reintroducing the drug. There is no specific time frame in which DTMA develops after introducing the medication. It could range from days to years after the initial dose [5].

The literature describes two main mechanisms causing DTMA which are immune-mediated and dose-dependent toxicity [5, 6, 20]. Immune-mediated reactions are also called idiosyncratic reactions as it involves the formation of reactive antibodies against drugs that cause damage to the endothelium leading to TMA [20]. DTMA due to an idiosyncratic reaction has been mostly reported with quinidine [21] and quetiapine [22]. However, DTMA occurring due to a toxic reaction is usually a dose-dependent toxicity, and results from either direct toxicity of the drug to microvasculature or inhibition of VEGF leading to endothelial damage [6, 20]. Most case reports linking DTMA to PIs favor immune-mediated mechanism as the cause of DTMA (Table 1) although drug-dependent antibodies were not documented.

Eleven cases of DTMA have been reported with bortezomib and carfilzomib [5]. To the best of our knowledge, it has been reported only once with ixazomib due to immune-mediated mechanism [6]. In this case report, we report the second case of DTMA caused by ixazomib. Contrary to the first case report, ixazomib-induced DTMA in our case is likely due to cumulative toxicity. Lack of improvement with plasmapheresis in our case makes immune-mediated mechanism less likely. According to pharmacokinetic data, 99% of ixazomib is plasma protein bound, and the mean area under the curve (AUC) could be 39% higher in patients with severe renal impairment (creatinine clearance <30 ml/min) [18]. We assume that severe renal impairment and hypoproteinemia (total protein: 4.9 g/dl; albumin: 2.4 g/dl) from persistent diarrhea and malnutrition might have precipitated the cumulative toxicity of ixazomib in our case.

TMA could be also caused by malignancies including multiple myeloma [23, 24]. It is important to differentiate between cancer-related TMA and DTMA in cancer patients receiving chemotherapeutic agents such as in multiple myeloma patients receiving PIs. TMA caused by multiple myeloma is usually treated with chemotherapy including PIs. Previous case reports suggest that TMA caused by monoclonal gammopathy resolved with bortezomib. This contrasts with cases of DTMA caused by bortezomib in which TMA resolved after stopping the medication. In our case, paraproteins were close to the normal limit at the time of TMA occurrence. Hemolytic anemia and thrombocytopenia resolved after stopping ixazomib and never reoccurred after that, suggesting TMA was caused by ixazomib rather than multiple myeloma itself.

One of the most commonly reported side effects of ixazomib is thrombocytopenia [15]. It is also crucial to differentiate between cyclic thrombocytopenia and thrombocytopenia due to DTMA. In general, cyclic thrombocytopenia related to PIs is caused by a direct effect on megakaryocyte function and the platelet budding from bone marrow rather than direct damage to the bone marrow with a nadir platelet count at day 11 of the cycle and resolving just before the next cycle [19], as seen in this case (Figure 1). This coincides with the elimination half-life of ixazomib of 7.5 days [15]. Cyclic thrombocytopenia is rarely severe and usually does not require platelet transfusion. This contrasts to the dramatic thrombocytopenia seen in DTMA. In our case, the patient developed cyclic thrombocytopenia after introducing ixazomib with a nadir platelet count of 75000/dl which usually improved before the next cycle of chemotherapy. The dramatic decrease in the platelet count during this hospitalization raised the concern for DTMA especially in the presence of conclusive hemolysis workup with profound schistocytes and acute renal dysfunction.

Pathophysiology behind which PIs cause DTMA is still unclear. The most reported theory in the literature suggests that PIs stabilize and inhibit NF-kB which decreases the production of VEGF leading to microvascular injury. This theory supports cumulative dose-dependent toxicity of PIs. Other theories suggest that PIs act as proinflammatory agents leading to production of TNF and IL-6 which induce the production of autoantibodies against ADAMTS13 [6, 25]. However, the latter theory is unlikely to be the cause of DTMA in our case as our patient had normal levels of ADAMTS13, and also platelet count did not improve with plasmapheresis. Current data report more cases of DTMA with carfilzomib than bortezomib, as carfilzomib irreversibly inhibits proteasomes while bortezomib causes reversible inhibition of proteasomes [20]. The only treatment of DTMA is immediate withdrawal of the implicated agent [2]. In our case, thrombocytopenia did not improve despite 5 days of plasmapheresis. It improved independently about 20 days after stopping ixazomib, which reflects approximately three elimination half-lives of ixazomib. Outpatient records showed that the patient never developed TMA after stopping ixazomib.

The question of whether to reintroduce PIs after causing DTMA depends on the mechanism of DTMA. If DTMA is caused by immune-mediated mechanism, the implicated PI should never be reintroduced again, even with lower doses. However, if DTMA is mediated by dose-dependent cumulative toxicity as in our case, it could be reintroduced with caution. The decision must balance the potential risk of recurrent DTMA and the potential benefits of restarting the medication [26]. Based on our experience from this case, medication dosage, renal function, and total protein/albumin levels should also be taken into consideration in the decision-making process. After the resolution of DTMA, our patient has regular follow-up visits every two months for a year till now. Her blood counts have been stable and paraproteins have not been elevated, indicating nonprogressive disease. Hence, ixazomib is not reintroduced again.

4. Conclusion

DTMA is a very rare side effect of PIs. Ixazomib is indicated in the treatment of refractory and relapsing multiple myeloma. DTMA due to ixazomib should be suspected in the setting of TMA occurring after introducing ixazomib with no evidence of other causes of TMA. The literature reported only one case of ixazomib-induced DTMA due to immune-mediated mechanism, whereas this case highlights the cumulative toxicity of ixazomib causing DTMA. Clinicians should pay attention to changes in renal function, nutrition status, and total protein/albumin level in addition to side effect profile in the management of patients being treated with PIs to prevent cumulative toxicity which could lead to DTMA. It is also important to differentiate DTMA from malignancy-induced TMA especially in multiple myeloma patients treated with PIs such as ixazomib, as both are treated differently.

Conflicts of Interest

The authors declare that they have no conflicts of interest.

References

[1] A. Lodhi, A. Kumar, M. U. Saqlain et al., "Thrombotic microangiopathy associated with proteasome inhibitors," *Clinical Kidney Journal*, vol. 8, no. 5, pp. 632–636, 2015.

[2] J. N. George and C. M. Nester, "Syndromes of thrombotic microangiopathy," *New England Journal of Medicine*, vol. 371, no. 7, pp. 654–666, 2014.

[3] K. Lechner and H. L. Obermeier, "Cancer-related microangiopathic hemolytic anemia: clinical and laboratory features in 168 reported cases," *Medicine*, vol. 91, no. 4, pp. 195–205, 2012.

[4] J. A. Reese, D. W. Bougie, B. R. Curtis et al., "Drug induced thrombotic microangiopathy: experience of the Oklahoma registry and the blood center of Wisconsin," *American Journal of Hematology*, vol. 90, no. 5, pp. 406–410, 2015.

[5] J. C. Yui, K. J. Van, B. M. Weiss et al., "Proteasome inhibitor associated thrombotic microangiopathy," *American Journal of Hematology*, vol. 91, no. 9, pp. E348–E352, 2016.

[6] J. C. Yui, A. Dispenzieri, and N. Leung, "Ixazomib-induced thrombotic microangiopathy," *American Journal of Hematology*, vol. 92, no. 4, pp. E53–E55, 2017.

[7] Z. L. Al-Nouri, J. A. Reese, D. R. Terrell et al., "Drug-induced thrombotic microangiopathy: a systematic review of published reports," *Blood*, vol. 125, no. 4, pp. 616–618, 2015.

[8] J. N. George, *Platelets on the Web*, http://www.ouhsc.edu/platelets/.

[9] J. S. Thrower, L. Hoffman, M. Rechsteiner, and C. M. Pickart, "Recognition of the polyubiquitin proteolytic signal," *EMBO Journal*, vol. 19, no. 1, pp. 94–102, 2000.

[10] J. S. Gelman, J. Sironi, I. Berezniuk et al., "Alterations of the intracellular peptidome in response to the proteasome inhibitor bortezomib," *PLoS One*, vol. 8, no. 1, Article ID e53263, 2013.

[11] P. G. Richardson, P. Sonneveld, M. W. Schuster et al., "Bortezomib or high-dose dexamethasone for relapsed multiple myeloma," *New England Journal of Medicine*, vol. 352, no. 24, pp. 2487–2498, 2005.

[12] P. G. Richardson, B. Barlogie, J. Berenson et al., "A phase 2 study of bortezomib in relapsed, refractory myeloma," *New England Journal of Medicine*, vol. 348, no. 26, pp. 2609–2617, 2003.

[13] R. Vij, D. S. Siegel, S. Jagannath et al., "An openlabel, single-arm, phase 2 study of single-agent carfilzomib in patients with relapsed and/or refractory multiple myeloma who have been previously treated with bortezomib," *British Journal of Haematology*, vol. 158, no. 6, pp. 739–748, 2012.

[14] D. S. Siegel, T. Martin, M. Wang et al., "A phase 2 study of single-agent carfilzomib (PX-171-003A1) in patients with relapsed and refractory multiple myeloma," *Blood*, vol. 120, no. 14, pp. 2817–2825, 2012.

[15] P. G. Richardson, R. Baz, M. Wang et al., "Phase 1 study of twice-weekly ixazomib, an oral proteasome inhibitor, in relapsed/refractory multiple myeloma patients," *Blood*, vol. 124, no. 7, pp. 1038–1046, 2014.

[16] D. Chauhan, Z. Tian, B. Zhou et al., "In vitro and in vivo selective antitumor activity of a novel orally bioavailable proteasome inhibitor MLN9708 against multiple myeloma cells," *Clinical Cancer Research*, vol. 17, no. 16, pp. 5311–5321, 2011.

[17] P. G. Richardson, R. Baz, L. Wang et al., "Investigational agent MLN9708, an oral proteasome inhibitor, in patients (Pts) with relapsed and/or refractory multiple myeloma (MM): results from the expansion cohorts of a phase 1 dose-escalation study," *Blood*, vol. 118, no. 21, p. 140, 2011.

[18] Ninlaro, ixazomib, *Prescribing Information*, Takeda Pharmaceutical Company Limited, Cambridge, MA, USA, 2016.

[19] S. Lonial, E. K. Waller, P. G. Richardson et al., "Risk factors and kinetics of thrombocytopenia associated with bortezomib for relapsed, refractory multiple myeloma," *Blood*, vol. 106, no. 12, pp. 3777–84, 2005.

[20] I. R. Edwards and J. K. Aronson, "Adverse drug reactions: definitions, diagnosis, and management," *Lancet*, vol. 356, no. 9237, pp. 1255–1259, 2000.

[21] K. Kojouri, S. K. Vesely, and J. N. George, "Quinine-associated thrombotic thrombocytopenic purpura–hemolytic uremic syndrome: frequency, clinical features, and long-term outcomes," *Annals of Internal Medicine*, vol. 135, no. 12, pp. 1047–1051, 2001.

[22] M. Huynh, K. Chee, and D. H. M. Lau, "Thrombotic thrombocytopenic purpura associated with quetiapine," *Annals of Pharmacotherapy*, vol. 39, no. 7-8, pp. 1346–1348, 2005.

[23] X. Xiao, H. Y. Zhong, G. S. Zhang, and M.-Y. Deng, "Thrombotic thrombocytopenic purpura as initial and major presentation of multiple myeloma," *Journal of Thrombosis and Thrombolysis*, vol. 36, no. 4, pp. 422-423, 2013.

[24] H. Yao, M. Monge, M. Renou et al., "Thrombotic thrombocytopenic purpura due to anti-ADAMTS13 antibodies in multiple myeloma," *Clinical Nephrology*, vol. 81, no. 3, pp. 210–215, 2014.

[25] H. Moore and K. Romeril, "Multiple myeloma presenting with a fever of unknown origin and development of thrombotic thrombocytopenic purpura post-bortezomib," *Internal Medicine Journal*, vol. 41, no. 4, pp. 348–350, 2011.

[26] J. N. George and A. Cuker, *Drug Induced Thrombotic Microangiopathy*, Uptodate, Waltham, MA, USA, 2017.

10

Iatrogenic Spinal Subdural Hematoma due to Apixaban

Alba Colell,[1] Adrià Arboix ⓘ,[1] Francesco Caiazzo,[2] and Elisenda Grivé[3]

[1]*Cerebrovascular Division, Department of Neurology, Hospital Universitari del SagratCor, Universitat de Barcelona, Barcelona, Catalonia, Spain*
[2]*Department of Neurosurgery, Hospital Universitari del SagratCor, Universitat de Barcelona, Barcelona, Catalonia, Spain*
[3]*Department of Neuroradiology, Hospital Universitari del SagratCor, Universitat de Barcelona, Barcelona, Catalonia, Spain*

Correspondence should be addressed to Adrià Arboix; aarboix@hscor.com

Academic Editor: Kate Khair

In the last decade, the clinical relevance for developing safer oral anticoagulants prompted the development of new classes of drugs that have shown a lower risk of life-threatening bleeding events as compared to standard warfarin. Nontraumatic spinal subdural hematoma is an uncommon urgent complication that can be associated with the use of these agents. An unusual case of spinal subdural hematoma related to apixaban treatment for nonrheumatic atrial fibrillation is reported here.

1. Introduction

Over more than 50 years, warfarin has been the only oral anticoagulant. Warfarin is a vitamin K antagonist with well-documented therapeutic efficacy, despite potential limitations including drug interactions, delayed effect onset of action, narrow therapeutic window, regular measurement of the international normalized ration (INR), and a number of associated hemorrhagic adverse events. For this reason, there has been a great interest in the last decade for developing novel oral anticoagulants to reduce bleeding risks. The new generation of nonvitamin K antagonist oral anticoagulants (NOACs) such as dabigatran, apixaban, and rivaroxaban has more predictable anticoagulant responses and has been shown to be effective in the prevention and treatment of venous thromboembolism and in the prevention of stroke and systemic embolism in patients with nonvalvular atrial fibrillation [1].

Intracranial hemorrhage is one of the most severe complications associated with NOACs as well as post-traumatic spinal hematoma. By contrast, development of a nontraumatic spinal hematoma as a consequence of anticoagulant treatment is an exceptional complication, the natural history of which has been poorly described. Only a few cases of nontraumatic spinal subdural hematoma

related to treatment with NOACs have been reported in the literature [2–4]. We report what appears to be the first case of nontraumatic spinal subdural hematoma in a woman with atrial fibrillation during treatment with apixaban. In all previous cases, rivaroxaban was the drug involved in the hemorrhagic adverse effect. The case described here adds further evidence to the development of this life-threatening neurosurgical entity in the context of treatment with the new oral anticoagulants.

2. Case Presentation

A previously healthy 75-year-old woman with paraparesis was referred to our hospital for diagnostic studies based on tentative diagnoses of low spinal vascular malformation or secondary spinal bleeding. She had a history of hypertension treated with enalapril 5 mg/daily and atrial fibrillation treated with NOACs. Ten days before admission to the hospital, she presented to the emergency room of a regional hospital with abdominal pain. On physical examination, a spontaneous hematoma 3×4 cm in diameter in the left iliac muscle was found. The patient was taking dabigatran at the dose of 150 mg twice a day. Change of dabigatran to apixaban (2.5 mg twice a day) was recommended because of the high cardioembolic risk associated with underlying atrial

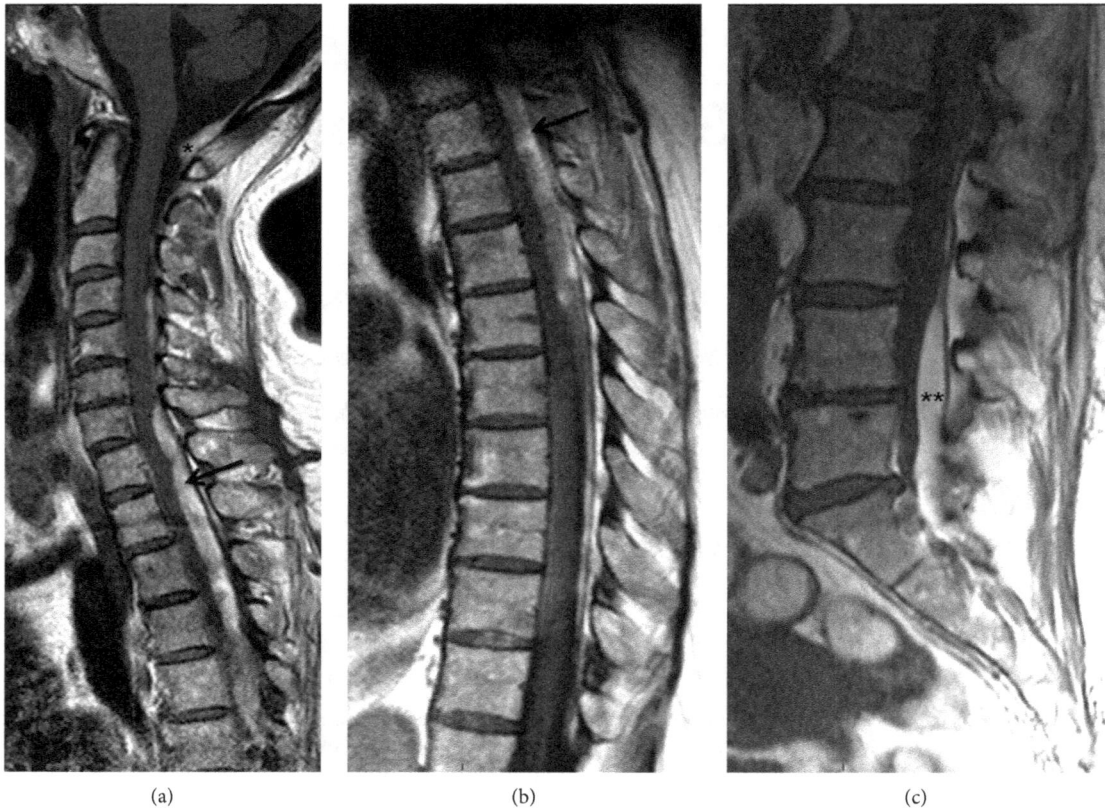

(a)   (b)   (c)

FIGURE 1: MRI scans: T1 sagittal view of the cervical (a), dorsal (b), and sacral (c) column showing a large subacute intraspinal extramedular hematoma from the craniocervical (*) region to the sacral (**) region, with spinal cord compression at the dorsal level (→). It was not possible to study the whole column in one sequence due to clinically silent dorsolumbar scoliosis.

fibrillation. The dose of apixaban was reduced because of bleeding risk. No other risk factors such as hemostatic or spinal disorders were present. Results of laboratory tests including coagulation tests and renal function tests were unrevealing. Ten days after discharge from the emergency room, she developed multiple cutaneous hematomas in the upper extremities and a sudden onset of predominantly distal bilateral crural motor deficit. She was admitted to the hospital where a predominantly left paraparesis was confirmed. A spinal magnetic resonance imaging (MRI) revealed a hemorrhagic focus suggestive of spinal vascular malformation, which was not confirmed at operation.

On admission to the Department of Neurology of our hospital, neurological examination showed paraparesis, predominantly distal and of the left side, with discrete hyperreflexia, hypoesthesia of the low dorsal deep sensitivity, indifferent left plantar reflex, and normal response on the right side. MRI of the spine revealed a large subdural hemorrhage with discontinuous cervical-dorsal-lumbar-sacral involvement with secondary spinal cord compression but without signs of associated vascular malformation (Figures 1 and 2). The patient was treated surgically, and D1 to D3 vertebral laminectomy was performed. The subdural hematoma was evacuated (36 hours after hospital admission), and the diagnosis of subacute spinal hematoma was confirmed. Postoperatively, she was treated with increasing

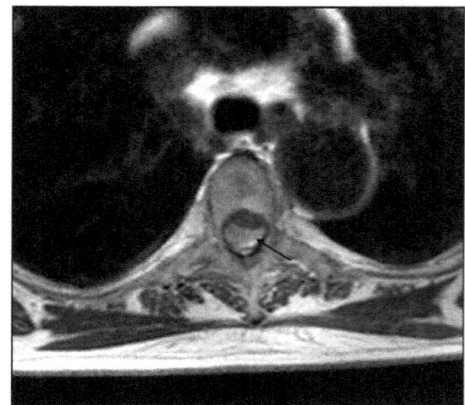

FIGURE 2: MRI scan: T1 transversal view of the dorsal column. Subacute subdural hematoma (→) with anterior displacement and compression of the spinal cord.

doses of dexamethasone 12 mg/24 h and standard analgesic medication. The clinical course was satisfactory, but a control MRI scan performed one week after surgery showed persistence of subdural hemorrhage and spinal compression at D4 to D7 segments with resolution of hematoma at D1–D3 (Figure 3). The patient was reoperated and underwent D4 and D7 partial laminectomy and D5 to D7

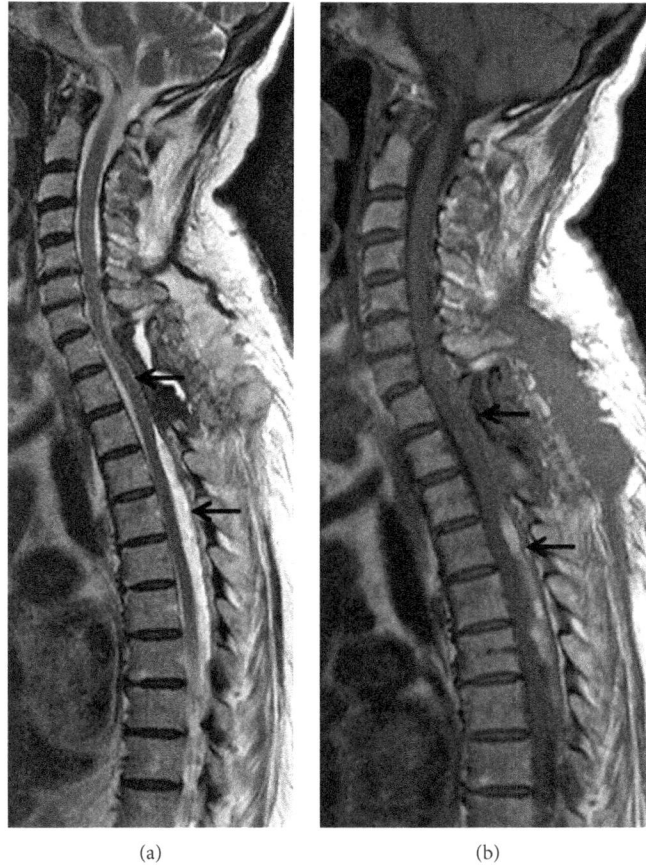

(a)   (b)

FIGURE 3: Postsurgical MRI scan. Sagittal views: T2 (a) and T1 (b). Resolution of spinal cord compression in the operated segment (D1–D3) upper arrows, with persistence of cord compression at the D4–D7 level (lower arrows).

complete vertebral laminectomy. Postoperatively, paraparesis improved slowly, and the patient was discharged 3 weeks after the last surgical procedure with assisted standing and initiation of walking with aids. Six months after the hospital discharge, the patient's clinical condition had largely improved. She was able to walk alone with the aid of a stick, with mild weakness graded 4/5. A control MRI scan showed D1–D3 and D5–D7 laminectomies without hemorrhagic signs in the spinal cord.

3. Discussion

Spinal hematoma is an uncommon clinical entity that can cause sudden and sometimes irreversible neurological impairment if diagnosis and treatment are not promptly established. Apparently, the first clinical case of spinal hematoma was reported by Jackson in 1869 under the term of "case of spinal apoplexy" [5], and the first case of spinal hematoma, which was successfully evacuated by a surgical operation, was reported in 1911 [6]. Depending on its location, the bleeding can be classified as epidural, intradural (subdural), subarachnoid, or intramedullary. Epidural hematomas are the most frequent (75% of cases), with subdural hematomas being extremely rare.

The exact underlying mechanism leading to spontaneous nontraumatic subdural hematoma remains controversial. It is postulated that sudden increases of pressure in the thoracic and/or abdominal cavities can raise the pressure inside the subdural vessels, with rupture of these vessels and subsequent formation of the hematoma [6]. Haines et al. [7] studied the dura-arachnoid junction with electron microscopy. The dura is composed of elongated, flattened fibroblasts and copious amounts of extracellular collagen, whereas the dural border layer (dura-arachnoid junction) is characterized by flattened fibroblasts, no extracellular collagen, extracellular spaces, and few cell junctions. Under normal conditions, there is no evidence of a naturally occurring space at the dura-arachnoid junction, but a space may appear at this point subsequent to pathological/traumatic processes that result in tissue damage with a cleavage opening of the structurally weakest plane in the dural border cell layer. Therefore, subdural hematomas should be considered intradural or hematomas of the dural inner cell border.

Spinal subdural hematomas, as in the case reported here, are usually secondary to vascular lesions, underlying tumors, or result from invasive procedures, such as lumbar puncture and spinal anaesthesia (or even acupuncture) [8], associated with blood dyscrasias and coagulation defects [9]. In a review of 106 cases of nontraumatic acute subdural spinal hematoma, there was a defect in the hemostatic mechanism in 57 patients (54%) and a history of spinal puncture in 50

TABLE 1: Characteristics of the cases of nontraumatic spontaneous spinal subdural hematoma secondary to NOACs.

Author [reference]	Sex, age	Topography	Type of drug, dose	Indication of anticoagulation	Symptom	Treatment	Outcome
Castillo et al. [2]	M, 69 yrs	Thoracolumbar	Rivaroxaban, 20 mg/day	Atrial fibrillation	Lumbar pain, paraplegia, sphincter dysfunction	Cervical and lumbar drainage	No improvement
Dargazanli et al. [3]	M, 72 yrs	Thoracic	Rivaroxaban, 20 mg/day	Atrial fibrillation	Acute interscapular pain, paraplegia	Prothrombin complex, surgery	No improvement at 6 months
Zaarour et al. [4]	F, 58 yrs	Cervicothoracic	Rivaroxaban, 20 mg/day	Atrial fibrillation	Acute interscapular pain, weakness of lower extremities	High-dose steroids, surgery	Important improvement but not complete
Present case	F, 75 yrs	Cervical-dorsal-lumbar-sacral	Apixaban 2.5 mg/12 h	Atrial fibrillation	Acute paraparesis (left side predominant)	High-dose steroids, two surgical operations	Partial improvement at 1 month after the second operation

patients (47%) [10]. Primary or spontaneous nontraumatic spinal hematomas are very uncommon.

A few cases of spinal hematoma directly related to anticoagulant treatment have been reported, most of them presenting as epidural hematomas [11]. Only three cases of spontaneous spinal subdural hematoma associated with the use of rivaroxaban have been reported in the literature [2–4], but to our knowledge, no case due to apixaban has been described. Salient features of these cases including the present case are summarized in Table 1.

Acute and sudden onset of symptoms, with dorsolumbar pain followed by symptoms of spinal cord compression, is characteristic clinical manifestations [11], although multiple neurological deficits have been reported, such as sensory and motor deficits, sphincter dysfunction, and Brown-Séquard syndrome. Our patient did not have dorsal pain, and her clinical picture was mostly a mixed motor-sensory deficit.

MRI is the technique of choice for diagnosis and preferable to computed tomography (CT) [12]. MRI has a high sensitivity for defining the type of bleeding and assessing the craniocaudal extension of the hematoma. Changes in the intensity of MRI signal after development of spinal hematoma are similar to those of cerebral hematomas, although it seems that metabolism of hemoglobin in the spinal canal is faster than that in the intracranial space. Thus, T1-isointense foci and T2-hyperintense lesions due to the presence of oxyhemoglobin can be seen during the first 24 hours, followed by hypointense T1 and T2 signals on the second and third days and subsequent greater signal intensity in both sequences due to the appearance of methemoglobin. Cervicodorsal and dorsolumbar levels are the most frequently affected regions, with predominantly cervical and dorsal involvement in young patients, whereas dorsolumbar involvement is more common in adults. Our patient showed extensive involvement especially in the D1 to D7 region.

The management of nontraumatic spontaneous spinal subdural hematoma has not been definitively established, probably because of the rarity of this condition. The management usually includes emergent surgical evacuation and discontinuation of NOACs. Conservative management may be considered in cases with mild neurological deficits, early spontaneous recovery, or high surgical risk [4]. Prognosis is poor in the presence of associated subarachnoid hemorrhage with spinal arachnoiditis as a potential complication [13].

4. Conclusion

Nontraumatic spontaneous spinal subdural hematoma is a potential complication of the use of apixaban, and this appears to be the first case reported in the literature. This entity should be distinguished from spinal subarachnoid hemorrhage, spinal epidural hemorrhage, or intraspinal hemorrhage [14]. Physicians should be aware of the increasing incidence of severe bleeding complications associated with the increasing use of NOACs. Serious spinal hematomas secondary to rivaroxaban and apixaban therapy are a devastating complication for the patient and the family. Recovery of the neurological deficit depends on prompt diagnosis with MRI scans and early surgical evacuation of the hematoma.

Conflicts of Interest

The authors declare that they have no conflicts of interest regarding the publication of this paper.

Authors' Contributions

Alba Colell participated in background research, literature review, care of the patient, and writing of this manuscript. Adrià Arboix assisted in literature review, diagnosis of the patient, and writing of the manuscript. Francesco Caiazzo and Elisenda Grivé participated in the care of the patient and review of the manuscript for intellectual content.

Acknowledgments

The authors thank Marta Pulido, MD, for editing the manuscript and editorial assistance.

References

[1] Y. M. Mekaj, A. Y. Mekaj, S. B. Duci, and E. I. Miftari, "New oral anticoagulants: their advantages and disadvantages compared with vitamin K antagonists in the prevention and treatment of patients with thromboembolic events," *Therapeutics and Clinical Risk Management*, vol. 11, pp. 967–977, 2015.

[2] J. M. Castillo, H. F. Afanador, E. Manjarrez, and X. A. Morales, "Non-traumatic spontaneous spinal subdural hematoma in a patient with non-valvular atrial fibrillation during treatment

with rivaroxaban," *American Journal of Case Reports*, vol. 16, pp. 377–381, 2015.

[3] C. Dargazanli, N. Lonjon, and G. Gras-Combe, "Non-traumatic spinal subdural hematoma complicating direct factor Xa inhibitor treatment (rivaroxaban): a challenging management," *European Spine Journal*, vol. 25, no. 1, pp. 1–4, 2016.

[4] M. Zaarour, S. Hassan, N. Thumallapally, and Q. Dai, "Rivaroxaban-induced nontraumatic spinal subdural hematoma: an uncommon yet life-threatening complication," *Case Reports in Hematology*, vol. 2015, Article ID 275380, 5 pages, 2015.

[5] R. Jackson, "Case of spinal apoplexy," *The Lancet*, vol. 94, no. 2392, pp. 5-6, 1869.

[6] D. Kreppel, G. Antoniadis, and W. Seeling, "Spinal hematoma: a literature survey with meta-analysis of 613 patients," *Neurosurgery Reviews*, vol. 26, no. 1, pp. 1–46, 2013.

[7] D. E. Haines, H. L. Harkey, and O. Al-Mefty, "The "subdural" space: a new look at an updated concept," *Neurosurgery*, vol. 32, no. 1, pp. 111–120, 1991.

[8] J. Park, R. Ahn, D. Son, B. Kang, and D. Yang, "Acute spinal subdural hematoma with hemiplegia after acupuncture: a case report and review of the literature," *Spine Journal*, vol. 13, no. 10, pp. e59–e63, 2013.

[9] P. Varela Rois, J. González Garcia, M. Regueira Portas, P. Martínez Cueto, and E. Azevedo González, "Hematomas espinales: la apoplejía espinal," *Neurología*, vol. 25, no. 2, pp. 96–103, 2010.

[10] M. Domenicucci, A. Ramieri, P. Ciappetta, and R. Delfini, "Nontraumatic acute spinal subdural hematoma: report of five cases and review of the literature," *Journal of Neurosurgery*, vol. 91, no. 1, pp. 65–73, 1999.

[11] M. Jaeger, B. Jeanneret, and S. Schaeren, "Spontaneous spinal epidural haematoma during Xa inhibitor treatment (rivaroxaban)," *European Spine Journal*, vol. 21, no. 4, pp. 433–435, 2012.

[12] M. Boukobza, D. Haddar, M. Boissonet, and J. J. Merland, "Spinal subdural hematoma: a study of three cases," *Clinical Radiology*, vol. 65, no. 6, pp. 475–480, 2001.

[13] A. J. Kok, W. I. Verhagen, R. H. Bartels, R. van Dijk, and M. J. Prick, "Spinal arachnoiditis following subarachnoid haemorrhage: report of two cases and review of the literature," *Acta Neurochirurgica*, vol. 142, no. 7, pp. 795–799, 2000.

[14] J. G. Heckmann, "Spinal subarachnoid haemorrhage in cortical superficial siderosis after apixaban and clopidogrel therapy," *Journal of Thrombosis and Thrombolysis*, vol. 41, no. 4, pp. 654-655, 2016.

11

Acute Myeloid Leukemia with Basophilic Differentiation Transformed from Myelodysplastic Syndrome

Yasuhiro Tanaka,[1] **Atsushi Tanaka,**[1] **Akiko Hashimoto,**[1]
Kumiko Hayashi,[2] **and Isaku Shinzato**[1]

[1]*Department of Hematology and Clinical Immunology, Nishi-Kobe Medical Center, Hyogo, Japan*
[2]*Molecular Genetic Analysis Department, LSI Medience Corporation, Tokyo, Japan*

Correspondence should be addressed to Yasuhiro Tanaka; ytanaka77@nmc-kobe.org

Academic Editor: Ramon Tiu

Myelodysplastic syndrome (MDS) terminally transforms to acute myeloid leukemia (AML) or bone marrow failure syndrome, but acute myeloid leukemia with basophilic differentiation has been rarely reported. An 81-year-old man was referred to our department for further examination of intermittent fever and normocytic anemia during immunosuppressive treatment. Chromosomal analysis showed additional abnormalities involving chromosome 7. He was diagnosed as having MDS. At the time of diagnosis, basophils had not proliferated in the bone marrow. However, his anemia and thrombocytopenia rapidly worsened with the appearance of peripheral basophilia three months later. He was diagnosed as having AML with basophilic differentiation transformed from MDS. At that time, monosomy 7 was detected by chromosomal analysis. We found that basophils can be confirmed on the basis of the positivity for CD203c and CD294 by flow cytometric analysis. We also found by cytogenetic analysis that basophils were derived from myeloblasts. He refused any chemotherapy and became transfusion-dependent. He died nine months after the transformation. We should keep in mind that MDS could transform to AML with basophilic differentiation when peripheral basophilia in addition to myeloblasts develops in patients with MDS.

1. Introduction

Myelodysplastic syndrome (MDS) is a clonal disorder of hematopoietic stem cells and is characterized by bone marrow failure of normal hematopoietic cells and a dysplastic change of trilineage cells [1]. Some cases of MDS show basophilia or eosinophilia in the bone marrow, which indicates a poor prognosis [2, 3]. MDS often develops into acute leukemia, which is termed transformation. Many cases of MDS transform to acute myeloid leukemia (AML) [1], but AML with basophilic differentiation has been rarely reported. On the other hand, acute basophilic leukemia (ABL) was originally reported over one hundred years before and classified as a distinct entity by the World Health Organization (WHO) classification in 2008 [4].

We report a case of AML with basophilic differentiation transformed from MDS. To the best of our knowledge, this is the fifth case of ABL or AML with basophilic differentiation

transformed from MDS. We also reviewed here the other four cases in the literature.

2. Case Presentation

An 81-year-old man was admitted to our hospital because of bilateral pitting edema of his legs for about one month in October 2015. He was operated on for prostate cancer twelve years ago and also for Vater papilla cancer five years ago. He did not receive any further treatment. Physical examinations revealed only bilateral pitting edema of his legs, and no abnormalities of his thorax and abdomen were found. He was diagnosed as having minimal change nephrotic syndrome (MCNS) on the basis of his renal biopsy results in November 2015. He started immunosuppressive treatment with cyclosporine (CsA) and prednisolone (PSL), and he achieved complete remission for MCNS about one month later. Thus, CsA was stopped and his PSL dose was gradually tapered.

During immunosuppressive treatment, he occasionally had fever of more than 38°C and felt general malaise due to normocytic anemia, as shown by laboratory tests. Thus, he was referred to our department for further examinations. Laboratory examinations revealed the following: white blood cell (WBC) count, 4.2×10^9/L with no abnormal cells; hemoglobin (Hb) level, 9.2 g/dL; platelet (Plt) count, 53.6 $\times 10^{10}$/L. A bone marrow smear showed 6.4% blasts and marked dysplasia of neutrophils and erythroid precursor cells. Flow cytometric analysis showed that the blasts were positive for CD13, CD33, CD34, CD56, and HLA-DR, which was consistent with myeloblasts. Chromosomal analysis by G banding showed additional add(7)(q22) in 2 out of 20 metaphase cells analyzed. These findings led to the diagnosis of myelodysplastic syndrome (MDS, refractory anemia with excess of blast-1) in accordance with the WHO 2008 classification [1] and MDS with multilineage dysplasia in accordance with the 2016 revision of WHO classification [6]. On the basis of revised international prognostic scoring system [7], he was classified as high risk. At that time, basophils were only 2.0% of all nucleated cells in the bone marrow. He received only one pack of red blood cell (RBC) transfusion as palliative therapy and felt better during oral PSL therapy.

In February 2016, he complained again of general malaise. Some abnormal cells with many basophilic granules appeared in his peripheral blood and then gradually increased in number (Figure 1(a)). One month later, anemia and thrombocytopenia rapidly developed. Laboratory examinations revealed the following: WBC count, 2.5×10^9/L with 2% myeloblasts and 47% abnormal cells; Hb level, 5.1 g/dL; Plt count, 4.8×10^{10}/L. Flow cytometric analysis of abnormal cells showed that these cells were positive for CD11b, CD13, CD33, CD38, CD123, CD203c, and CD294 and negative for CD34 and HLA-DR, which was consistent with basophils (Figure 1(b)). Serum histamine (8.67 ng/ml; normal range, 0.15–1.23) and tryptase (6.6 μg/L; normal range, 1.2–5.7) levels were slightly elevated. The bone marrow smear showed 30.4% myeloblasts and 16.8% mature basophils (Figure 2(a)). Flow cytometric analysis showed that the myeloblasts were positive for CD13, CD33, CD34, CD56, CD117, and HLA-DR (Figure 2(b)), which indicated the same phenotype as the blasts in the initial bone marrow examination. Fluorescence in situ hybridization (FISH) analysis showed neither fusion signals of the BCR and ABL genes nor those of the DEK and NUP214 genes. Chromosomal analysis by G banding showed monosomy 7 in 14 out of 20 metaphase cells and additional add(1)(q21) in 4 out of 20 metaphase cells analyzed (Figure 2(c)). Monosomy 7 was confirmed by FISH analysis (Figure 2(d)). The loss of chromosome 7 was found in myeloblasts and basophils of the bone marrow (Figure 1(c)), which showed that basophils were derived from myeloblasts. These findings indicated the diagnosis of AML with basophilic differentiation transformed from MDS. We did not check for basophilic granules by electron microscopy. He refused intensive chemotherapy and azacitidine treatment, and he was RBC-transfusion-dependent with 10 mg of oral PSL per day. In August 2016, he developed *Klebsiella pneumoniae* bacteremia complicated by solitary liver abscess.

His bacteremia was treated with intravenous administration of tazobactam/piperacillin for six weeks. After his discharge, he had continued to receive regular RBC transfusion, but he suddenly died of bronchopneumonia at home in November 2016. An autopsy was not carried out. One week before his death, a laboratory examination showed the following: WBC count, 5.9×10^9/L with 3% myeloblasts and 49% mature basophils; Hb level, 7.0 g/dL; Plt count, 4.0×10^{10}/L. These findings did not change over nine months after the transformation.

3. Discussion

Here, we report the case of a patient with AML with basophilic differentiation transformed from MDS. We diagnosed him as having AML with basophilic differentiation on the basis of the results of flow cytometric analysis. More than 30% of blasts occupied the bone marrow and were positive for CD13, CD33, CD34, CD56, CD117, and HLA-DR, which was consistent with myeloblasts. Some mature basophils were found in the same bone marrow sample. On the other hand, in peripheral blood, many basophils were found. They were positive for CD11b, CD13, CD33, CD38, CD123, CD203c, and CD294 and negative for CD34 and HLA-DR. Both CD203c and CD294 are specific markers of basophils [8]. Thus, myeloblasts and basophils express different markers. We also showed by FISH analysis that basophils were derived from myeloblasts. FISH analysis showed the loss of chromosome 7 in myeloblasts and basophils in the bone marrow. This is the first case study by FISH analysis confirming that basophils were derived from myeloblasts. The origin of basophils in ABL has been shown by electron microscopy and chromosomal analysis by G banding thus far. These methods do not directly show the cell origin. Thus, FISH analysis was very useful for detecting the cell origin of basophils.

ABL is a very rare disease characterized by the proliferation of blasts containing basophilic granules in the cytoplasm. Although almost all cases of ABL were de novo [4], some cases of ABL transformed from myeloproliferative neoplasms (MPNs) have been reported thus far. The representative case of transformed ABL is the basophilic blast crisis of chronic myeloid leukemia (CML). In the case of the basophilic crisis of CML, although a very rare type of blast crisis, the basophils are derived from a CML clone, which is shown by chromosomal analysis by G banding [9]. Among MPNs except CML, only two cases of ABL transformed from MPNs were reported. One case was ABL transformed from essential thrombocytosis reported by Shah et al. [10], and the other was that transformed from primary myelofibrosis reported by Sugimoto et al. [11]. Thus, reports of cases of basophilic leukemia transformed from MPNs are relatively rare in the literature.

To the best of our knowledge, four other cases of ABL or AML with basophilic differentiation transformed from MDS have been reported (Table 1). Shirakawa et al. reported a case of a 52-year-old woman admitted for further examination of anemia [12]. She was diagnosed as having MDS (refractory anemia with excess of blast, RAEB). About two months later, her blood examinations showed

(a)

(b)

(c)

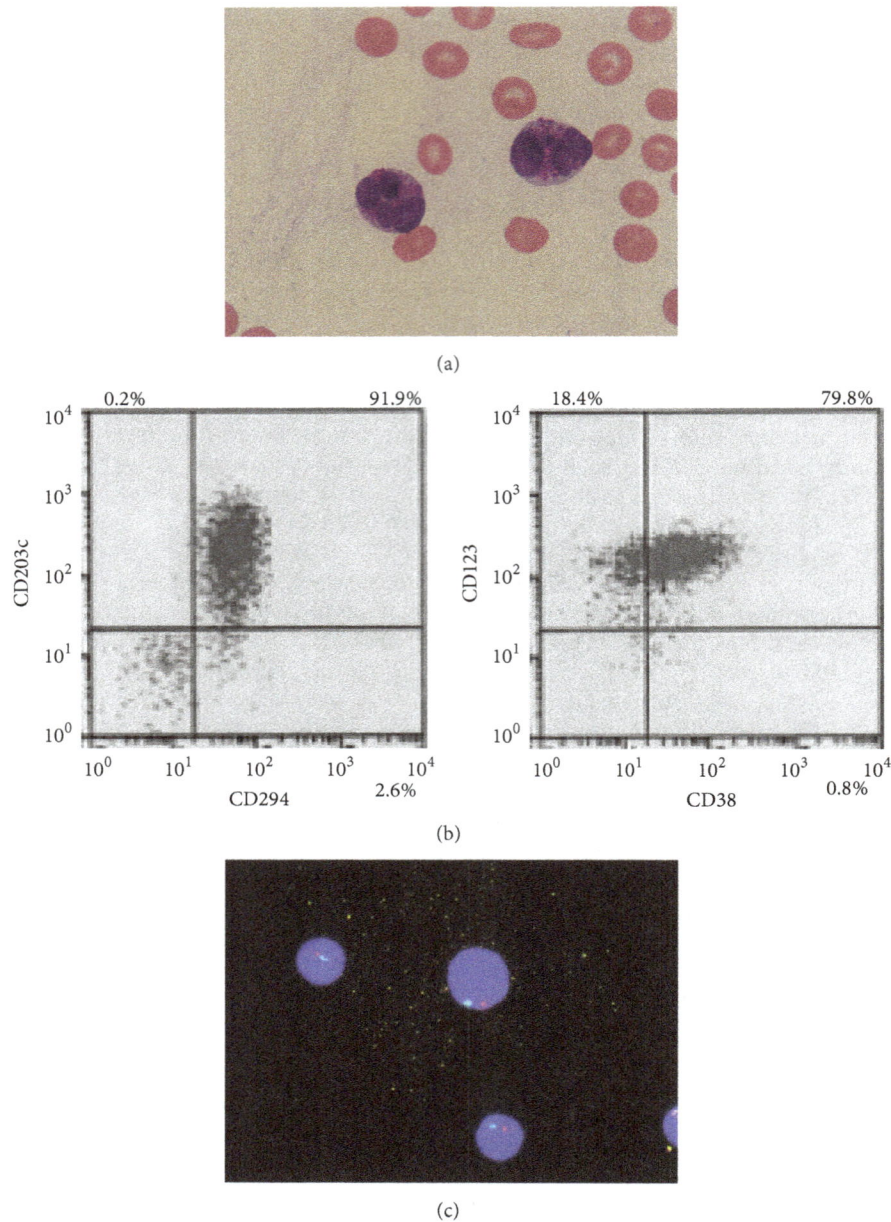

FIGURE 1: The characterization of basophils in peripheral blood. (a) Peripheral blood smear showed some medium- to large-sized abnormal cells with lobulated nucleus, and many basophilic granules were observed (May-Giemsa staining, original magnification, ×1000). (b) Flow cytometric analysis showed that abnormal cells were positive for CD38, CD123, CD203c, and CD294, which was consistent with basophils. (c) Dual-color FISH analysis using chromosome 7 probes showed that abnormal cell with many granules contained one red signal and one green signal, which indicated monosomy 7 (D7S486 probe, red signal; D7Z1 probe, green signal). Other cells without any granules also showed monosomy 7.

increased severity of leukocytosis. Chromosomal analysis showed a complex karyotype including monosomy 7. She died of respiratory failure and bacteremia six months after the transformation. Yamagata et al. reported the case of a 52-year-old woman presenting with general malaise [13]. She was diagnosed as having MDS (refractory anemia, RA). Chromosomal analysis showed del(5)(q31q35). About two years later, bone marrow examination showed normocellularity with 42.8% blasts and 26.6% basophils. Chromosomal

analysis revealed the same abnormalities as those in the initial diagnosis of MDS. She died of severe interstitial pneumonia two months after the transformation. Wells et al. reported the case of an 84-year-old woman presenting with general deterioration of her health [14]. She showed pancytopenia with peripheral blasts. Her neutrophils were almost dysplastic, and the blasts contained basophilic granules. She was diagnosed as having AML with myelodysplasia-related changes showing basophilic differentiation. Chromosomal

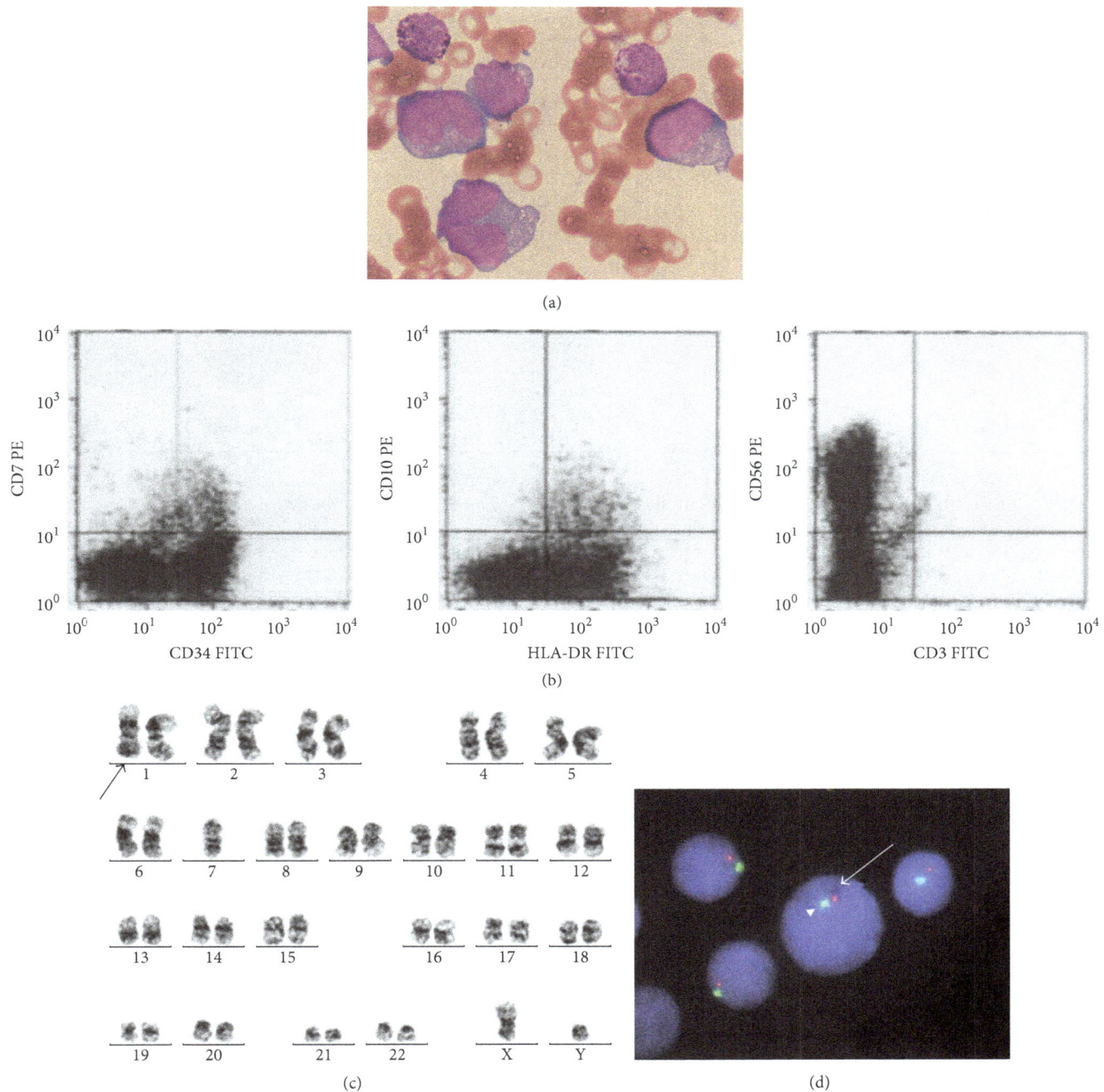

(a)

(b)

(c)

(d)

FIGURE 2: The characterization of myeloblasts in bone marrow. (a) Bone marrow smear showed some large-sized myeloblasts with clear nucleoli, basophilic cytoplasm, and some vacuoles. Some mature basophils were observed (May-Giemsa staining, original magnification, ×1000). (b) Flow cytometric analysis showed blasts positive for CD34, CD56, and HLA-DR. (c) Chromosomal analysis by G banding showed 45, XY, -7 [5]/45, idem, add(1)(q21) [4]/46, XY [2]. (d) Dual-color FISH analysis using chromosome 7 probes showed that myeloblasts contained one red signal and one green signal, which indicated monosomy 7 (D7S486 probe, red signal, arrow; D7Z1 probe, green signal, arrow head).

analysis showed a complex karyotype including monosomy 7. This case was consistent with AML with myelodysplasia-related changes and basophilic differentiation transformed from MDS, which was not diagnosed previously. Bahmanyar and Chang reported the case of a 64-year-old man who presented with increased shortness of breath due to pancytopenia [5]. He was diagnosed as having MDS (refractory anemia with multilineage dysplasia, RCMD). Chromosomal analysis showed a complex karyotype including monosomy 7. Two months later, his MDS transformed to AML with

TABLE 1: Previous reports of patients with acute basophilic leukemia or acute myeloid leukemia with basophilic differentiation transformed from myelodysplastic syndrome. M, male; F, female; RA, refractory anemia; RAEB, refractory anemia with excess blasts; RCMD, refractory cytopenia with multilineage dysplasia; ND, not described; IP, interstitial pneumonia.

Case	Age/sex	Diagnosis	Interval from diagnosis to transformation	Karyotype at transformation	Outcome	prognosis from transformation	Reference
1	52/F	RAEB	2 months	Complex karyotype including -7	Death of disease	6 months	Shirakawa et al., 1992
2	52/F	RA	2 years	del(5)(q31q35)	Death due to IP	2 months	Yamagata et al., 1995
3	84/F	ND	2 months	Complex karyotype including -7	ND	ND	Wells et al., 2014
4	64/M	RCMD	2 months	Complex karyotype including -7	ND	ND	Bahmanyar and Chang, 2016
5	81/M	RAEB-1	3 months	-7, add(1)(q21)	Death of bronchopneumonia	6 months	This case

myelodysplasia-related changes and prominent basophilic differentiation. Chromosomal analysis revealed the same abnormalities as those in the initial diagnosis of MDS. Clinical characteristics of ABL or AML with basophilic differentiation transformed from MDS were the very short interval (within six months) from the diagnosis of MDS to the transformation, monosomy 7 detected in 3 out of 5 cases by chromosomal analysis, and very poor outcome (i.e., death) in 3 out of 5 cases. These clinical features might be due to the monosomy 7 abnormality. Thus, we should keep in mind that MPNs could transform to ABL or AML with basophilic differentiation.

The normal range of basophils in the bone marrow was below 1% [15]. Our patient showed a slightly elevated basophil count in the bone marrow at the time of the diagnosis of MDS. Regarding the two cases in Japan previously reported [12, 13], we found that the percentage of basophils at the time of the diagnosis of MDS was slightly high in the bone marrow. We speculated that the increased percentage of basophils in the bone marrow at the time of the diagnosis of MDS would be a predictor of the transformation to ABL or AML with basophilic differentiation. The mechanism by which basophils differentiate from myeloblasts has not been clarified so far, and no mechanism has been proposed to the best of our knowledge. Collection of more cases of ABL or AML with basophilic differentiation transformed from MDS may clarify this mechanism.

In conclusion, we here reported the case of AML with basophilic differentiation transformed from MDS. The combination of flow cytometry and FISH analysis is useful easily for the diagnosis of AML with basophilic differentiation.

Competing Interests

The authors declare no conflict of interests.

References

[1] R. D. Brunning, A. Orazi, U. Germing et al., "Myelodysplastic syndrome/neoplasms, overview," in WHO Classification of Tumors of Haematopoietic and Lymphoid Tissues, pp. 88–93, IARC, Lyon, France, 2008.

[2] T. Matsushima, H. Handa, A. Yokohama et al., "Prevalence and clinical characteristics of myelodysplastic syndrome with bone marrow eosinophilia or basophilia," Blood, vol. 101, no. 9, pp. 3386–3390, 2003.

[3] F. Wimazal, U. Germing, M. Kundi et al., "Evaluation of the prognostic significance of eosinophilia and basophilia in a larger cohort of patients with myelodysplastic syndromes," Cancer, vol. 116, no. 10, pp. 2372–2381, 2010.

[4] D. A. Arber, R. D. Brunning, A. Orazi et al., "Acute myeloid leukemia, not otherwise specified," in WHO Classification of Tumors of Haematopoietic and Lymphoid Tissues, pp. 130–139, IARC, Lyon, France, 2008.

[5] M. Bahmanyar and H. Chang, "Acute myeloid leukemia with myelodysplasia-related changes demonstrating prominent basophilic differentiation," Blood, vol. 127, no. 20, article 2503, 2016.

[6] D. A. Arber, A. Orazi, R. Hasserjian et al., "The 2016 revision to the World Health Organization classification of myeloid neoplasms and acute leukemia," Blood, vol. 127, no. 20, pp. 2391–2405, 2016.

[7] P. L. Greenberg, H. Tuechler, J. Schanz et al., "Revised international prognostic scoring system for myelodysplastic syndromes," Blood, vol. 120, no. 12, pp. 2454–2465, 2012.

[8] Y. Gernez, R. Tirouvanziam, G. Yu et al., "Basophil CD203c levels are increased at baseline and can be used to monitor omalizumab treatment in subjects with nut allergy," International Archives of Allergy and Immunology, vol. 154, no. 4, pp. 318–327, 2011.

[9] J. Pidala, J. Pinilla-Ibarz, and H. D. Cualing, "A case of acute basophilic leukemia arising from chronic myelogenous leukemia with development of t(7;8)(q32;q13)," Cancer Genetics and Cytogenetics, vol. 182, no. 1, pp. 46–49, 2008.

[10] I. Shah, L. M. Lewkow, and F. Koppitch, "Acute basophilic leukemia," The American Journal of Medicine, vol. 76, no. 6, pp. 1097–1099, 1984.

[11] N. Sugimoto, T. Ishikawa, S. Gotoh et al., "Primary myelofibrosis terminated in basophilic leukemia and successful allogeneic bone marrow transplantation," International Journal of Hematology, vol. 80, no. 2, pp. 183–185, 2004.

[12] C. Shirakawa, M. Ohno, H. Sugishima et al., "Overt leukemia from MDS associated with marked basophilia," *The Japanese Journal of Clinical Hematology*, vol. 33, no. 8, pp. 1031–1035, 1992.

[13] T. Yamagata, A. Miwa, M. Eguchi et al., "Transformation into acute basophilic leukaemia in a patient with myelodysplastic syndrome," *British Journal of Haematology*, vol. 89, no. 3, pp. 650–652, 1995.

[14] R. Wells, B. Williams, and B. J. Bain, "Acute myeloid leukemia with myelodysplasia-related changes showing basophilic differentiation," *American Journal of Hematology*, vol. 89, no. 11, p. 1082, 2014.

[15] D. H. Ryan, "Examination of the marrow," in *Williams Hematology*, pp. 17–25, McGraw-Hill, New York, NY, USA, 2001.

12

A Case of Blastic Plasmacytoid Dendritic Cell Neoplasm Extensively Studied by Flow Cytometry and Immunohistochemistry

Martina Pennisi,[1] **Clara Cesana,**[2] **Micol Giulia Cittone,**[1] **Laura Bandiera,**[2] **Barbara Scarpati,**[2] **Valentina Mancini,**[1] **Silvia Soriani,**[2] **Silvio Veronese,**[2] **Mauro Truini,**[2] **Silvano Rossini,**[2] **and Roberto Cairoli**[1]

[1]*Division of Hematology, Niguarda Ca' Granda Hospital, Milan, Italy*
[2]*Department of Laboratory Medicine, Niguarda Ca' Granda Hospital, Milan, Italy*

Correspondence should be addressed to Martina Pennisi; pennisi.marti@gmail.com

Academic Editor: Yusuke Shiozawa

Blastic plasmacytoid dendritic cell neoplasm (BPDCN) is a rare hematologic malignancy with aggressive clinical course and poor prognosis. Diagnosis is based on detection of CD4$^+$ CD56$^+$, CD123^{high}, TCL-1$^+$, and blood dendritic cell antigen-2/CD303$^+$ blasts, together with the absence of lineage specific antigens on tumour cells. In this report we present a case of BPDCN presenting with extramedullary and bone marrow involvement, extensively studied by flow cytometry and immunohistochemistry, who achieved complete remission after acute lymphoblastic leukemia like chemotherapy and allogeneic hematopoietic stem cell transplantation.

1. Introduction

Blastic plasmacytoid dendritic cell neoplasm (BPDCN) is a rare aggressive hematologic neoplasm, included among acute myeloid leukemia (AML) and related precursor disorders in the 2008 World Health Organization (WHO) classification of hematological diseases and then classified as a distinct entity among myeloid neoplasms in the 2016 revision [1, 2].

Clinical presentation is characterized by an indolent onset of the disease, with extramedullary involvement and tropism towards skin and lymph nodes, followed by systemic dissemination and bone marrow (BM) infiltration [3]. The diagnosis is mainly provided by detection of CD4$^+$ CD56$^+$, CD123^{high}, TCL-1$^+$, and blood dendritic cell antigen-2 (BDCA2)/CD303$^+$ Lin$^-$ blasts [3].

Despite the increasing number of reports and biologic insights about BPDCN, early recognition of the disease still remains a challenge, because its phenotype largely overlaps that displayed by other hematologic malignancies. In this report we present a case of BPDCN, in which extensive flow cytometry (FCM) and immunohistochemistry (IHC) analyses allowed a prompt and accurate diagnosis.

2. Case Presentation

A 37-years-old man was referred to our hospital for a two months' history of skin lesions, followed by moderate hearing loss and nosebleed and, lately, by sudden onset of visual impairment and headache. No B symptoms were complained of. Physical exam showed conjunctival bleeding, brown nodular bruise-like lesions on the scalp, neck, and back (Figures 1(a), 1(b), 1(c), and 1(d)), and bilateral cervical and submandibular lymph nodes enlargement. No hepatosplenomegaly was found. At otolaryngology inspection, hypertrophic obstruction of the rhinopharyngeal tract was observed. Ophthalmologic evaluation revealed reduced visual acuity, without retinal or lenses abnormality. Laboratory exams showed white blood cell (WBC) count 6.0 × 10^9/L (neutrophils 59%, lymphocytes 31%, monocytes 9%, and eosinophils 1%), hemoglobin 14.6 g/dL, and platelet count 92 × 10^9/L. Blood chemistry and coagulation tests were unremarkable, except for increased lactate dehydrogenase levels (348 U/L, normal < 225 U/L). Anti-DNA/antinuclear antibodies, circulating immune complexes, were absent and serologic tests for hepatitis B and C viruses were negative.

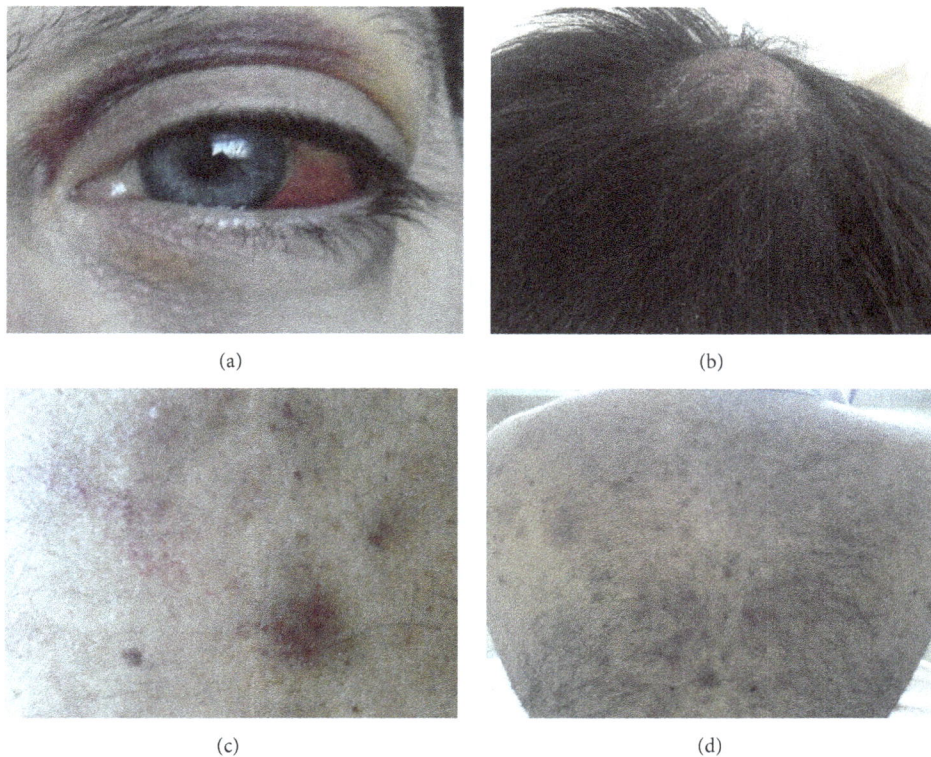

(a) (b) (c) (d)

FIGURE 1: Clinical presentation: close view picture of conjunctival bleeding with eyelid hemorrhage and periorbital edema (a); voluminous infiltrative and erythematous nodule localized on the scalp (b); detailed view of bruise-like brown cutaneous nodules and plaques (c); multiple bruise-like brown cutaneous nodules and plaques localized on the back (d).

Computed tomography scan displayed rhinopharyngeal obstruction by pathological tissue, 2–2.5 cm-sized laterocervical, axillary, abdominal, and inguinal lymph node enlargement, and no cerebral involvement. At positron emission tomography lymph nodes and skin lesions exhibited only a slight fluorodeoxyglucose uptake.

Skin biopsy showed a diffuse dermal and hypodermal infiltration by immature cells, with irregular nuclei and scant cytoplasm, with a perivascular and periadnexal pattern, involving nervous structures (Figures 2(a), 2(b), and 2(c)). A lymph node biopsy proved complete architectural effacement secondary to massive infiltration by analogous cells with the following IHC expression: $CD4^+$ $CD10^+$ $CD56^+$ $CD99^+$ $CD123^+$ $CD303^+$ TdT^+ $BCL2^+$; $CD68PGM1^{+/-}$ $CD7^{+/-}$ $CD43^{+/-}$ $CD2^{-/+}$; $CD3^-$ $CD5^-$ $CD8^-$ $CD20^-$ $CD30^-$ $CD34^-$ $CD79a^-$ $CD117^-$ $CD138^-$ MPO^- $TIA1^-$ $PAX5^-$ $CyclinD^-$ (Figures 3 and 4). Ki67 expression was 80%. T-cell receptor (TCR) gamma chain gene resulted monoclonal.

Few days after admission, sudden worsening of signs and symptoms and the development of peripheral cytopenias (WBC 2.1×10^9/L, Hb 10.3 g/dL, and platelets 36×10^9/L) were registered. Blood smear revealed the presence of blasts 7%, neutrophils 42%, lymphocytes 44%, and monocytes 7%. BM smear showed 78% middle-size blasts with occasional pseudopodia, characterized by the following antigen expression as detected by FCM: $CD45^{dim}$ $CD4^+$ $CD10^+$ $CD38^+$ $CD45RA^+$ $CD56^+$ $CD123^+$ $HLADR^+$; $CD2^{-/+}$ $CD7^{-/+}$

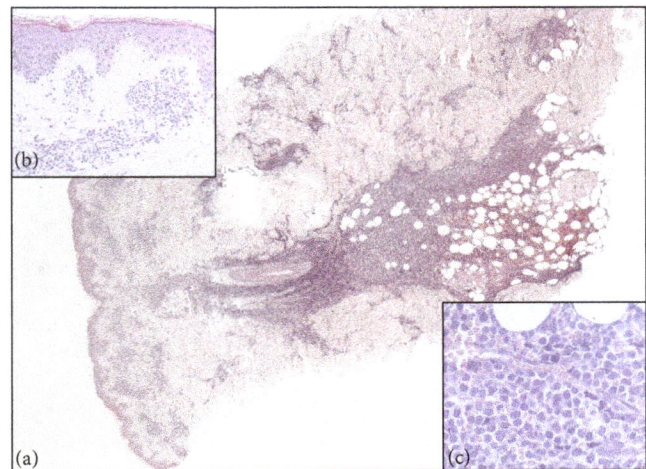

(b) (a) (c)

FIGURE 2: Biopsy of dorsal cutaneous nodule: EE20x dermal-hypodermal blast infiltration, disrupting collagen and muscle tissues, with nodular distribution, sparing epidermidis (a); EE 100x (b) and EE400x (c) dermal-hypodermal monomorphous infiltration by middle-sized blastic elements, with irregular nuclei, small nucleolus, and scant cytoplasm.

$TdT^{-/+}$; $CD1a^-$ $CD3^-$ $CD5^-$ $CD8^-$ $CD11b^-$ $CD11c^-$ $CD13^-$ $CD14^-$ $CD15^-$ $CD16^-$ $CD19^-$ $CD20^-$ $CD22^-$ $CD25^-$ $CD33^-$ $CD34^-$ $CD36^-$ $CD64^-$ $CD66c^-$ $CD117^-$ $CD138^-$ $CD235a^-$

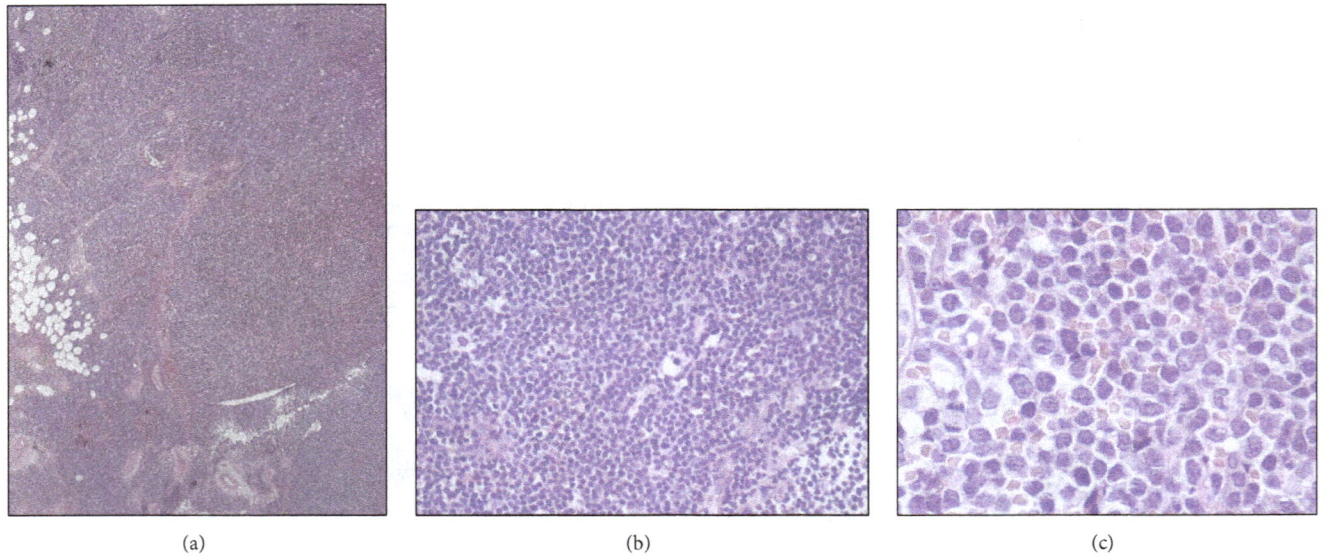

FIGURE 3: Laterocervical lymph node biopsy: EE20x (a), EE100x (b), and EE400x (c) diffuse and partially nodular infiltration by blast cells with complete effacement of lymph node architecture.

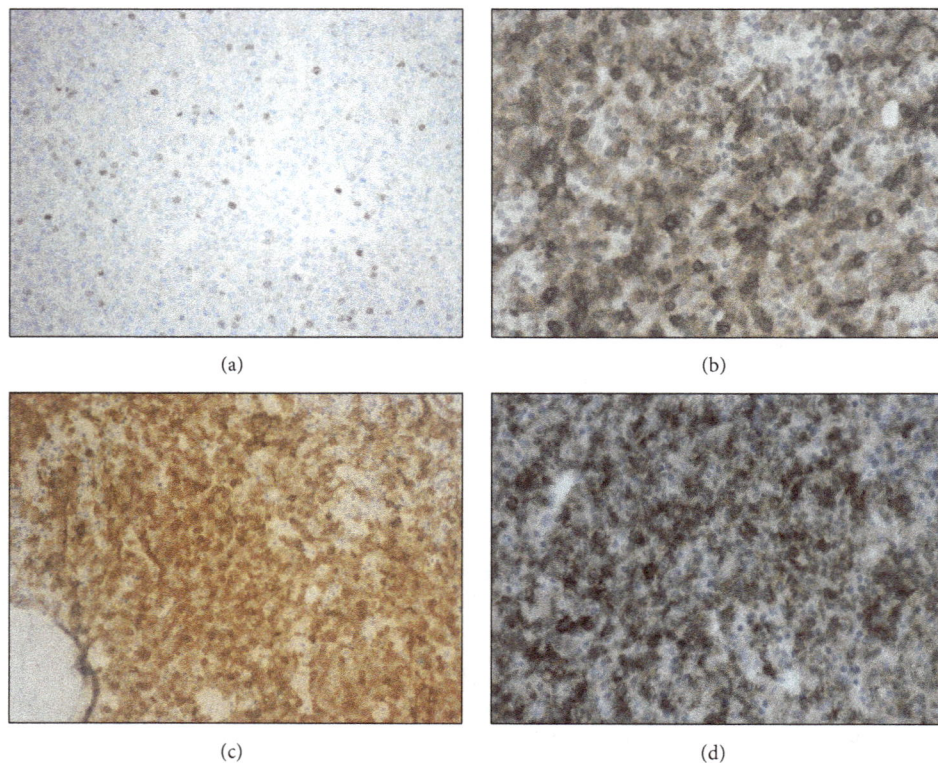

FIGURE 4: Lymph node immunohistochemistry analysis: immunostaining for TdT showing partial positivity (a); CD4 positive immunostaining (b); CD10 immunostaining on cell surface (c); CD56 positive immunostaining (d).

cytCD3⁻ cytCD22⁻ cytCD41⁻ cytCD61⁻ cytCD79a⁻ cytMPO⁻ (Figure 5). Conventional cytogenetics on BM showed normal karyotype, and no BCL2 rearrangement was detected by hybridization and molecular analyses; heavy chain immunoglobulin gene and TCR gamma chain gene showed polyclonal rearrangement. Cerebrospinal fluid FCM displayed a cluster of CD4⁺ CD10⁺ CD56⁺ CD123⁺ blast cells, coherent with occult central nervous system localization.

After an effective steroid debulking, the patient was started on acute lymphoblastic leukemia- (ALL-) like

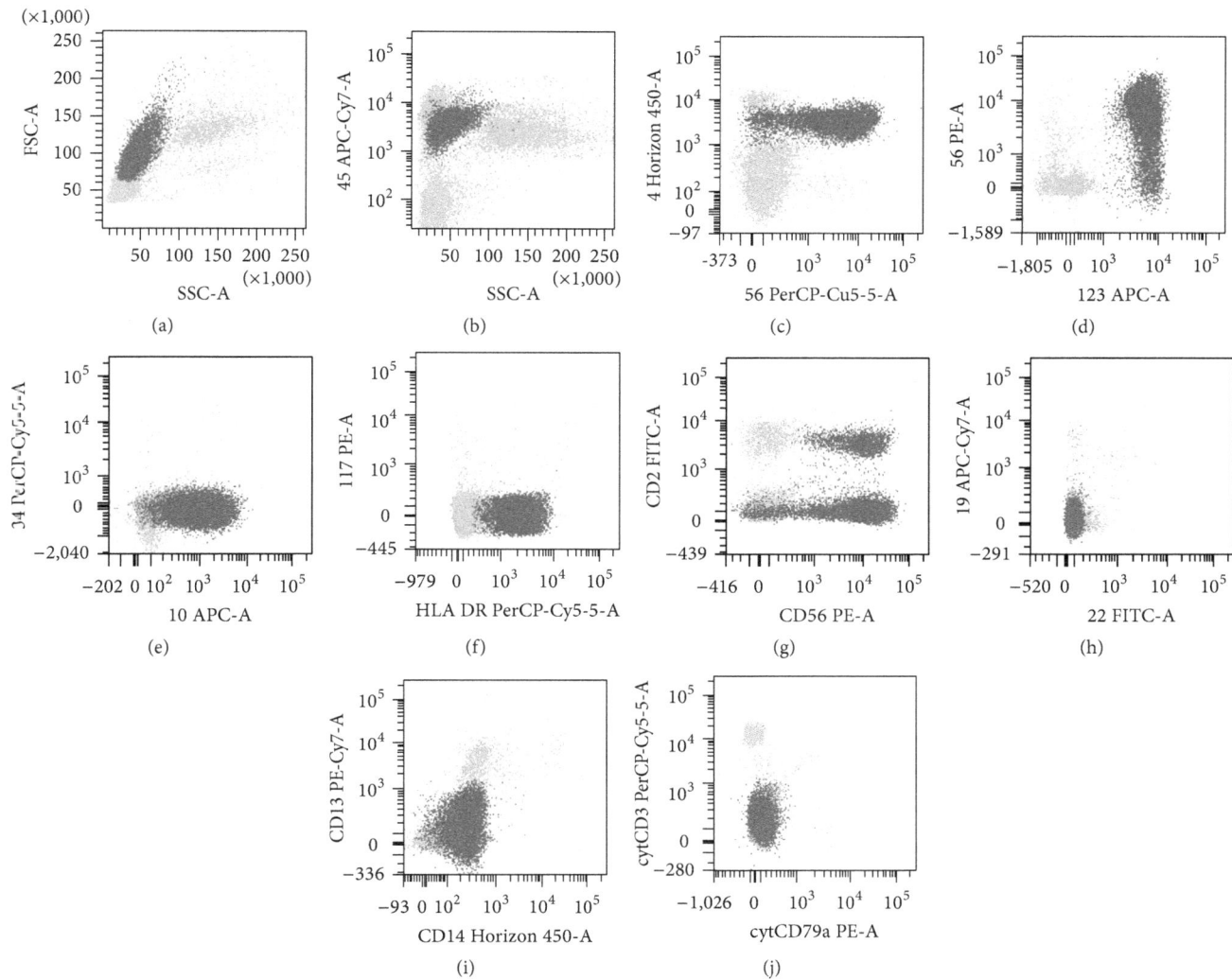

FIGURE 5: Immunophenotype of the bone marrow showing a large blastic plasmacytoid dendritic cell population (green): the blasts were large-sided cells with variable side scatter properties (a) and were weakly positive for CD45 (b); positive for CD4 (c), CD56 (c, d, e), CD123 (d), CD10 (e), and HLADR (f); partly positive for CD2 (g); and negative for CD34 (e), CD117 (f), CD19 (h), CD22 (h), CD13 (i), CD14 (i), cytCD3 (j), and cytCD79a (j).

treatment, with three courses of HyperCVAD chemotherapy (fractionated cyclophosphamide, vincristine, Adriamycin, and dexamethasone) and concomitant intrathecal prophylaxis (methotrexate, cytarabine, and methylprednisolone), and achieved complete remission (CR); afterwards he underwent consolidation with allogeneic hematopoietic stem cell transplantation (HSCT) from an unrelated matched donor. At present, thirteen months after diagnosis, he is still in CR.

3. Discussion

BPDCN is a very rare and aggressive hematologic malignancy, whose biologic insights and optimal treatment approach are still under investigation.

Different techniques have been employed to address the molecular basis for BPDCN. It has been recognized that the normal counterpart of BPDCN resides in plasmacytoid dendritic cells (pDCs), mononuclear cells produced in the BM and then circulating in blood, lymph nodes, and mucosal sites when an immune response is activated [4, 5]. Great emphasis has been placed on the origin of pDCs. A certain degree of developmental and functional heterogeneity exists within the pDCs population. Indeed, different studies proved evidence that pDCs originate from myeloid precursors, but the possibility of a partial lymphoid contribution to pDCs development has also been postulated [5–7]. Gene expression profiling and sequencing analysis showed that BPDCN shares deregulated genes with both AML and ALL, but it owns a unique molecular signature, distinct from myeloid or lymphoid neoplasms [8]. Conventional cytogenetic analysis shows frequent complex aberrations, often chromosomal losses such as 5q, 12p13, 13q21, 6q23-ter, 9, but no specific karyotypic abnormalities [9, 10]. Several studies identified inactivation of tumour suppressors (RB1, TP53, and CDKN2A), activation of oncogenes (NRAS, KRAS), and mutations in epigenetic regulators (TET2, TET1, DNMT3A, IDH1, and IHD2) that are also frequently mutated in AML and myelodysplastic syndromes; furthermore, mutations in the IKAROS family genes and ATM aberrations have been discovered that are commonly found in lymphoid neoplasms [11–15]. Collectively, these data support that the cell of origin of the tumour can be closer to a myeloid precursor, but a shared trait with lymphoid malignancies cannot be excluded.

Most patients exhibit an indolent onset, with peculiar skin tropism and lymph node involvement, followed by systemic dissemination and BM infiltration. A small percentage of BPDCN is conversely characterized by leukemic presentation at diagnosis [16–21]. Within the spectrum of the disease, different maturation stages of BPDCN have been postulated based on the expression of CD34 and CD117. The double negative subset with high frequency of extramedullary involvement, as in the case of our patient, has been defined as the "mature" one [22]. On the other hand, our patient showed partial TdT positivity. This finding conflicts with a previous BPDCN classification, identifying as more mature the TdT negative cases [23]. Indeed, TdT expression, which is registered in a third of BPDCN, can be regarded as a paramount marker of precursor differentiation [1]. Therefore, the CD34$^-$ CD117$^-$ TdT+ phenotype of our patient is not appropriately consistent with subgroup definition and suggests the need for further investigation on this matter.

At the screening, the immunophenotype of BPDCN largely overlaps that of other hematologic malignancies, such as AML, extranodal nasal type Natural Killer/T-cell lymphoma, and T-cell leukemia/lymphoma [9, 24]. In our case CD10 positivity was recorded. CD10 is commonly expressed on early, pro-/pre-B cells, but also on T/NK cell precursors, subsequently lost during lymphoid differentiation [25]. Even if commonly reported as a negative antigen, it has been observed in few reports in BPDCN and occasionally in acute myeloid leukemia [18, 26, 27]. Despite the absence of lineage antigen expression, CD10 positivity, together with TdT expression and lymphoid tissues involvement, might have been misleading for diagnosis in the absence of a comprehensive FCM and IHC characterization.

Several reports demonstrate that lymphoid-like chemotherapy is currently the best treatment option for BPDCN, achieving high response rates; the efficacy of ALL protocols might be sustained by deregulation of genes that herald sensitivity to methotrexate, prednisone, and vincristine. However, unlike the majority of lymphoid malignancies, conventional chemotherapy alone does not appear to be sufficient to ensure durable long-term remissions, with an early relapse rate of about 60% of patients achieving CR [17, 21, 28]. As such, our patient demonstrated an excellent response to HyperCVAD chemotherapy that was further consolidated with allogeneic HSCT. In fact, available information derived from retrospective case reports and single-institution experiences suggests that adults may benefit from allogeneic HSCT in first CR, achieving long-term survival with both myeloablative and reduced intensity conditioning regimens [17, 29–31]. Moreover, novel potential therapeutic targets have been identified, such as BCL-2, an antiapoptotic protein

commonly overexpressed in BPDCN, as in our case [8, 16, 32, 33]. The chance to find effective targeted therapies furtherly strengthens the need for complete characterization of this neoplasm.

Conflicts of Interest

The authors declare that there are no conflicts of interest regarding the publication of this paper.

References

[1] F. Facchetti, D. Jones, and T. Petrella, "Blastic plasmacytoid dendritic cell neoplasm," in *WHO Classification of Tumors of Haematopoietic and Lymphoid Tissues*, S. H. Swerdlow, E. Campo, N. L. Hazzis et al., Eds., pp. 145–147, IARC press, Lyon, France, 2008.

[2] D. A. Arber, A. Orazi, R. Hasserjian et al., "The 2016 revision to the World Health Organization classification of myeloid neoplasms and acute leukemia," *Blood*, vol. 127, no. 20, pp. 2391–2405, 2016.

[3] F. Facchetti, M. Cigognetti, S. Fisogni, G. Rossi, S. Lonardi, and W. Vermi, "Neoplasms derived from plasmacytoid dendritic cells," *Modern Pathology*, vol. 29, no. 2, pp. 98–111, 2016.

[4] A. G. Jegalian, F. Facchetti, and E. S. Jaffe, "Plasmacytoid dendritic cells physiologic roles and pathologic states," *Advances in Anatomic Pathology*, vol. 16, no. 6, pp. 392–404, 2009.

[5] M. Swiecki and M. Colonna, "The multifaceted biology of plasmacytoid dendritic cells," *Nature Reviews Immunology*, vol. 15, no. 8, pp. 471–485, 2015.

[6] G. Breton, J. Lee, K. Liu, and M. C. Nussenzweig, "Defining human dendritic cell progenitors by multiparametric flow cytometry," *Nature Protocols*, vol. 10, no. 9, pp. 1407–1422, 2015.

[7] N. Onai, K. Kurabayashi, M. Hosoi-Amaike et al., "A clonogenic progenitor with prominent plasmacytoid dendritic cell developmental potential," *Immunity*, vol. 38, no. 5, pp. 943–957, 2013.

[8] M. R. Sapienza, F. Fuligni, C. Agostinelli et al., "Molecular profiling of blastic plasmacytoid dendritic cell neoplasm reveals a unique pattern and suggests selective sensitivity to NF-κB pathway inhibition," *Leukemia*, vol. 28, no. 8, pp. 1606–1616, 2014.

[9] R. Dijkman, R. Van Doorn, K. Szuhai, R. Willemze, M. H. Vermeer, and C. P. Tensen, "Gene-expression profiling and array-based CGH classify CD4$^+$CD56$^+$ hematodermic neoplasm and cutaneous myelomonocytic leukemia as distinct disease entities," *Blood*, vol. 109, no. 4, pp. 1720–1727, 2007.

[10] M. Lucioni, F. Novara, G. Fiandrino et al., "Twenty-one cases of blastic plasmacytoid dendritic cell neoplasm: focus on biallelic locus 9p21.3 deletion," *Blood*, vol. 118, no. 17, pp. 4591–4594, 2011.

[11] F. Jardin, M. Callanan, D. Penther et al., "Recurrent genomic aberrations combined with deletions of various tumour suppressor genes may deregulate the G1/S transition in CD4+CD56+ haematodermic neoplasms and contribute to the aggressiveness of the disease," *Leukemia*, vol. 23, no. 4, pp. 698–707, 2009.

[12] O. Abdel-Wahab and R. L. Levine, "Mutations in epigenetic modifiers in the pathogenesis and therapy of acute myeloid leukemia," *Blood*, vol. 121, no. 18, pp. 3563–3572, 2013.

[13] K. Alayed, K. P. Patel, S. Konoplev et al., "TET2 mutations, myelodysplastic features, and a distinct immunoprofile characterize blastic plasmacytoid dendritic cell neoplasm in the bone

marrow," *American Journal of Hematology*, vol. 88, no. 12, pp. 1055–1061, 2013.

[14] J. Menezes, F. Acquadro, M. Wiseman et al., "Exome sequencing reveals novel and recurrent mutations with clinical impact in blastic plasmacytoid dendritic cell neoplasm," *Leukemia*, vol. 28, no. 4, pp. 823–829, 2014.

[15] A. Stenzinger, V. Endris, N. Pfarr et al., "Targeted ultra-deep sequencing reveals recurrent and mutually exclusive mutations of cancer genes in blastic plasmacytoid dendritic cell neoplasm," *Oncotarget*, vol. 5, no. 15, pp. 6404–6413, 2014.

[16] C. Cota, E. Vale, I. Viana et al., "Cutaneous manifestations of blastic plasmacytoid dendritic cell neoplasm-morphologic and phenotypic variability in a series of 33 patients," *The American Journal of Surgical Pathology*, vol. 34, no. 1, pp. 75–87, 2010.

[17] L. Pagano, C. G. Valentini, A. Pulsoni et al., "Blastic plasmacytoid dendritic cell neoplasm with leukemic presentation: an italian multicenter study," *Haematologica*, vol. 98, no. 2, pp. 239–246, 2013.

[18] K. Laribi, N. Denizon, H. Ghnaya et al., "Blastic plasmacytoid dendritic cell neoplasm: the first report of two cases treated by 5-Azacytidine," *European Journal of Haematology*, vol. 93, no. 1, pp. 81–85, 2014.

[19] J. Ferreira, M. G. Gasparinho, and R. Fonseca, "Cytomorphological features of blastic plasmacytoid dendritic cell neoplasm on FNA and cerebrospinal fluid cytology: a review of 6 cases," *Cancer Cytopathology*, vol. 124, no. 3, pp. 196–202, 2016.

[20] J.-H. Kim, H.-Y. Park, J.-H. Lee, D.-Y. Lee, J.-H. Lee, and J.-M. Yang, "Blastic plasmacytoid dendritic cell neoplasm: analysis of clinicopathological feature and treatment outcome of seven cases," *Annals of Dermatology*, vol. 27, no. 6, pp. 727–737, 2015.

[21] U. Deotare, K. W. L. Yee, L. W. Le et al., "Blastic plasmacytoid dendritic cell neoplasm with leukemic presentation: 10-Color flow cytometry diagnosis and HyperCVAD therapy," *American Journal of Hematology*, vol. 91, no. 3, pp. 283–286, 2016.

[22] L. Martín-Martín, A. López, B. Vidriales et al., "Classification and clinical behavior of blastic plasmacytoid dendritic cell neoplasms according to their maturation-associated immunophenotypic profile," *Oncotarget*, vol. 6, no. 22, pp. 19204–19216, 2015.

[23] D. L. Jaye, C. M. Geigerman, M. Herling, K. Eastburn, E. K. Waller, and D. Jones, "Expression of the plasmacytoid dendritic cell marker BDCA-2 supports a spectrum of maturation among CD4+ CD56+ hematodermic neoplasms," *Modern Pathology*, vol. 19, no. 12, pp. 1555–1562, 2006.

[24] C. Assaf, S. Gellrich, S. Whittaker et al., "CD56-positive haematological neoplasms of the skin: a multicentre study of the Cutaneous Lymphoma Project Group of the European Organisation for Research and Treatment of Cancer," *Journal of Clinical Pathology*, vol. 60, no. 9, pp. 981–989, 2007.

[25] A. Galy, M. Travis, D. Cen, and B. Chen, "Human T, B, natural killer, and dendritic cells arise from a common bone marrow progenitor cell subset," *Immunity*, vol. 3, no. 4, pp. 459–473, 1995.

[26] N. R. Bavikatty, C. W. Ross, W. G. Finn, B. Schnitzer, and T. P. Singleton, "Anti-CD10 immunoperoxidase staining of paraffin-embedded acute leukemias: comparison with flow cytometric immunophenotyping," *Human Pathology*, vol. 31, no. 9, pp. 1051–1054, 2000.

[27] F. Garnache-Ottou, J. Feuillard, C. Ferrand et al., "Extended diagnostic criteria for plasmacytoid dendritic cell leukaemia," *British Journal of Haematology*, vol. 145, no. 5, pp. 624–636, 2009.

[28] N. Pemmaraju, D. A. Thomas, H. Kantarjian et al., "Analysis of outcomes of patients (pts) with blastic plasmacytoid dendritic cell neoplasm (BPDCN)," *Journal of Clinical Oncology*, vol. 30, supplement, abstract 6578, 2012, Proceedings of the 2012 ASCO Annual Meeting.

[29] D. Roos-Weil, S. Dietrich, A. Boumendil et al., "Stem cell transplantation can provide durable disease control in blastic plasmacytoid dendritic cell neoplasm: A Retrospective Study from The European Group for Blood and Marrow Transplantation," *Blood*, vol. 121, no. 3, pp. 440–446, 2013.

[30] M. Leclerc, R. Peffault de Latour, M. Michallet et al., "Can reduced intensity conditioning regimen cure blastic plasmacytoid dendritic cell neoplasm?" *Blood*, vol. 129, pp. 1227–1230, 2017.

[31] T. Aoki, R. Suzuki, Y. Kuwatsuka et al., "Long-term survival following autologous and allogeneic stem cell transplantation for blastic plasmacytoid dendritic cell neoplasm," *Blood*, vol. 125, no. 23, pp. 3559–3562, 2015.

[32] M. Ceribelli, Z. E. Hou, P. N. Kelly et al., "A druggable TCF4- and BRD4-dependent transcriptional network sustains malignancy in blastic plasmacytoid dendritic cell neoplasm," *Cancer Cell*, vol. 30, no. 5, pp. 764–778, 2016.

[33] E. M. Carrington, J.-G. Zhang, R. M. Sutherland et al., "Prosurvival Bcl-2 family members reveal a distinct apoptotic identity between conventional and plasmacytoid dendritic cells," *Proceedings of the National Academy of Sciences of the United States of America*, vol. 112, no. 13, pp. 4044–4049, 2015.

13

EBV-Negative Monomorphic B-Cell Posttransplant Lymphoproliferative Disorder with Marked Morphologic Pleomorphism and Pathogenic Mutations in *ASXL1*, *BCOR*, *CDKN2A*, *NF1*, and *TP53*

Agata M. Bogusz

Department of Pathology and Laboratory Medicine, Hospital of the University of Pennsylvania, Philadelphia, PA 19104-4283, USA

Correspondence should be addressed to Agata M. Bogusz; agata.bogusz@uphs.upenn.edu

Academic Editor: Yusuke Shiozawa

Posttransplant lymphoproliferative disorders (PTLDs) are a diverse group of lymphoid or plasmacytic proliferations frequently driven by Epstein-Barr virus (EBV). EBV-negative PTLDs appear to represent a distinct entity. This report describes an unusual case of a 33-year-old woman that developed a monomorphic EBV-negative PTLD consistent with diffuse large B-cell lymphoma (DLBCL) 13 years after heart-lung transplant. Histological examination revealed marked pleomorphism of the malignant cells including nodular areas reminiscent of classical Hodgkin lymphoma (cHL) with abundant large, bizarre Hodgkin-like cells. By immunostaining, the malignant cells were immunoreactive for CD45, CD20, CD79a, PAX5, BCL6, MUM1, and p53 and negative for CD15, CD30, latent membrane protein 1 (LMP1), and EBV-encoded RNA (EBER). Flow cytometry demonstrated lambda light chain restricted CD5 and CD10 negative B-cells. Fluorescence *in situ* hybridization studies (FISH) were negative for *cMYC*, *BCL2*, and *BCL6* rearrangements but showed deletion of *TP53* and monosomy of chromosome 17. Next-generation sequencing studies (NGS) revealed numerous genetic alterations including 6 pathogenic mutations in *ASXL1*, *BCOR*, *CDKN2A*, *NF1*, and *TP53*(x2) genes and 30 variants of unknown significance (VOUS) in *ABL1*, *ASXL1*, *ATM*, *BCOR*, *BCORL1*, *BRNIP3*, *CDH2*, *CDKN2A*, *DNMT3A*, *ETV6*, *EZH2*, *FBXW7*, *KIT*, *NF1*, *RUNX1*, *SETPB1*, *SF1*, *SMC1A*, *STAG2*, *TET2*, *TP53*, and *U2AF2*.

1. Introduction

Posttransplant lymphoproliferative disorders (PTLDs) are lymphoid and plasmacytic proliferations that arise in the setting of immunosuppression in a recipient of a solid organ transplant (SOT) or hematopoietic stem cell transplant (HSCT) [1]. PTLDs affect 1–25% of posttransplant patients, with the highest incidents for intestinal and multiorgan transplant, followed by heart and lung transplants [2]. The revised 2016 World Health Organization (WHO) categorizes PTLDs into the following categories: plasmacytic hyperplasia PTLD, infectious mononucleosis PTLD, florid follicular hyperplasia PTLD, polymorphic PTLD, monomorphic PTLD (B- and T-/NK-cell types), and classical Hodgkin (cHL) lymphoma PTLD [3]. The vast majority of PTLDs are of B-cell origin and are usually associated with Epstein-Barr virus (EBV) infection; however a significant subset are EBV-negative [1,

4, 5]. Early onset PTLDs are typically Epstein-Barr virus- (EBV-) driven lymphoproliferations and may be polyclonal or oligoclonal, whereas late onset ones are typically monoclonal lymphoid malignancies that can lack EBV association. The pathogenesis of non-EBV-related PTLD may be similar to non-Hodgkin's lymphomas (NHL) [6]. EBV-negative PTLD has been proposed to be a distinct entity and typically presents as a late complication of transplantation with a median of 50–60 months [5, 7–10]. EBV-negative PTLDs typically display monomorphic morphology [1]. Here we present a rare case of EBV-negative PTLD occurring more than a decade after solid organ transplant (SOT) and presenting with a large variety of morphologies of the malignant cells and numerous genetic alterations comprising 6 pathogenic mutations (*ASXL1*, *BCOR*, *CDKN2A*, *NF1*, and *TP53*x2) and 30 variants of unknown significance (VOUSs).

2. Materials and Methods

2.1. Histology and Immunohistochemistry. Formalin-fixed paraffin-embedded (FFPE) tissue sections were stained with hematoxylin and eosin (H&E) according to manufacturer's instructions. Immunohistochemical staining was performed on 4 μm tissue sections using an Autostainer (Leica BOND platform, Buffalo Grove, IL) according to manufacturer's instructions. Briefly, sections were deparaffinized in xylene and graded alcohols. Detection of the antibodies was performed using a chromogenic substrate, diaminobenzene (Dako).

2.2. Molecular Analysis for Clonality. DNA was extracted from FFPE small bowel tumor tissue and analyzed for clonality as described previously [11]. Briefly, PCR amplification was performed with two sets of fluorescently labeled primers (InVivoScribe Technologies) that hybridize to a conserved V-framework, framework 2 (FR2), and framework 3 (FR3) regions and the conserved J-region of immunoglobulin heavy chain *(IGH)* gene. The PCR products were subsequently size-separated by capillary electrophoresis on a 3500xL Genetic Analyzer (Life Technologies). Data were analyzed (GeneMapper v5.0 software) and examined for peak patterns consistent with a clonal expansion.

2.3. Fluorescence In Situ Hybridization (FISH) Analysis. FISH was performed on 3 μm FFPE tissue sections using the MYC break-apart probe, BCL6 break-apart probe, BCL2 break-apart probe, and TP53/NF1 probes (all from Metasystems Group, Inc.) according to the manufacturers' instructions. Briefly, slides were deparaffinized using xylene incubation (×3), followed by ethanol wash steps (100%, 70%). The slides were treated with Dako pretreatment solution (Dako, Inc., K5799) prior to hybridization, followed by digestion with pepsin (37°C, 15 min). Slides were then dehydrated in ethanol (70, 85, and 100%) and dried and the FISH probes were added for incubation overnight. The next day, the slides were washed, counterstained with DAPI, manually visualized, and scored.

2.4. Gene Mutation Analysis. Mutational analysis of FFPE tissue samples was performed by the University of Pennsylvania at the Center for Personalized Diagnostics as described previously [11]. The genes sequenced were part of a custom, targeted next-generation sequencing amplicon panel testing for 68 hematologic malignancy-associated genes *(ABL1, ASXL1, ATM, BCOR, BCORL1, BIRC3, BRAF, CALR, CBL, CDKN2A, CEBPA, CSF1R, CSF3R, DDX3X, DNMT3A, ETV6, EZH2, FAM5C, FBXW7, FLT3, GATA2, GNAS, HNRNPK, IDH1, IDH2, IL7R, JAK2, KIT, KLHL6, KRAS, MAP2K1, MAPK1, MIR142, MPL, MYC, MYCN, MYD88, NF1, NOTCH1, NOTCH2, NPM1, NRAS, PDGFRA, PHF6, POT1, PRPF40B, PTEN, PTPN11, RAD21, RIT1, RUNX1, SETBP1, SF1, SF3A1, SF3B1, SMC1A, SRSF2, STAG2, TBL1XR1, TET2, TP53, TPMT, U2AF1, U2AF2, WT1, XPO1, ZMYM3, and ZRSR2)* (TruSeq Custom Amplicon, Illumina Inc.) based on previously described analyses [12, 13]. A custom bioinformatics pipeline was utilized to detect alterations

[14] and manual data review was performed with variants compared with our knowledgebase and online databases for further curation, using human reference sequence UCSC build hg 19 (NCBI build 37.1) for comparison. Single nucleotide polymorphisms (SNPs) with a minor allele frequency (MAF) > 0.1% were classified as benign and were not reported based on the Exome Variant Server (http://evs.gs .washington.edu/EVS), the ExAC browser (http://exac.broad-institute.org), and dbSNP. Reported variants used nomenclature that is based on the Human Genome Variation Society nomenclature guidelines (http://www.hgvs.org/mutnomen) and internally categorized into five categories (benign, likely benign, variant of uncertain significance, likely pathogenic, and pathogenic); the categories "likely benign," "variant of uncertain significance," and "likely pathogenic" were reported as variants of uncertain significance (VOUSs).

3. Case Presentation

A 33-year-old female presented with progressive cramps, emesis, and alternating constipation and diarrhea. The patient received a heart and unilateral lung transplant 13 years prior to presentation for treatment of end-stage congenital heart disease (single ventricle, dextrocardia, and severe pulmonary stenosis). Her posttransplant course was complicated by severe cytomegalovirus (CMV) pneumonia and allograft dysfunction, including an acute rejection of her heart within three months and an episode of lung rejection seven years after transplant. The patient was subsequently stable on immunosuppression (azathioprine, 50 mg oral, 3 times a day, and prednisone, 5 mg oral, once a day). The patient was referred for evaluation at our institution. A computed tomography (CT) scan of the abdomen showed thickening of the jejunum. Surgical resection revealed a 9 cm exophytic tumor in the small bowel.

4. Pathologic Findings

Histological examination by hematoxylin and eosin (H&E) staining (Figure 1) revealed a large morphologic heterogeneity in this specimen. Under low power there were present nodular cellular areas intercepted by thick bands of fibrosis (Figure 1(a)) reminiscent of nodular sclerosis type cHL, areas with more monomorphic large immunoblast-like cells and foci of necrosis (Figure 1(b)) and areas with monomorphic appearance with admixed abundant eosinophils (Figure 1(c)). Higher power examination of the nodular areas revealed numerous large, highly atypical cells (Figure 1(d)) with a variety of morphologies (Figures 1(j)–1(r)) including lacunar cells, multinucleated cells, markedly hyperchromatic cells, mummified cells, Reed-Sternberg-like cells, and popcorn cells. Higher power examination of the monomorphic appearing areas revealed a remarkable diversity of morphology, including areas with monotonous medium to large cells (Figure 1(e)), increased infiltrating eosinophils (Figure 1(f)), prominence of plasmacytoid cells (Figure 1(g)), clear large cells (Figure 1(h)), and spindle-shaped cells (Figure 1(i)).

Immunohistochemistry revealed that the malignant cells, including the very large atypical cells, were immunoreactive

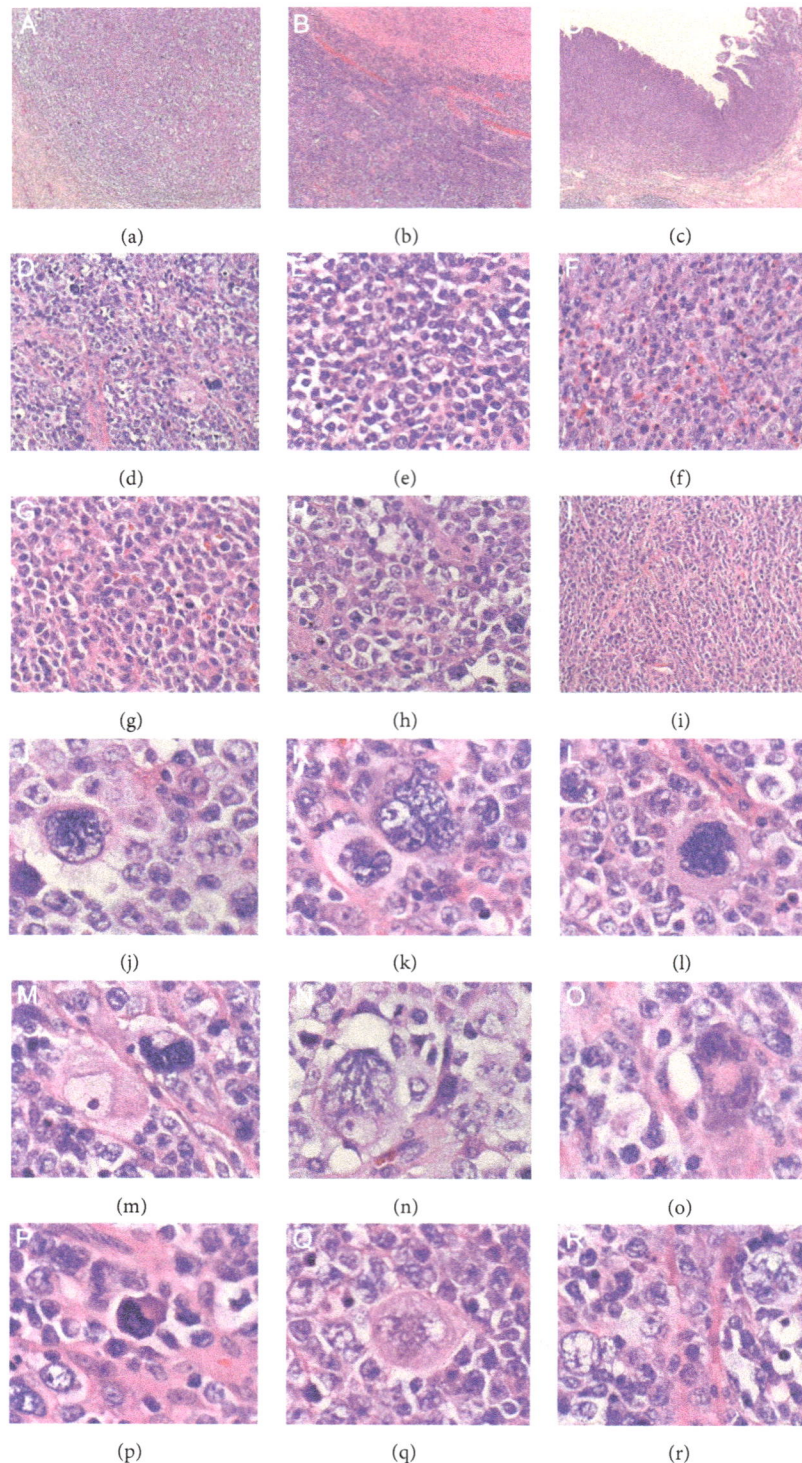

FIGURE 1: Histological findings of the small bowel tumor. Low power examination (50x) shows (a) nodular cellular areas with scattered large atypical cells surrounded by thick bands of fibrosis as well as (b) monomorphic areas with dense blue cells and more clear areas and foci of necrosis and (c) monomorphic areas with increased eosinophils in the lamina propria. Higher power examination (200x) of the different areas of the specimen reveal a variety of morphologies with (d) pleomorphic areas with many bizarre large atypical cells, (e) areas with monotonous medium- to large-sized cells, (f) areas with increased infiltrating eosinophils, (g) cells with plasmacytoid appearance, (h) areas with clear large cells, and (i) areas with spindle-shaped cells with somewhat plasmacytoid features. High power examination (400x) of areas seen in (i) and (d) shows the variety of morphologies of the large atypical cells (j-r) with (j) lacunar cells, (k) multinucleated cells, (l) markedly hyperchromatic cells with dense eosinophilic cytoplasm, (m,n) bizarre cells with eosinophilic nucleoli, (o) Reed-Sternberg-like cells with smudgy eosinophilic nucleoli and dense ampophilic cytoplasm, (p) mummified cells, (q) large atypical cells with multiple clear nuclei, and (r) popcorn-like cells with small nucleoli.

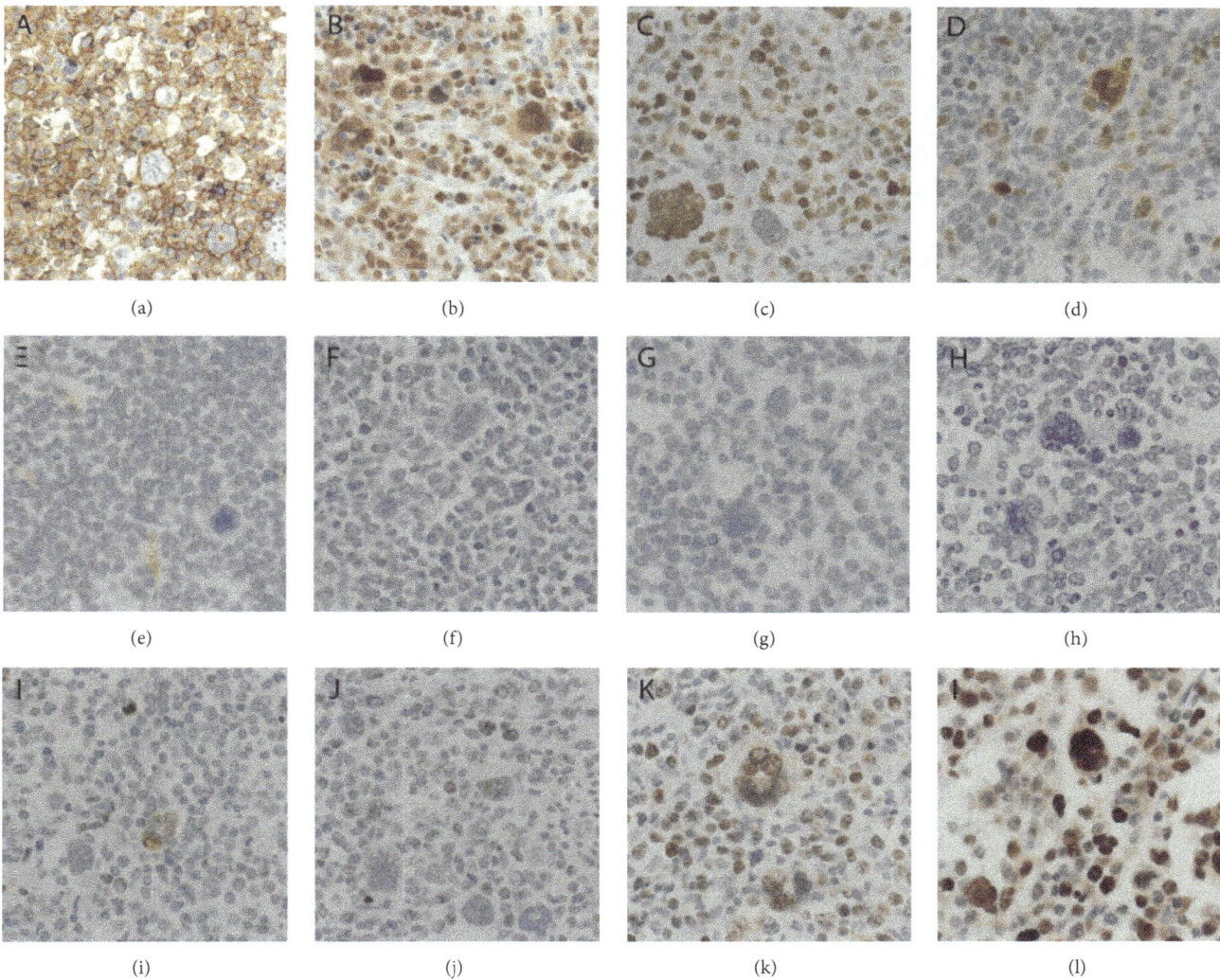

FIGURE 2: Immunophenotypic findings of the small bowel tumor. The tumor cells are immunoreactive for (a) CD20, (b) PAX5, (c) MUM1, and (d) BCL6 (major subset). The tumor cells are negative for (e) CD10, (f) CD30, (g) CD15, and (h) EBER. (i) Staining for BCL2 and (j) cMYC shows only occasional positive cells. (k) Ki67 staining reveals that high proliferation index is approximately 70%. (l) The staining for p53 was strongly positive.

for CD45, CD20 (Figure 2(a)), CD79a, PAX5 (Figure 2(b)), BCL6 (Figure 2(c)), and MUM1 (predominantly in the larger cells, Figure 2(d)) and were negative for CD3, CD5, CD10 (Figure 2(e)), CD30 (Figure 2(f)), CD15 (Figure 2(g)), LMP1, EBER (Figure 2(h)), and CMV. BCL2 was positive only in rare cells (Figure 2(i)) and cMYC (Figure 2(j)) was only focally positive but was overall negative (<40% positive cells, Figure 2(j)). The proliferation index as determined by Ki67 staining was high at 70% (Figure 2(k)). Staining for p53 was strongly and diffusely positive (Figure 2(l)).

Flow cytometry demonstrated a population of variably sized surface lambda light chain restricted CD5 and CD10 negative B-cells that represented the predominant population of monotonous large immunoblast-like B-cells. A diagnosis was rendered of monomorphic PTLD (B-cell type) with features of a diffuse large B-cell lymphoma, EBV-negative with pleomorphic, HL/RS-like cells.

Fluorescence *in situ* hybridization studies (FISH) were negative for *cMYC*, *BCL2*, and *BCL6* rearrangements but revealed deletion of *TP53* in 14/100 cells (Figure 3(a)) and monosomy of chromosome 17 in 20/100 cells (although these results fall within the range of the cutoff of 20–30% on paraffin tissue) (Figure 3(b)) as compared to normal cells (Figure 3(c)).

Molecular studies for *IGH* gene rearrangement performed on the DNA extracted from the small bowel tumor revealed a 163.85-base pair (bp) peak and a 243.99 bp peak in framework 2 (FR2) as well as a 78 bp peak in framework 3 (FR3) (Figure 4) confirming a clonal process.

Next-generation sequencing (NGS) studies revealed numerous genetic alterations including 6 pathogenic mutations in *ASXL1, BCOR, CDKN2A, NF1,* and *TP53*(x2) genes and 30 variants of unknown significance (VOUSs) in *ABL1, ASXL1, ATM, BCOR, BCORL1, BRNIP3, CDH2, CDKN2A,*

(a)   (b)   (c)

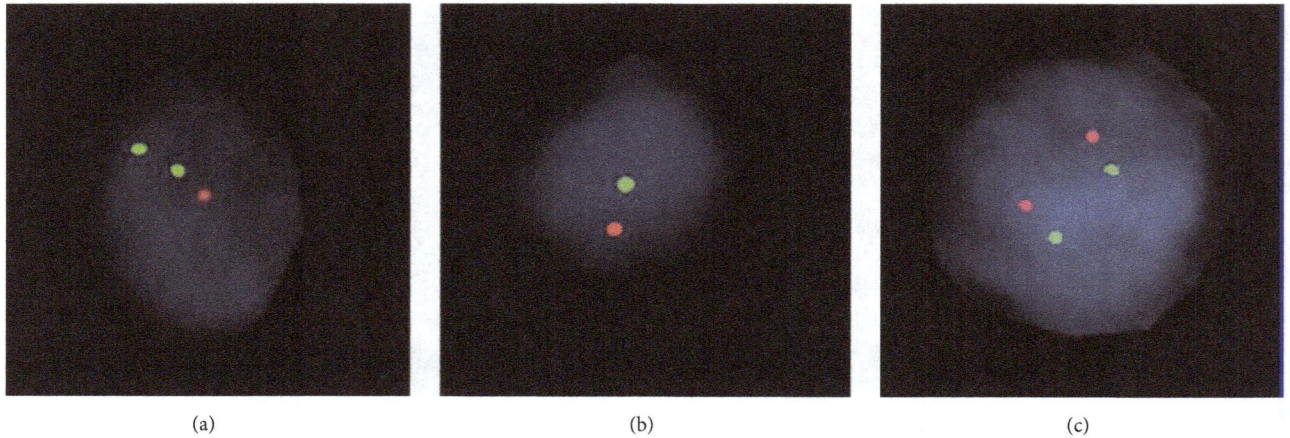

FIGURE 3: FISH analysis for *TP53* deletion. FISH studies performed on formalin-fixed paraffin-embedded sections of the small bowel tumor using TP53/NF1 probe revealed (a) deletion of *TP53* in 14/100 cells and (b) monosomy of chromosome 17 in 20/100 cells. (c) Normal cell.

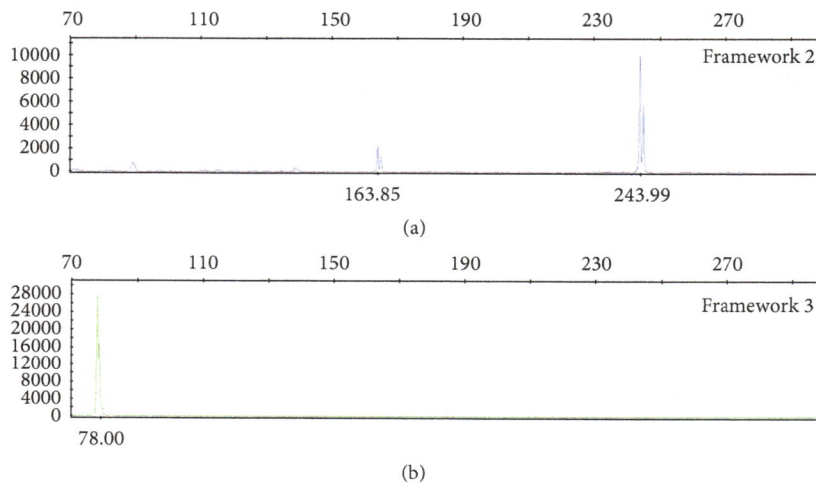

(a)

(b)

FIGURE 4: *IGH* PCR analysis of the small bowel tumor. *IGH* PCR analysis using primers for framework 2 (FR2) region identified two clonal peaks at approximately 163.85 bp and 243.99 bp (a). Primers targeting framework 3 (FR3) region identified a 78 bp peak (b).

DNMT3A, ETV6, EZH2, FBXW7, KIT, NF1, RUNX1, SETPB1, SF1, SMC1A, STAG2, TET2, TP53, and *U2AF2* (Table 1).

5. Clinical Follow-Up

Staging of the patient confirmed that her disease was confined to the small bowel. The patient's immunosuppression was decreased and following recovery from surgery she received rituximab and R-CY/VP16 (rituximab-cyclophosphamide/ etoposide) with no response and subsequently responded to R-CHOP (4 cycles). The patient appeared in complete remission by CT scan ten months after surgery but developed pleural effusion following the 4th cycle of R-CHOP and was also found to have retraction of the transplanted lung and anemia (Hg 9.5 g/dL). While receiving the next cycle of R-CHOP and transfusion 4 weeks later, the patient went into cardiac arrest and expired at the hospital. An autopsy was not requested. The cause of death was listed as shock, respiratory

failure, hypotension, and asystole related to acute transplant rejection.

6. Discussion

PTLDs are a clinically and morphologically heterogeneous group of diseases that occur after organ transplant. Histologically, PTLDs comprise a spectrum of lymphoid proliferations that range from polyclonal expansions to overt lymphomas [3]. This case is characterized by very late onset and EBV negativity. EBV-negative PTLDs typically present years after transplantation and display monomorphic morphology [15]. In rare cases a progression from an EBV-positive to EBV-negative neoplasm has been suspected [16]. The prognosis of EBV-negative PTLD appears to be similar to EBV-positive cases [17]. The reduction of immunosuppressive therapy is considered the first step in treating PTLD; however patients with poor prognostic factors, such as late onset

TABLE 1: Genetic alterations comprising pathogenic mutations and VOUSs (variants of unknown significance) detected in the patient's PTLD specimen.

Gene	Protein change	cDNA change	Categorization	Allele frequency
ABL1	p.G882Afs*12	c.2648delG	VOUS	36.3
ASXL1	**p.G645Vfs*58**	**c.1934delG**	**Pathogenic**	**18.63**
ASXL1	p.A1016V	c.C3047T	VOUS	32.09
ASXL1	p.C1240F	c.G3719T	VOUS	42.79
ATM	p.E871K	c.G2611A	VOUS	37.24
BCOR	**p.P1621Qfs*53**	**c.4862delC**	**Pathogenic**	**31.07**
BCOR	p.L1333M	c.C3997A	VOUS	57.17
BCOR	p.P407L	c.C1220T	VOUS	52.6
BCOR	p.P178L	c.C533T	VOUS	19.94
BCORL1	p.T39M	c.C116T	VOUS	23.36
BCORL1	p.R500H	c.G1499A	VOUS	63.21
BRINP3	p.A437T	c.G1309A	VOUS	36.36
CDH2	p.L870M	c.T2608A	VOUS	34.9
CDKN2A	**p.R58***	**c.C172T**	**Pathogenic**	**38.3**
DNMT3A	p.A70V	c.C209T	VOUS	35.05
ETV6	p.R259W	c.C775T	VOUS	38.87
EZH2	p.Y330C	c.A989G	VOUS	53.56
FBXW7	p.R441Q	c.G1322A	VOUS	45.79
KIT	p.P468L	c.C1403T	VOUS	36.26
KIT	p.N564D	c.A1690G	VOUS	35.63
NF1	p.P464L	c.C1391T	VOUS	38.12
NF1	**p.Q2147***	**c.6439_6441delinsTAG**	**Pathogenic**	**35.66**
RUNX1	p.R250C	c.C748T	VOUS	38.67
SETBP1	p.R54H	c.G161A	Likely benign	45.23
SETBP1	p.G1392S	c.G4174A	VOUS	39.64
SETBP1	p.R589*	c.C1765T	VOUS	38.75
SF1	p.N200Y	c.A598T	VOUS	39.27
SMC1A	p.R1066H	c.G3197A	VOUS	25.34
STAG2	p.S853R	c.T2559A	VOUS	14.12
TET2	p.A347V	c.C1040T	VOUS	38.03
TET2	p.V1900I	c.G5698A	VOUS	36.76
TP53	**p.G245S**	**c.G733A**	**Pathogenic**	**38.4**
TP53	p.E56K	c.G166A	VOUS	40.77
TP53	**p.R306***	**c.C916T**	**Pathogenic**	**40.02**
U2AF2	p.R44H	c.G131A	VOUS	20.15

ABL1: Abelson Tyrosine Kinase; ASXL1: Additional Sex Combs-Like 1; BCOR: BCL6 Corepressor; BCORL1: BCL6 Corepressor-Like 1; BRINP3: BMP/Retinoic Acid Inducible Neural Specific 3; CDH2: Cadherin 2; CDKN2A: cyclin-dependent kinase inhibitor 2A; DNMT3A: DNA methyltransferase 3 alpha; ETV6: ETS (erythroblast transformation-specific) variant 6; EZH2: enhancer of zeste 2 polycomb repressive complex 2 subunit; FBXW7: F-Box and WD Repeat Domain Containing 7; KIT: KIT Protooncogene Receptor Tyrosine Kinase; NF1: Neurofibromin 1; RUNX1: Runt Related Transcription Factor 1; SETBP1: SET Binding Protein 1; SF1: Splicing Factor 1: SMC1A: Structural Maintenance of Chromosomes 1A; STAG2: Stromal Antigen 2: TET2: Tet Methylcytosine Dioxygenase 2: TP53: Tumor Protein P53; U2AF2: U2 Small Nuclear RNA Auxiliary Factor 2.

disease and EBV negativity, typically require chemotherapy and immunotherapy [15]. It has been postulated that EBV-negative PTLD represents a distinct entity [5, 8]. In support of this hypothesis, gene expression profiling studies have revealed clear differences between EBV-positive and EBV-negative PTLDs [10, 18].

This case is unique in that several distinct morphologies coexist within this monomorphic PTLD including a nodular sclerosis Hodgkin lymphoma- (HL-) like component and large B-cell lymphoma component with diverse morphology (Figure 1). The large atypical HL/RS-like cells within the HL-like component were negative for CD15 and CD30 and immunoreactive for CD45 and CD20 (Figure 2) ruling out cHL PTLD and supporting the diagnosis of PTLD, DLBCL type. Since the patient's tumor was negative for CD10 and positive for BCL6 and MUM1, it can be classified as the more aggressive non-GCB (germinal center B-cell) type DLBCL [19].

NGS studies revealed a large number of genetic alterations in the patient's tumor (Table 1) with most of the altered genes involved in chromatin remodeling and DNA repair. This included 2 pathogenic mutations and 1 VOUS in *TP53*. A recent paper demonstrates that EBV-negative PTLDs frequently contain *TP53* mutations implicating p53 role in the disease process [9]. The pathogenesis of EBV-negative PTLD is not well understood but frequent *TP53* mutations might be one of the contributory factors [9]. Staining for p53 protein was uniformly strong in the tumor, correlating well with the presence of mutations. Expression of p53 in de novo DLBCL was shown to be correlated with inferior outcome [20, 21]. In addition to *TP53* mutations, FISH studies of the patient's tumor showed deletion of *TP53* in 14/100 cells and monosomy of chromosome 17 in 20/100 cells (Figure 3).

Other pathogenic mutations in this tumor affected *ASXL1*, *BCOR*, *CDKN2A*, and *NF1* genes (Table 1). *ASXL1* is one of the most mutated genes in myeloid neoplasms including chronic myelomonocytic leukemia (CMML), acute myeloid leukemia (AML), myelodysplastic syndrome (MDS), and myelodysplastic/myeloproliferative neoplasm (MDS/MPN) [22] and only rare mutations have been reported in lymphoid malignancies such as chronic lymphocytic leukemia (CLL) [23]. Mutations in *ASXL1* are generally associated with poor prognosis in myeloid malignancies [24]. *BCOR* encodes BCL6 interacting corepressor. BCL6 is a zinc-finger transcriptional repressor and key regulator of germinal center reaction that is frequently translocated and hypermutated in DLBCL [25]. However, NGS studies of 388 cases of B-cell lymphomas revealed only one Burkitt lymphoma case with a missense *BCOR* mutation (S1295T) [26]. Interestingly, frequent *BCOR* aberrations were reported in extranodal NK/T-cell lymphoma, nasal type [26]. In addition to one pathogenic mutation in *BCOR*, we have detected three VOUSs in *BCOR* and two VOUSs in *BCORL1* gene. *BCOR* and *BCORL1* are homologous X-linked genes that act as corepressors that were found to be recurrently mutated in AML. About 50% of *BCOR/BCORL1*-mutated cases also carry *DNTM3A* mutations and we have detected a VOUS in *DNTM3A* gene (Table 1). *CDKN2A* mutations have been previously reported in DLBCL [27]. Interestingly, proteins encoded by *TP53* and *CDKN2A* are components of the p53 pathway and it has been previously reported that alterations in these genes are independent in DLBCL, providing additional tumor growth advantage [28]. *NF1* mutations have been reported in rare cases of orbital DLBCL [29].

The VOUSs detected in this patient's sample (Table 1) included many genes that are typically mutated in myeloid malignancies (*ABL1*, *ASXL1*, *BCOR*, *BCORL1*, *BRNIP3*, *DNMT3A*, *ETV6*, *EZH2*, *KIT*, *RUNX1*, *SETPB1*, *SF1*, *SMC1A*, *STAG2*, *TET2*, and *U2AF2*) and not commonly seen in lymphoid malignancies. The significance of these findings is unclear but may suggest the pathogenesis of EBV-negative monomorphic PTLD is much more complex than that of EBV-driven PTLD. It has been proposed to stratify PTLD according to the histological subtype and EBV status in future clinical trials so as to better understand the mechanisms underlying the PTLD lymphomagenesis [30].

Conflicts of Interest

The author declares that there are no conflicts of interest regarding the publication of this paper.

Acknowledgments

The author is grateful to David Lieberman (University of Pennsylvania) for performing the NGS analysis, to April Schrank-Hacker (University of Pennsylvania) for performing FISH studies, and to Dr. Vivianna Van Deerlin (University of Pennsylvania) for performing *IGH* clonality analysis.

References

[1] S. H. Swerdlow, E. Campo, N. L. Harris et al., *WHO Classsification of Tumours of Haematopoietic and Lymphoid Tissues*, IARC Press, Lyon, France, 2008.

[2] J. Morscio, D. Dierickx, and T. Tousseyn, "Molecular pathogenesis of B-cell posttransplant lymphoproliferative disorder: what do we know so far?" *Clinical and Developmental Immunology*, vol. 2013, Article ID 150835, 2013.

[3] S. H. Swerdlow, E. Campo, S. A. Pileri et al., "The 2016 revision of the World Health Organization classification of lymphoid neoplasms," *Blood*, vol. 127, no. 20, pp. 2375–2390, 2016.

[4] D. A. Thorley-Lawson and A. Gross, "Persistence of the Epstein-Barr virus and the origins of associated lymphomas," *New England Journal of Medicine*, vol. 350, no. 13, pp. 1328–1337, 2004.

[5] B. P. Nelson, M. A. Nalesnik, D. W. Bahler, J. Locker, J. J. Fung, and S. H. Swerdlow, "Epstein-Barr virus-negative post-transplant lymphoproliferative disorders: a distinct entity?" *American Journal of Surgical Pathology*, vol. 24, no. 3, pp. 375–385, 2000.

[6] A. L. Taylor, R. Marcus, and J. A. Bradley, "Post-transplant lymphoproliferative disorders (PTLD) after solid organ transplantation," *Critical Reviews in Oncology/Hematology*, vol. 56, no. 1, pp. 155–167, 2005.

[7] G. Dotti, R. Fiocchi, T. Motta et al., "Epstein-Barr virus-negative lymphoproliferate disorders in long-term survivors after heart, kidney, and liver transplant," *Transplantation*, vol. 69, no. 5, pp. 827–833, 2000.

[8] V. Leblond, F. Davi, F. Charlotte et al., "Posttransplant lymphoproliferative disorders not associated with Epstein-Barr virus: a distinct entity?" *Journal of Clinical Oncology*, vol. 16, no. 6, pp. 2052–2059, 1998.

[9] E. L. Courville, S. Yohe, D. Chou et al., "EBV-negative monomorphic B-cell post-transplant lymphoproliferative disorders are pathologically distinct from EBV-positive cases and frequently contain TP53 mutations," *Modern Pathology*, vol. 29, pp. 1200–1211, 2016.

[10] J. Finalet Ferreiro, J. Morscio, D. Dierickx et al., "EBV-positive and EBV-negative posttransplant diffuse large B cell lymphomas have distinct genomic and transcriptomic features," *American Journal of Transplantation*, vol. 16, no. 2, pp. 414–425, 2016.

[11] J. Hatem, A. M. Schrank-Hacker, C. D. Watt et al., "Marginal zone lymphoma-derived interfollicular diffuse large B-cell lymphoma harboring 20q12 chromosomal deletion and missense mutation of BIRC3 gene: a case report," *Diagnostic Pathology*, vol. 11, no. 1, article 137, 2016.

[12] C. E. Sloan, M. R. Luskin, A. M. Boccuti et al., "A modified integrated genetic model for risk prediction in younger patients

with acute myeloid leukemia," *PLoS ONE*, vol. 11, no. 4, Article ID e0153016, 2016.

[13] J. P. Patel, M. Gönen, M. E. Figueroa et al., "Prognostic relevance of integrated genetic profiling in acute myeloid leukemia," *New England Journal of Medicine*, vol. 366, no. 12, pp. 1079–1089, 2012.

[14] R. Daber, S. Sukhadia, and J. J. D. Morrissette, "Understanding the limitations of next generation sequencing informatics, an approach to clinical pipeline validation using artificial data sets," *Cancer Genetics*, vol. 206, no. 12, pp. 441–448, 2013.

[15] Z. Al-Mansour, B. P. Nelson, and A. M. Evens, "Post-transplant lymphoproliferative disease (PTLD): risk factors, diagnosis, and current treatment strategies," *Current Hematologic Malignancy Reports*, vol. 8, no. 3, pp. 173–183, 2013.

[16] M. R. Ambrosio, B. J. Rocca, A. Ginori et al., "A look into the evolution of Epstein-Barr virus-induced lymphoproliferative disorders: a case study," *American Journal of Clinical Pathology*, vol. 144, no. 5, pp. 817–822, 2015.

[17] M. R. Luskin, D. S. Heil, K. S. Tan et al., "The Impact of EBV status on characteristics and outcomes of posttransplantation lymphoproliferative disorder," *American Journal of Transplantation*, vol. 15, no. 10, pp. 2665–2673, 2015.

[18] F. E. Craig, L. R. Johnson, S. A. K. Harvey et al., "Gene expression profiling of epstein-barr virus-positive and -negative monomorphic B-cell posttransplant lymphoproliferative disorders," *Diagnostic Molecular Pathology*, vol. 16, no. 3, pp. 158–168, 2007.

[19] C. P. Hans, D. D. Weisenburger, T. C. Greiner et al., "Confirmation of the molecular classification of diffuse large B-cell lymphoma by immunohistochemistry using a tissue microarray," *Blood*, vol. 103, no. 1, pp. 275–282, 2004.

[20] X. J. Wang, L. Jeffrey Medeiros, C. E. Bueso-Ramos et al., "P53 expression correlates with poorer survival and augments the negative prognostic effect of MYC rearrangement, expression or concurrent MYC/BCL2 expression in diffuse large B-cell lymphoma," *Modern Pathology*, vol. 30, no. 2, pp. 194–203, 2016.

[21] Y. Xie, M. Ajaz Bulbul, L. Ji et al., "P53 expression is a strong marker of inferior survival in de novo diffuse large B-cell lymphoma and may have enhanced negative effect with MYC coexpression: A Single Institutional Clinicopathologic Study," *American Journal of Clinical Pathology*, vol. 141, no. 4, pp. 593–604, 2014.

[22] J. Alvarez Argote and C. A. Dasanu, "*ASXL1* mutations in myeloid neoplasms: pathogenetic considerations, impact on clinical outcomes and survival," *Current Medical Research and Opinion*, 2017.

[23] V. Quesada, L. Conde, N. Villamor et al., "Exome sequencing identifies recurrent mutations of the splicing factor SF3B1 gene in chronic lymphocytic leukemia," *Nature Genetics*, vol. 44, no. 1, pp. 47–52, 2012.

[24] V. Gelsi-Boyer, M. Brecqueville, R. Devillier, A. Murati, M.-J. Mozziconacci, and D. Birnbaum, "Mutations in ASXL1 are associated with poor prognosis across the spectrum of malignant myeloid diseases," *Journal of Hematology and Oncology*, vol. 5, article 12, 2012.

[25] K. Basso and R. Dalla-Favera, "Roles of BCL6 in normal and transformed germinal center B cells," *Immunological Reviews*, vol. 247, no. 1, pp. 172–183, 2012.

[26] A. Dobashi, N. Tsuyama, R. Asaka et al., "Frequent BCOR aberrations in extranodal NK/T-Cell lymphoma, nasal type," *Genes Chromosomes and Cancer*, vol. 55, no. 5, pp. 460–471, 2016.

[27] S. Dubois, P.-J. Viailly, S. Mareschal et al., "Next-generation sequencing in diffuse large B-cell lymphoma highlights molecular divergence and therapeutic opportunities: A LYSA Study," *Clinical Cancer Research*, vol. 22, no. 12, pp. 2919–2928, 2016.

[28] M. B. Møller, Y. Ino, A.-M. Gerdes, K. Skjødt, D. N. Louis, and N. T. Pedersen, "Aberrations of the p53 pathway components p53, MDM2 and CDKN2A appear independent in diffuse large B cell lymphoma," *Leukemia*, vol. 13, no. 3, pp. 453–459, 1999.

[29] A. K. Cani, M. Soliman, D. H. Hovelson et al., "Comprehensive genomic profiling of orbital and ocular adnexal lymphomas identifies frequent alterations in MYD88 and chromatin modifiers: new routes to targeted therapies," *Modern Pathology*, vol. 29, no. 7, pp. 685–697, 2016.

[30] J. Morscio and T. Tousseyn, "Recent insights in the pathogenesis of post-transplantation lymphoproliferative disorders," *World Journal of Transplantation*, vol. 6, no. 3, pp. 505–516, 2016.

14

Rivaroxaban Treatment for Warfarin-Refractory Thrombosis in a Patient with Hereditary Protein S Deficiency

Koken Ameku ⓘD and Mariko Higa

Department of Respiratory Medicine, Okinawa Prefectural Nanbu Medical Center & Children's Medical Center, Okinawa, Japan

Correspondence should be addressed to Koken Ameku; ameqcoke@live.jp

Academic Editor: Simon Davidson

Protein S (PS) deficiency, an autosomal dominant hereditary thrombophilia, is more prevalent in East Asian populations than in Caucasians. PS-deficient patients have historically been administered a heparin product followed by warfarin for the treatment and secondary prevention of venous thromboembolism (VTE). However, warfarin can be ineffective or causes detrimental effects in rare cases. While direct oral anticoagulants (DOACs) are being increasingly used for the treatment and prevention of VTE, their efficacy in PS-deficient patients has not been established. We describe a 91-year-old woman who presented with chronic bilateral lower leg swelling with VTE that was refractory to warfarin anticoagulation therapy for over 1 year. Her recurrent VTE was diagnosed as quantitative hereditary PS deficiency. Rivaroxaban was administered as maintenance therapy instead of warfarin; after 8 weeks, the severities of the patient's leg swelling and venous ulcerations were significantly reduced with rivaroxaban compared to warfarin, thus demonstrating the efficacy of rivaroxaban for warfarin-refractory chronic VTE associated with hereditary PS deficiency. This case illustrates that rivaroxaban can potentially serve as therapeutic agents to treat warfarin-refractory VTE in PS-deficient patients. Further investigations are required to confirm the efficacy of rivaroxaban on the long term in this regard.

1. Introduction

Venous thromboembolism (VTE) develops from interactions between multiple genetic and environmental risk factors [1]. Hereditary thrombophilia that is common in East Asian populations involves dysfunction of the activated protein C anticoagulant system caused by protein S (PS) and protein C (PC) deficiencies [2]. The prevalence of PS deficiency is 0.03–0.13% among Caucasians, whereas it is 1-2% in the Japanese population [3]. PS and PC are vitamin K-dependent glycoproteins that act as natural anticoagulants. PS-deficient patients have historically been administered a heparin product, followed by warfarin, for the treatment and secondary prevention of VTE. Warfarin not only functions as an anticoagulant by inhibiting vitamin K-dependent procoagulant factors (II, VII, IX, and X) but also inhibits the body's own production of the vitamin K-dependent natural anticoagulants, PS and PC. Since, in

PS-deficient patients, warfarin can further decrease these natural anticoagulants, PS and PC, this may in turn offset the anticoagulant effects of warfarin to exacerbate clotting or even precipitate new clots in certain cases. Since direct oral anticoagulants (DOACs) act by directly inhibiting thrombin or factor Xa without affecting the synthesis of PS and PC, and because they have fewer drug-drug, drug-food, and drug-disease interactions compared to warfarin, they can be feasible alternatives for the treatment of warfarin-refractory patients [4]. In this case report, we describe the successful use of rivaroxaban in the treatment of a 91-year-old woman with chronic bilateral lower leg swelling and recurrent warfarin-refractory VTE with hereditary PS deficiency.

2. Case Presentation

A 91-year-old woman experienced chronic bilateral lower leg swelling with VTE. She was admitted to the hospital with

TABLE 1: Coagulation studies of the patient and her two daughters.

| | | | Patient (91 years) | | | | Daughter 1 (66 years) | Daughter 2 (54 years) |
| | | Normal range | Period after warfarin cessation | | | Period after rivaroxaban | | |
			2 weeks	4 weeks	5 weeks	2 weeks	3 weeks		
Total PS antigen	%	65–135	—	52	54	57	54	62	53
Free PS antigen	%	60–150	—	25	30	27	27	29	25
PS activity	%	56–126	<10	—	—	—	—	—	—
PC activity	%	64–146	40	120	—	—	—	156	131
PT-INR			1.11	0.96	1.00	0.89	0.85	1.02	1.10
II	%	75–135	—	76	—	—	—	—	—
VII	%	75–140	—	146	—	—	—	—	—
IX	%	70–130	—	105	—	—	—	—	—
X	%	70–130	—	85	—	—	—	—	—

PS: protein S; PC: protein C; PT-INR: prothrombin time-international normalized ratio.

swollen lower legs with exudate and venous ulcerations that were diagnosed as chronic lower extremity deep venous disease. Before admission to the current hospital, she had previously undergone repeated hospitalization elsewhere for recurrent leg swelling with VTE 4 times within 1 year, for a total of 6 months. During each hospitalization, she was extensively treated with anticoagulation therapy and had shown temporary improvement. While the bilateral/unilateral leg edema and thrombosis had improved on heparin treatment, it recurred repeatedly under warfarin anticoagulation maintenance therapy after discharge. Furthermore, the patient had a medical history of subtotal gastrectomy, cholecystectomy, and chronic kidney disease (CKD), but had no history of miscarriage, thrombosis during pregnancy, or venous thrombosis until the age of 90 years. The patient's lead surgeon from her previous hospital had reported that her prothrombin time-international normalized ratio (PT-INR) was unstable owing to CKD. Current laboratory tests revealed decreased renal function, proteinuria (creatinine (Cre): 1.69 mg/dL; urine protein: 1-2 g/g Cre), and elevated levels of D-dimer (12.4 μg/mL), which is a coagulation and fibrinolysis marker. PT-INR values measured on different days during treatment with 1 mg/day warfarin were 1.56, 2.39, and 4.31; they did not stabilize because of the patient's low food intake and antibiotic use for a urinary tract infection. Warfarin therapy was temporarily suspended; 2 weeks afterwards, plasma PC and PS activities were 40% (reference range, 64–146%) and <10% (reference range, 56–126%), respectively (Table 1). A PC or PS deficiency was suspected, and she was administered unfractionated heparin without warfarin. Decreased plasma levels of both total PS (52%; reference range, 65–135%) and free PS (25%; reference range, 60–150%) antigens were noted after 4 weeks of warfarin cessation and vitamin K supplementation, along with normal levels of other vitamin K-dependent coagulation proteins (factors II, VII, IX, X, and PC) (Table 1). Five weeks after warfarin cessation, decreased levels of total PS (54%) and free PS (30%) were maintained (Table 1). Anticardiolipin antibodies and lupus anticoagulant tests yielded negative results. The patient's 2 daughters,

aged 66 and 54 years, also showed decreased levels of total PS (62% and 53%, resp.) and free PS (29% and 25%, resp.) antigens; furthermore, the patient's older sister had a history of refractory VTE (Table 1). Repeated VTE observed in the patient was diagnosed as quantitative hereditary PS deficiency. Intravenous administration of unfractionated heparin was continued for 7 weeks with a small amount of a diuretic (spironolactone 25 mg/day) and 10 mg/day prednisolone for chronic glomerulonephritis with proteinuria, upon which the leg swelling completely resolved and renal function was slightly improved (Cre: 1.0 mg/dL). As her past clinical course suggested the ineffectiveness of warfarin, rivaroxaban was administered as maintenance therapy (15 mg/day, which is the approved dose in Japan for long-term treatment and prevention of VTE) for 8 weeks. The patient was followed during 8 weeks of treatment; her condition improved without any major side effects. While her leg swelling and venous ulcerations were not completely cured, the reduction in their severity compared to that under warfarin therapy was notable (Figure 1).

3. Discussion

This patient's course revealed 3 important clinical findings. First, the DOAC rivaroxaban was effective for the treatment of warfarin-refractory chronic VTE associated with hereditary PS deficiency. Warfarin is commonly used for the long-term treatment and prevention of VTE associated with PS deficiency. However, warfarin decreases the body's production of the natural anticoagulant PS owing to its vitamin K dependency. Additionally, thrombosis may worsen in some patients with PS deficiency, as also occurs in cases of warfarin-induced skin necrosis [5]. As rivaroxaban does not decrease the production of PS, it can be more effective in cases of PS deficiency [6]. In fact, rivaroxaban did not decrease the levels of total and free PS antigen at 2 and 3 weeks of administration in our patient. Rivaroxaban had comparable efficacy and better safety when compared to warfarin in the treatment and prevention of VTE in phase 3 trial [7]. However, as patients with inherited thrombophilia

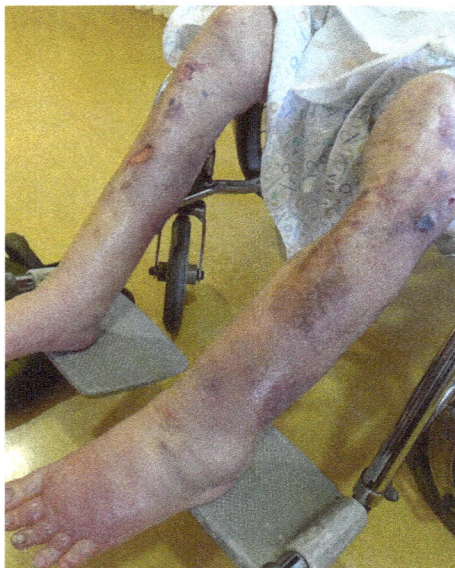

FIGURE 1: Chronic deep venous disease of the lower extremities. Leg swelling and venous ulcerations remained but were reduced in their severity after rivaroxaban therapy.

presenting with VTE were not distinguished in the trials, data regarding the efficacy of DOACs for PS deficiency are limited. Additionally, the efficacy of DOACs for inherited thrombophilia is not clear and their use remains controversial [8], although some reports of positive efficacy have been published [9]. Our patient provides an important example regarding the efficacy of rivaroxaban.

Second, VTE due to PS deficiency in our patient was refractory to warfarin therapy; however, as mentioned above, warfarin may not be the best anticoagulant for patients with PS deficiency. The patient showed decreased PC and PS activities even 2 weeks after warfarin cessation. Decreased levels of PC and PS activities as a result of vitamin K suppression by warfarin might have contributed to hypercoagulation in the patient. Several incidents of ineffective treatment or detrimental effects with warfarin have been reported in patients with PS deficiency [10–12]. Moreover, it is often difficult to achieve and maintain the target PT-INR using warfarin, especially in the elderly, because of its variable response, higher sensitivity, association with comorbidities, and interactions with concomitant medications. Therefore, when using warfarin in the elderly, lower doses and more intensive monitoring are required [13, 14]. As DOACs do not decrease PS and PC and have fewer drug-drug, drug-food, and drug-disease interactions compared to warfarin, they might have a therapeutic advantage over warfarin for the treatment of patients with PS or PC deficiency [4, 6, 8].

Third, our patient had familial quantitative heterozygous PS deficiency that produced a mild phenotype. This highlights the existence of a mild form of PS deficiency that may not manifest with a thrombotic event until a well-advanced age. Neither of the patient's two daughters who had decreased levels of total and free PS antigens, the older of whom was 66 years, had developed thrombotic events. It is previously reported that 50% of patients with heterozygous

PS deficiency develop VTE by the age of 55 years [3]. In contrast, only 38% of relatives of patients with PS deficiency who do not exhibit additional thrombotic deficiencies or defects (such as factor V Leiden, prothrombin G20210A, or hyperhomocysteinemia) develop VTE by the age of 65 years [1]. Even in hereditary thrombophilia, it is thought that VTE does not develop solely because of genetic risk factors. As such, our patient's VTE may have partially been attributed to additional acquired environmental risk factors or to old age, CKD, and proteinuria.

In the Japanese population, the most prevalent genetic risk factor for VTE is identified as qualitative PS deficiency caused by the K196E mutation within the PROS1 gene (PS Tokushima) [2, 15]; approximately 1 in 58 Japanese individuals is a heterozygous carrier (1.72%). Despite the high prevalence of PS Tokushima among Japanese individuals, our patient's family likely harbors other genetic mutations that manifest as quantitative PS deficiency [16]. We did not perform genetic analysis on our patient, as the technique was not readily available. An enzyme-linked immunosorbent assay (ELISA) system using the PS K196E mutation-specific antibody is now being developed for rapid identification of PS Tokushima carriers and will be available in the near future [17].

The efficacy and safety of DOACs in patients who are elderly, have renal impairment, or have low body weight are important to note, as all the DOACs are dependent on renal clearance to varying extents [18]. These patient subgroups have elevated risks of both embolic and bleeding events. Even in these subgroups, anticoagulant therapy has antithrombotic benefits that outweigh the risk of bleeding [13]. In so far as using rivaroxaban for VTE treatment, pooled and subgroup analyses of the phase III EINSTEIN DVT [7] and EINSTEIN PE [19] studies were conducted. In the pooled analysis, similar efficacy (hazard ratio (HR): 0.68), a significantly lower rate of major bleeding (HR: 0.27), and a significantly more favorable net clinical benefit (HR: 0.51) were reported in fragile patients who were over 75 years, or creatinine clearances (CrCl) < 50 mL/min or body weights < 50 kg [20]. In the prespecified subgroup analysis, although both VTE recurrence and major bleeding events increased according to the severity of renal impairment following enoxaparin/vitamin K antagonist (VKA) treatment, only increased VTE recurrence with similar efficacy to enoxaparin/VKA was observed using rivaroxaban treatment. However, major bleeding was not increased by renal impairment and occurred less frequently compared with enoxaparin/VKA (HR: 0.79 in patients with CrCl > 80 mL/min; HR: 0.44 in those with CrCl 50–79 mL/min; and HR: 0.25 in those with CrCl 30–49 mL/min) [21]. Of note, patients with severe renal impairment (CrCl < 30 mL/min) were excluded from these 2 studies. Furthermore, noninferior efficacy and a lower incidence of primary adverse events were shown when using both apixaban and edoxaban compared to warfarin in the elderly [13, 22]. Our patient was 91 years old with a CrCl of 30 mL/min and a low body weight of 35 kg. Among the 3 DOACs (rivaroxaban, apixaban, and edoxaban) currently available to treat VTE in Japan, we chose rivaroxaban because it better assured compliance among the elderly as it is administered once daily (compared to apixaban which is administered twice daily) and has a relatively smaller fraction of renal clearance as an unchanged drug (36%) than edoxaban (50%). Plasma rivaroxaban concentration-time profiles for patients of extremely old age (90 years), renal function (CrCl: ~30 mL/min), and body weight (~45 kg) were simulated using pharmacokinetic data collected from the 2 phase II studies of rivaroxaban for the treatment of acute deep vein thrombosis. The C_{max} values in all simulations were within the 5th to 95th percentile ranges of the population's mean values, showing that age and renal function had a moderate influence on rivaroxaban exposure and that the influence of body weight was small. Thus, fixed dosing of rivaroxaban was considered feasible for a broad segment of the patient population [23]. These predictable pharmacokinetic profiles could be associated with the efficacy and safety of rivaroxaban as shown in the phase III studies, and also in our patient. Owing to the different regimens used for VTE treatment in Japan (low-molecular-weight heparins are not used, and the PT-INR target when administering warfarin is 1.5–2.5), Japanese patients were not enrolled in the global EINSTEIN DVT and PE trials. Instead, the domestic J-EINSTEIN DVT and PE programs were performed and, as with the 2 global trials, showed similar efficacy and safety with rivaroxaban [24]. In Japan, the approved dose of rivaroxaban for VTE is 15 mg twice daily for 3 weeks followed by 15 mg once daily. Anticoagulation therapy requires long-term administration for patients with inherited thrombophilia. Rivaroxaban therapy was also demonstrated to be safe when administered for as long as 1 year in the EINSTEIN EXTENSION [7] and EINSTEIN CHOICE [25] studies. Overall, data for elderly patients, those with renal impairment, those with low body weight, and the effect of extended-term treatment remain scarce; hence, additional research is required in the real-world setting.

In conclusion, our patient demonstrated the efficacy of rivaroxaban for warfarin-refractory chronic VTE associated with hereditary PS deficiency. DOACs may therefore be therapeutic alternatives for warfarin-refractory VTE in PS-deficient patients. Further investigations are required to confirm the efficacy of rivaroxaban on the long term in this patient population.

Conflicts of Interest

The authors declare that they have no conflicts of interest regarding the publication of this article.

Acknowledgments

The authors would like to thank Editage (http://www.editage.com) for English language editing.

References

[1] J. L. Brouwer, N. J. Veeger, H. C. Kluin-Nelemans, and J. van der Meer, "The pathogenesis of venous thromboembolism: evidence for multiple interrelated causes," *Annals of Internal Medicine*, vol. 145, no. 11, pp. 807–815, 2006.

[2] N. Hamasaki, H. Kuma, and H. Tsuda, "Activated protein C anticoagulant system dysfunction and thrombophilia in Asia," *Annals of Laboratory Medicine*, vol. 33, no. 1, pp. 8–13, 2013.

[3] M. K. ten Kate and J. van der Meer, "Protein S deficiency: a clinical perspective," *Haemophilia*, vol. 14, no. 6, pp. 1222–1228, 2008.

[4] A. E. Burnett, C. E. Mahan, S. R. Vazquez, L. B. Oertel, D. A. Garcia, and J. Ansell, "Guidance for the practical management of the direct oral anticoagulants (DOACs) in VTE treatment," *Journal of Thrombosis and Thrombolysis*, vol. 41, no. 1, pp. 206–232, 2016.

[5] B. Lipe and D. L. Ornstein, "Deficiencies of natural anticoagulants, protein C, protein S, and antithrombin," *Circulation*, vol. 124, no. 14, pp. e365–e368, 2011.

[6] J. W. Skelley, C. W. White, and A. R. Thomason, "The use of direct oral anticoagulants in inherited thrombophilia," *Journal of Thrombosis and Thrombolysis*, vol. 43, no. 1, pp. 24–30, 2017.

[7] EINSTEIN Investigators, R. Bauersachs, S. D. Berkowitz, and B. Brenner, "Oral rivaroxaban for symptomatic venous thromboembolism," *New England Journal of Medicine*, vol. 363, no. 26, pp. 2499–2510, 2010.

[8] A. Undas and T. Góralczyk, "Direct oral anticoagulants in patients with thrombophilia: challenges in diagnostic evaluation and treatment," *Advances in Clinical and Experimental Medicine*, vol. 25, no. 6, pp. 1321–1330, 2016.

[9] I. Martinelli, P. Bucciarelli, A. Artoni et al., "Anticoagulant treatment with rivaroxaban in severe protein S deficiency," *Pediatrics*, vol. 132, no. 5, pp. e1435–e1439, 2013.

[10] M. Z. Haran, I. Lichman, A. Berebbi, E. Weinmann, and N. Rosenberg, "Unbalanced protein S deficiency due to warfarin treatment as a possible cause for thrombosis," *British Journal of Haematology*, vol. 139, no. 2, pp. 310-311, 2007.

[11] O. R. Odegaard, A. K. Lindahl, K. Try, G. Kvalheim, and J. Hjalmar Sørbø, "Recurrent venous thrombosis during warfarin treatment related to acquired protein S deficiency," *Thrombosis Research*, vol. 66, no. 6, pp. 729–734, 1992.

[12] S. Sallah, J. M. Abdallah, and G. A. Gagnon, "Recurrent warfarin-induced skin necrosis in kindreds with protein S deficiency," *Haemostasis*, vol. 28, no. 1, pp. 25–30, 1998.

[13] F. Andreotti, B. Rocca, S. Husted et al., "Antithrombotic therapy in the elderly: expert position paper of the European Society of Cardiology Working Group on Thrombosis," *European Heart Journal*, vol. 36, no. 46, pp. 3238–3249, 2015.

[14] N. Karamichalakis, S. Georgopoulos, K. Vlachos et al., "Efficacy and safety of novel anticoagulants in the elderly," *Journal of Geriatric Cardiology*, vol. 13, no. 8, pp. 718–723, 2016.

[15] T. Miyata, K. Maruyama, F. Banno, and R. Neki, "Thrombophilia in East Asian countries: are there any genetic differences in these countries?," *Thrombosis Journal*, vol. 14, p. 25, 2016.

[16] P. García de Frutos, P. Fuentes-Prior, B. Hurtado, and N. Sala, "Molecular basis of protein S deficiency," *Thrombosis and Haemostasis*, vol. 98, no. 3, pp. 543–556, 2007.

[17] K. Maruyama, M. Akiyama, K. Kokame, A. Sekiya, E. Morishita, and T. Miyata, "ELISA-based detection system for protein S K196E Mutation, a genetic risk factor for venous thromboembolism," *PLoS One*, vol. 10, no. 7, Article ID e0133196, 2015.

[18] A. G. G. Turpie, D. Purdham, and A. Ciaccia, "Nonvitamin K antagonist oral anticoagulant use in patients with renal impairment," *Therapeutic Advances in Cardiovascular Disease*, vol. 11, no. 9, pp. 243–256, 2017.

[19] EINSTEIN–PE Investigators, H. R. Büller, M. H. Prins, and A. W. Lensin, "Oral rivaroxaban for the treatment of symptomatic pulmonary embolism," *New England Journal of Medicine*, vol. 366, no. 14, pp. 1287–1297, 2012.

[20] M. H. Prins, A. W. Lensing, R. Bauersachs et al., "Oral rivaroxaban versus standard therapy for the treatment of symptomatic venous thromboembolism: a pooled analysis of the EINSTEIN-DVT and PE randomized studies," *Thrombosis Journal*, vol. 11, no. 1, p. 21, 2013.

[21] R. M. Bauersachs, A. W. Lensing, M. H. Prins et al., "Rivaroxaban versus enoxaparin/vitamin K antagonist therapy in patients with venous thromboembolism and renal impairment," *Thrombosis Journal*, vol. 12, p. 25, 2014.

[22] V. Geldhof, C. Vandenbriele, P. Verhamme, and T. Vanassche, "Venous thromboembolism in the elderly: efficacy and safety of non-VKA oral anticoagulants," *Thrombosis Journal*, vol. 12, p. 21, 2014.

[23] W. Mueck, J. Stampfuss, D. Kubitza, and M. Becka, "Clinical pharmacokinetic and pharmacodynamic profile of rivaroxaban," *Clinical Pharmacokinetics*, vol. 53, no. 1, pp. 1–16, 2014.

[24] N. Yamada, A. Hirayama, H. Maeda et al., "Oral rivaroxaban for Japanese patients with symptomatic venous thromboembolism - the J-EINSTEIN DVT and PE program," *Thrombosis Journal*, vol. 13, p. 2, 2015.

[25] J. I. Weitz, A. W. A. Lensing, M. H. Prins et al., "Rivaroxaban or aspirin for extended treatment of venous thromboembolism," *New England Journal of Medicine*, vol. 376, no. 13, pp. 1211–1222, 2017.

15

A Rare Case of ALK-Positive Large B-Cell Lymphoma with CD33 Expression

Jessica Corean⑩ **and K. David Li**⑩

Department of Pathology, ARUP Laboratories, University of Utah, Salt Lake City, UT, USA

Correspondence should be addressed to K. David Li; david.li@hsc.utah.edu

Academic Editor: Sergio Storti

Anaplastic lymphoma kinase-positive large B-cell lymphoma (ALK+ LBCL) is a very rare and aggressive subtype of diffuse large B-cell lymphoma characterized by *ALK* rearrangement. Immunophenotypically, the tumor cells are typically negative for common B-cell markers, T-cell markers, and CD30; however, they express markers of terminally differentiated B cells/plasma cells such as CD38, CD138, and MUM-1/IRF4. The diagnosis of ALK+ LBCL can be challenging, and often a large panel of immunostains is required to exclude other hematopoietic and nonhematopoietic neoplasms. To date, approximately 130–140 cases have been reported, but here we report the first known case of ALK+ LBCL with unusual CD33 expression.

1. Introduction

Anaplastic lymphoma kinase-positive large B-cell lymphoma (ALK+ LBCL) is a rare hematopoietic neoplasm accounting for less than 1% of diffuse large B-cell lymphomas (DLBCL) [1]. The entity was first described in 1997, and to date, approximately 130–140 cases have been reported in the literature [2]. ALK+ LBCL affects both adult and pediatric populations and can present with nodal and/or extranodal involvement. Unfortunately, the tumor is frequently discovered at a higher stage and has been shown to demonstrate aggressive clinical behavior, high relapse rate, and poor response to standard treatments, such as cyclophosphamide, doxorubicin, vincristine, and prednisone (CHOP) and CHOP-derived regimens [2, 3]. Histologically, the lymphoma cells resemble plasmablast and/or immunoblast and frequently show nodal sinusoidal growth patterns [4, 5].

The most important distinguishing feature of ALK+ LBCL from DLBCL and other lymphomas is the *ALK* rearrangement. ALK is a tyrosine kinase receptor of the insulin receptor superfamily and plays an important role in neural development [2, 6–8]. The majority of ALK+ LBCL harbor the *t*(2;17)(p23;q23) with fusion of the *clathrin* gene

(*CLTC*) on chromosome 17q23 with the *ALK* gene on chromosome 2p23. Rare cases are associated with *t*(2;5)(p23; q35), as described in ALK-positive anaplastic large cell lymphoma [1]. *ALK* gene activation through point mutations and gene amplifications has also been described [6]. The classic *t*(2;17)(p23;q23) results in a unique restricted granular cytoplasmic staining pattern present by immunohistochemistry (IHC).

In addition to the characteristic ALK protein expression by IHC, the lymphoma has an immunophenotypic profile that includes expressions of terminally differentiated B-cell/plasma cell markers such as MUM-1, CD38, and CD138, but typically lack expression of CD20 (although weak expression has been reported) and CD30 [1–5]. EMA is typically positive in the tumor cells, and aberrant expression of T-cell markers has also been described. In contrast, myeloid lineage-associated markers such as CD13 and CD33 that are commonly expressed by myeloid neoplasms are not routinely performed as a part of lymphoma workup and have not been reported in ALK+ LBCL. However, CD33 has been reported in a high percentage of ALK+ anaplastic large cell lymphoma, rare cases of CLL/SLL, and Burkitt lymphoma [9–11]. To the best of our knowledge and based on literature review, we describe the first case of ALK+ LBCL with CD33 expression.

(a)

(b)

(c)

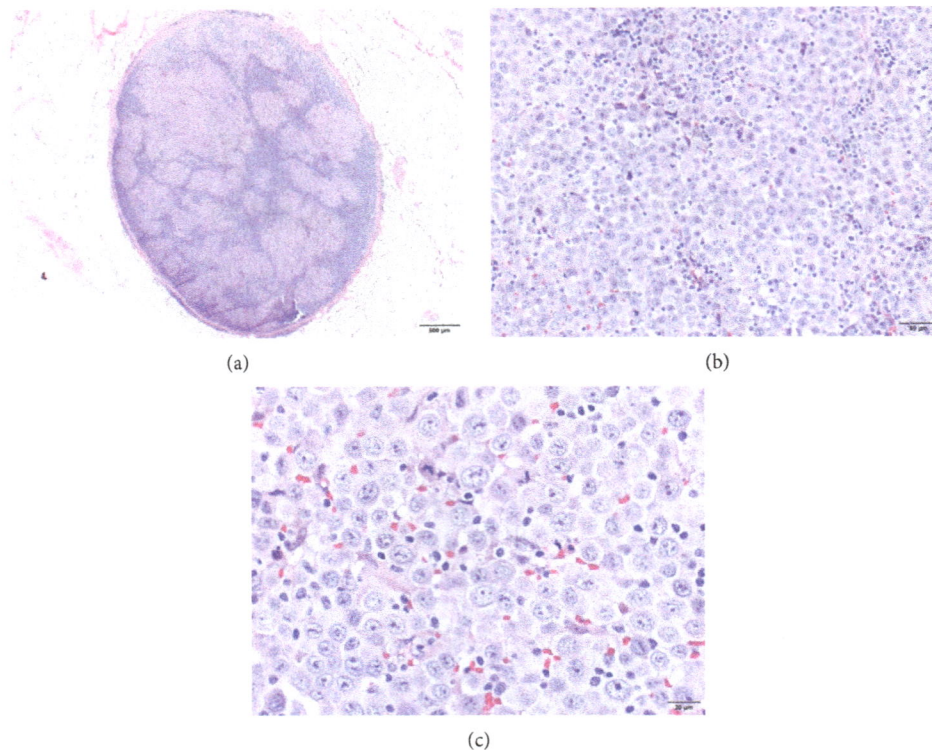

FIGURE 1: H&E sections of the biopsy specimen demonstrating an involved lymph node. Images (a), (b), and (c) are at 2x, 10x, and 40x magnifications, respectively. The tumor cells are large, monomorphic, immunoblast-like with oval nuclei, prominent nucleoli, and abundant cytoplasm. The background shows residual small lymphocytes.

2. Case Presentation

2.1. Clinical History. A 54-year-old Caucasian male presented with an enlarging right neck mass in November, 2015. Fine-needle aspiration (FNA) was performed on the mass at that time which showed malignant cells consistent with squamous cell carcinoma. The patient did not have follow-up or further treatment at that time due to socioeconomic issues. His past medical history is significant for alcoholism, tobacco abuse, noninsulin-dependent type 2 diabetes mellitus, and osteoarthritis. For the next sixteen months, he reported three flares of painful neck adenopathy. He sought treatment, and short courses of antibiotics and steroids were administered each time.

In March of 2017, his latest flare of right-sided neck adenopathy did not respond to antibiotics and steroid treatment course. He presented to the Emergency Department and found to have a grossly palpable mass in the right neck. He reported no symptoms of fevers, chills, night sweats, fatigue, or weight loss. Computed tomography (CT) revealed multiple low-density cystic structures in the right neck consistent with necrotic lymph nodes. The lymph nodes ranged in size from 1.4 cm to 2.9 cm in greatest dimension. No additional masses were detected in nasopharynx, oropharynx, or larynx. At this point, the patient was admitted for further workup and management. PET-CT showed right neck hypermetabolic uptake ranging from SUV of 4.3 to 4.5, and a CT of the chest showed no obvious disease and no evidence of lymphadenopathy. Following an

FNA suggestive of either an anaplastic carcinoma or a hematolymphoid neoplasm, an excisional biopsy of the neck mass was performed.

2.2. Pathology. Hematoxylin and eosin- (H&E-) stained right neck mass excisional biopsy material demonstrated lymph node and soft tissue with sinusoidal infiltration of large atypical monomorphic cells with round nuclei, occasional prominent central nucleoli, and abundant amphophilic cytoplasm. The lymph node was mostly effaced by tumor cells, but the uninvolved areas appeared unremarkable and showed residual small mature lymphocytes (Figure 1).

An extensive immunohistochemical panel was performed to aid the diagnosis with appropriate reactive controls (Figures 2 and 3). The tumor cells expressed CD45, weak CD38, CD138, and EMA. ALK-1 showed a restricted granular cytoplasmic staining pattern highly suggestive of CLTC-ALK fusion protein expression. MIB-1/Ki-67 was approximately 80%. Interestingly, the tumor cells also showed strong and diffuse CD33 expression. The tumor cells were negative for PAX-5, myeloperoxidase (MPO), TIA-1, EBV, HHV8, CD2, CD4, CD5, CD7, CD8, CD20, CD30, CD34, CD79a, and kappa/lambda light chains. Other nonhematopoietic immunostains including CK OSCAR, CK7, melan-A, CK5/6, p40, and p63 were negative. Flow cytometry, cytogenetics, and FISH studies were

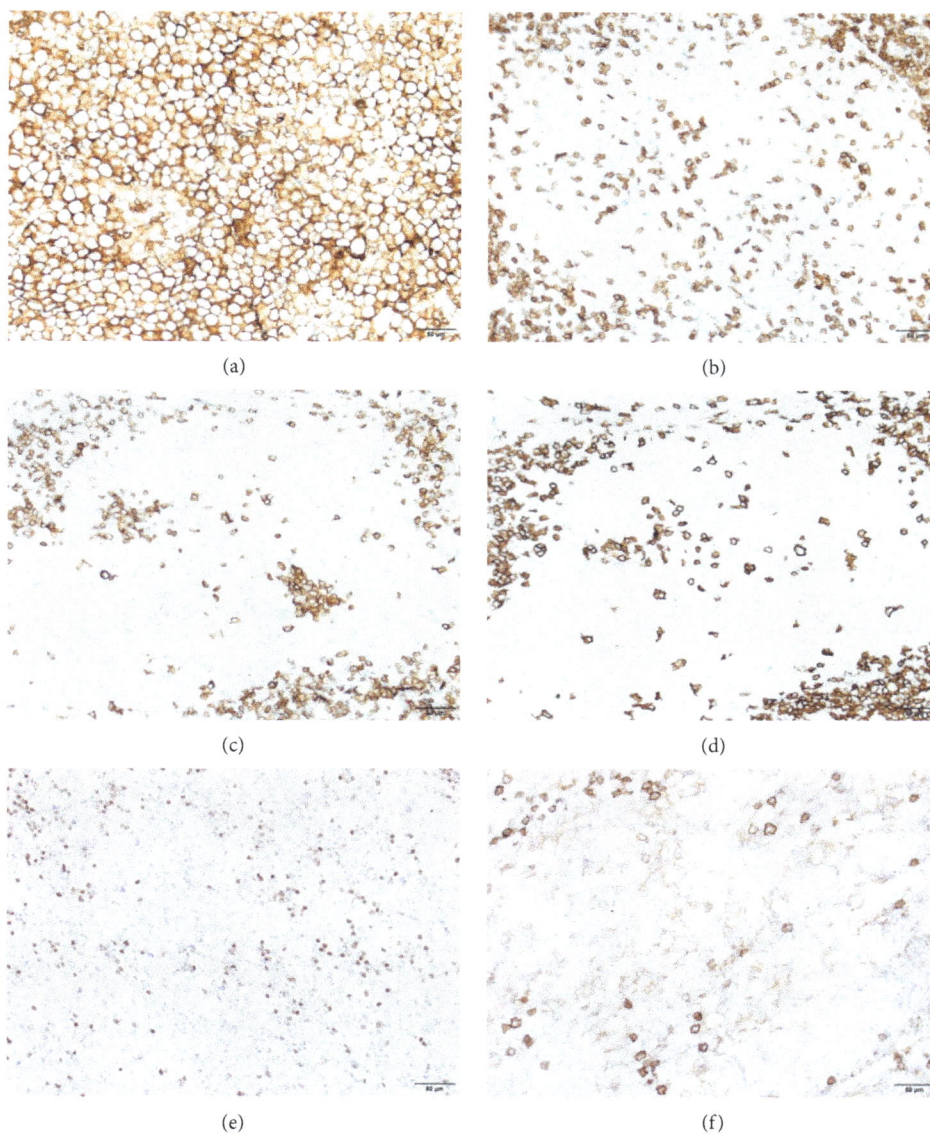

FIGURE 2: Immunohistochemical stains of the tumor cells. The tumor cells express CD45 (a) and weak CD38 (f) but are negative for CD3 (b), CD20 (c), CD79a (d), and PAX5 (e). All images are at 20x magnification.

not performed on the sample. Based on the morphology and immunohistochemistry, a diagnosis of ALK+ LBCL was rendered. The case was also reviewed at NIH, and the diagnosis was confirmed. Due to the aberrant CD33 expression, additional molecular studies were performed in an attempt to identify any myeloid malignancy-associated mutations. A myeloid malignancies mutation panel by next generation sequencing (NGS) was performed and did not reveal any significant mutations. Currently, the patient is under treatment protocol, which includes three cycles of CHOP chemotherapy to be followed by radiation therapy.

3. Discussion

ALK+ LBCL is a rare type of large cell lymphoma recognized by the World Health Organization's classification of tumors of hematopoietic and lymphoid tissue [1]. To date, less than 140 cases have been reported in the literature. ALK+ LBCL is generally considered an aggressive disease with approximately half of the reported patients dying within two years and a five-year overall survival rate of 34% [2]. Patients with stage I/II disease had significantly better overall survival at 76% and 66%, respectively [2]. Poor clinical response has been consistently reported to conventional therapies, such as CHOP and CHOP-derived treatments. New treatment options available such as ALK inhibitors have shown promising therapeutic activity in ALK+ ALCL, which could become a rationale therapy to be considered in ALK+ LBCL.

The diagnosis of ALK+ LBCL is challenging due to the rare incidence, morphology resembling DLBCL, plasma cell neoplasms, myeloid sarcomas, and epithelial neoplasms, and ALK immunostain is not routinely performed in practice.

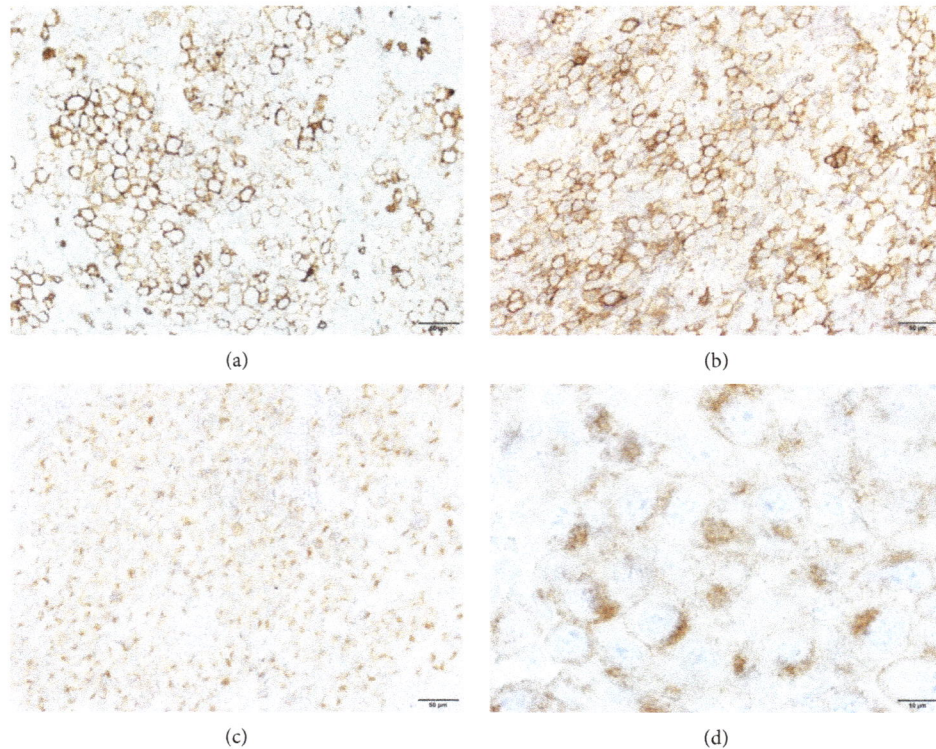

FIGURE 3: Additional immunohistochemical stains of tumor cells. The tumor cells also express CD138 (a), CD33 (b), and ALK (c). Higher magnification (100x, oil) of ALK in panel (d) demonstrates a cytoplasmic granular pattern highly suggestive of CLTC-ALK fusion protein expression. Images (a), (b), and (c) are all at 20x magnification.

Key differential diagnoses to be considered include ALK-positive anaplastic large cell lymphoma (ALK+ ALCL), plasmacytoma, immunoblastic/plasmablastic variants of DLBCL, plasmablastic lymphoma (PBL), and primary effusion lymphoma (PEL). ALK+ LBCL and ALK+ ALCL can show significant overlap in terms of clinical presentation, sinusoidal pattern of involvement, and markers such as CD45, EMA, and CD4. One important distinguishing feature is cytology where ALK+ LBCL shows plasmablastic morphology and ALK+ ALCL commonly shows anaplastic morphology with "hallmark cells." Additionally, CD30 is usually positive in ALK+ ALCL and negative in ALK+ LBCL. ALK+ LBCL can also share many similarities with other B-cell lymphomas such as PBL and PEL in terms of cytology and immunophenotypic features including expression of plasma cell markers and lack of conventional B-cell markers. PBL and PEL commonly occur in HIV-positive patients and are associated with EBV and HHV8, respectively. Other variants of DLBCL are less difficult to distinguish from ALK+ LBCL due to the presence of common B-cell markers such as CD20 and PAX5 and the lack of ALK expression. Plasmacytoma (primary bone and extraosseous forms), including morphologic variants such as anaplastic plasmacytoma, can often resemble ALK+ LBCL. There is significant immunophenotypic overlap including expressions of plasmacytic differentiation. However, features including the presence of bone involvement, myeloma component, and ALK immunohistochemistry can help distinguish plasmacytoma from ALK+ LBCL. In the workup

of a suspected case of ALK+ LBCL, the plasmblastic morphology/immunophenotype (CD38 and CD138), lack of CD30, expression of ALK, and the lack of confirmed viral associations (EBV, HHV8, and HIV) would aid the diagnosis of ALK+ LBCL.

Our case demonstrates the classic morphology and immunophenotypic profile of ALK+ LBCL but with aberrant CD33 expression. Since CD33 is not a commonly used marker in lymphoma workup, the rationale for its use in this case was based on the broad initial differential diagnosis, which included myeloid sarcoma and ALK+ ALCL. To the best of our knowledge, myeloid lineage expression has not been ever reported in the literature. In a fairly recent, large series study of ALK+ LBCL with literature review by Pan et al., myeloid lineage-associated markers were not reported [2]. Given the unusual CD33 expression, we performed NGS panel looking for common myeloid malignancy-associated mutations; however, the results were negative, and the significance of myeloid expression in our case is uncertain. MPO was also performed on the case and was negative. Although CD33 expression was an incidental finding in our case, it illustrates the fact that ALK+ LBCL is a rare entity, and when initial immunohistochemistry panels for T and B cells proved to be inconclusive, the differential diagnosis can expand to hematologic neoplasm of other lineages. Finally, the clinical significance of this finding is unknown.

In conclusion, we present a rare case of ALK+ LBCL with unusual CD33 expression that has not been reported in the literature. The pathologic significance of CD33 expression is unclear based on the lack of myeloid-associated mutations by molecular studies and whether there is a clinical significance is also uncertain. To the best of our knowledge, the patient is currently alive and undergoing therapy.

Conflicts of Interest

The authors have no conflicts of interest to disclose.

References

[1] S. Swerdlow, E. Campo, N. L. Harris et al., *WHO Classification of Tumours of Haematopoietic and Lymphoid Tissue*, WHO, Geneva, Switzerland, 4th edition, 2016.

[2] Z. Pan, S. Hu, M. Li et al., "ALK-positive large B-cell lymphoma: a clinicopathologic study of 26 cases with review of additional 108 cases in the literature," *American Journal of Surgical Pathology*, vol. 41, no. 1, pp. 25–38, 2017.

[3] C. Laurent, C. Do, R. D. Gascoyne et al., "Anaplastic lymphoma kinase-positive diffuse large B-cell lymphoma: a rare clinicopathologic entity with poor prognosis," *Journal of Clinical Oncology*, vol. 27, no. 25, pp. 4211–4216, 2009.

[4] H. Xiong, S. Y. Liu, Y. X. Yang et al., "An unusual case of anaplastic lymphoma kinase-positive large B-cell lymphoma in an elderly patient: a case report and discussion," *Experimental and Therapeutic Medicine*, vol. 11, no. 5, pp. 1799–1802, 2016.

[5] K. Li, A. M. Tipps, and H. Y. Wang, "Anaplastic lymphoma kinase-positive diffuse large B-cell lymphoma presenting as an isolated nasopharyngeal mass: a case report and review of literature," *International Journal of Clinical and Experimental Pathology*, vol. 4, no. 2, pp. 190–196, 2010.

[5] S. Li, "Anaplastic lymphoma kinase-positive large B-cell lymphoma: a distinct clinicopathological entity," *International Journal of Clinical and Experimental Pathology*, vol. 2, no. 6, pp. 508–518, 2009.

[7] Z. Zhao, V. Verma, and M. Zhang, "Anaplastic lymphoma kinase: role in cancer and therapy perspective," *Cancer Biology & Therapy*, vol. 16, no. 12, pp. 1691–1701, 2015.

[8] H. Sakr, M. Cruise, P. Chahal et al., "Anaplastic lymphoma kinase positive large B-cell lymphoma: literature review and report of an endoscopic fine needle aspiration case with tigroid backgrounds mimicking seminoma," *Diagnostic Cytopathology*, vol. 45, no. 2, pp. 148–155, 2017.

[9] I. M. Bovio and R. W. Allan, "The expression of myeloid antigens CD13 and/or CD33 is a marker of ALK+ anaplastic large cell lymphomas," *American Journal of Clinical Pathology*, vol. 130, no. 4, pp. 628–634, 2008.

[10] S. Casares, J. M. Rodríguez, A. Martin, and A. Parrado, "Rearrangements of c-myc and c-abl genes in tumour cells in Burkitt's lymphoma," *Journal of Clinical Pathology*, vol. 46, no. 8, pp. 778-779, 1993.

[11] B. Kampalath, M. P. Barcos, and C. Stewart, "Phenotypic heterogeneity of B cells in patients with chronic lymphocytic leukemia/small lymphocytic lymphoma," *American Journal of Clinical Pathology*, vol. 119, no. 6, pp. 824–832, 2003.

16

Splenic B-Cell Lymphomas with Diffuse Cyclin D1 Protein Expression and Increased Prolymphocytic Cells: A Previously Unrecognized Diagnostic Pitfall

Khaled Algashaamy,[1] Yaohong Tan,[1] Nicolas Mackrides,[1] Alvaro Alencar,[2] Jing-Hong Peng,[1] Joseph Rosenblatt,[2] Juan P Alderuccio,[2] Izidore S. Lossos,[2] Francisco Vega (ID),[1,2] and Jennifer Chapman (ID)[1]

[1]Department of Pathology, Division of Hematopathology, University of Miami, Sylvester Comprehensive Cancer Center and Jackson Memorial Hospital, Miami, Florida, USA
[2]Department of Medicine, Division of Hematology-Oncology, University of Miami, Sylvester Comprehensive Cancer Center and Jackson Memorial Hospital, Miami, Florida, USA

Correspondence should be addressed to Jennifer Chapman; jchapman@med.miami.edu

Academic Editor: Kostas Konstantopoulos

Prolymphocytic transformation is a concept usually applied in the context of chronic lymphocytic leukemia/small lymphocytic lymphoma to describe the presence of a high percentage of prolymphocytes in peripheral blood (usually more than 55%). Prolymphocytic transformation has also been reported in mantle cell lymphoma (MCL) but only rarely in splenic marginal zone lymphoma (SMZL). We present two splenic B-cell lymphomas presenting in the leukemic phase and with increased prolymphocytes, both classified as SMZL with prolymphocytic transformation. One case clinically simulated B-prolymphocytic leukemia (B-PLL). Both lymphomas were very unusual because the tumor cells diffusely and strongly expressed cyclin D1 despite lacking the t(11; 14)(q13; q32) as detected by several approaches including next-generation sequencing, fluorescence *in situ* hybridization using *CCND1* break apart probe and fusion probes for t(11; 14)(q13; q32), and conventional karyotyping. These cases therefore simulated prolymphocytic variants of MCL. The incidence of this phenomenon is unknown, and awareness of this potential alternate protein expression pattern is important in order to avoid diagnostic errors.

1. Introduction

Splenic marginal zone lymphoma (SMZL) is an indolent, extranodal mature B-cell lymphoma typically presenting with massive splenomegaly and bone marrow and peripheral blood involvement [1, 2]. Neoplastic lymphoid cells are predominantly small, mature B cells with abundant pale cytoplasm. In the spleen, the tumor cells involve the white pulp in a micronodular pattern, invade the red pulp, and exhibit marginal zone differentiation [1]. SMZL are most frequently CD20 positive B-cell lymphomas that lack expression of CD5, CD10, CD43, CD23, and cyclin D1. Scattered large lymphoid cells are typical,

particularly within the marginal zone of involved follicles. Additional features of SMZL include villous lymphocytes in the peripheral blood, intrasinusoidal infiltration of the bone marrow and, in a subset of cases, allelic loss of chromosome 7q22-36 [3].

SMZL is clinically characterized by a relatively indolent disease course unless adverse prognostic factors are present, such as poor performance status, high tumor burden, *TP53* abnormality, 7q deletion, and/or absence of *IgVH* somatic mutation [4]. A subset of SMZLs (~5-13%) progresses to diffuse large B-cell lymphoma (DLBCL), which can be identified at the time of initial diagnosis or years later [5–7]. The rate of histologic transformation of

SMZL to DLBCL is slightly higher than that of extranodal MZL and chronic lymphocytic leukemia/small lymphocytic lymphoma (CLL/SLL) (1–10%) but is less frequent than that of follicular lymphoma (25–60%). Although mantle cell lymphoma (MCL) does not undergo transformation to DLBCL per se, histologic progression to blastoid or pleomorphic variants can occur (11–39% of cases) [5, 6]. The mechanisms underlying histologic transformation of SMZL are poorly understood, but it is clear that this event is clinically relevant given its association with shorter time to progression and overall survival [7]. SMZLs have been described to have high genomic instability, in part related to loss of the *POT1* gene (at 7q31.32), which may contribute to progression to large cell lymphoma [3, 8].

As opposed to that in CLL/SLL and MCL, prolymphocytic transformation of SMZL is infrequently reported. One series of splenic lymphomas showing prolymphocytic transformation as defined by increased prolymphocytes in peripheral blood included 4 cases, 3 of which were classified as SMZL [9]. In this series, patients were elderly, presented with splenomegaly, marrow involvement, and leukocytosis with >55% prolymphocytes in peripheral blood. All cases in this previous report were negative for cyclin D1 protein. Deletion 7q was present in 3 of the cases, supporting the concept that this deletion is a risk factor for histologic transformation in the context of SMZL.

Similar to SMZL, B-cell prolymphocytic leukemia (B-PLL) is also a mature B-cell chronic leukemia presenting with peripheral blood, spleen, and bone marrow involvement. However, as opposed to SMZL, lymphoma cells with prolymphocytic morphologic features comprise >55% of tumor cells in peripheral blood, and patients typically present with B symptoms, massive splenomegaly, and markedly elevated white blood cell counts, usually $>100 \times 10^9$/L [1]. Similar to SMZL, B-PLL tumor cells are CD20 positive and usually negative for CD5, CD10, CD23, and cyclin D1. Rates of CD5 and CD23 expression in B-PLL are higher than those in SMZL with approximately 20–30% of B-PLL expressing CD5 and 10–20% expressing CD23 [1]. While initial reports of cytogenetic abnormalities in B-PLL identified a high rate of *IgH/CCND1* translocations, cases with this translocation are now classified as MCL. B-PLL lacking *IgH/CCND1* translocations frequently have complex karyotypes, but specific cytogenetic abnormalities are not known. Deletions at 17p13 and 13q14 are relatively frequent as are *TP53* mutations [1].

In this report, we present two unusual cases of non-MCL splenic B-cell leukemia/lymphoma that underwent prolymphocytic transformation or presented with increased prolymphocytes and showed diffuse cyclin D1 protein expression. These cases therefore simulated the prolymphocytic variant of MCL and represented an important diagnostic pitfall. To our knowledge, diffuse cyclin D1 protein expression has not been previously reported in SMZL or in its prolymphocytic transformation.

2. Case Presentations

2.1. Case 1

2.1.1. Clinical History. This patient was a 71-year-old male who presented with abdominal discomfort and was found to have significant splenomegaly upon physical exam, confirmed by imaging. He was diagnosed clinically with SMZL and underwent splenectomy to control his disease. We have not been able to determine whether he had peripheral blood lymphocytosis at that time of initial presentation.

Ten years after the initial diagnosis of lymphoma, he presented to our institution with weight loss and extensive anterior mediastinal, hilar, and retroperitoneal lymphadenopathy with an anterior mediastinal mass measuring 9.8×5.6 cm. Serum lactate dehydrogenase was elevated (281 U/L, reference range: 135–225 U/L). He was started on weekly rituximab with no response. In view of progressive symptoms, he was switched to R-CHOP (rituximab, cyclophosphamide, doxorubicin, vincristine, and prednisone) therapy at an outside institution. He presented to our institution after his first cycle of R-CHOP for additional recommendations. He felt dramatically better at that time. The clinical impression was that he had a large-cell transformation of his previously diagnosed low-grade SMZL.

2.1.2. Histopathologic, Immunophenotypic, and Molecular Findings. Laboratory analysis showed a white blood cell count of 9.4×10^3 cells/μL, hemoglobin level of 12.2 g/dL, platelet count of 242×10^3/μL, and absolute lymphocyte count of 1.33×103/μL. Peripheral smear was morphologically unremarkable. Peripheral blood flow cytometry showed a minor monotypic B-cell population, CD5, CD10, and CD23 negative, comprising 0.7% of analyzed events, consistent with minimal peripheral blood involvement by his previously diagnosed lymphoma. He was referred for lymph node biopsy to clarify the diagnosis.

Excisional biopsy of the axillary lymph node showed extensive involvement by lymphoma composed of both small, cytologically atypical lymphoid cells with abundant cytoplasm admixed with more predominant intermediate to large-sized lymphoma cells with variably abundant cytoplasm, large nuclei, and prominent, centrally located nucleoli, consistent with prolymphocytes (Figures 1(a) and 1(b)). The aggregates of prolymphocytes did not resemble proliferation centers seen in CLL/SLL as they were more discrete, monotonous, and expansile in nature. Transformed cells, defined as having intermediate to large-sized nuclei and central nucleoli, comprised more than 50% of all lymphoma cells. Sheets of large cells were not present; thus, designation as a large-cell transformation was not warranted [1, 10].

By immunohistochemistry, lymphoma cells were positive for CD20, CD5 (dim, subset), BCL2, and cyclin D1 (diffuse, positive in small lymphoma cells and those with prolymphocytic features), and negative for CD3, CD10,

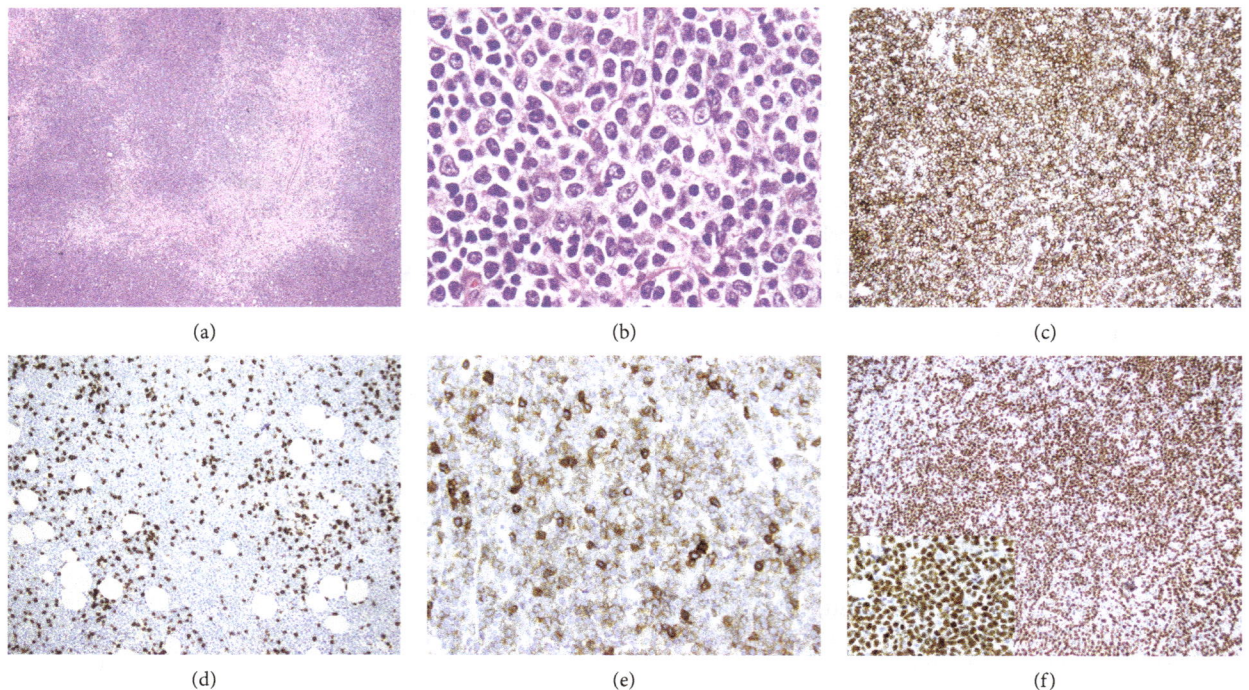

(a)   (b)   (c)

(d)   (e)   (f)

Figure 1: Case 1: lymph node biopsy showing relapsed splenic marginal zone lymphoma with prolymphocytic transformation and acquired CD5 (dim) and cyclin D1 (diffuse, strong) expression. Lymphoma cells consist of both small lymphoid cells with condensed nuclear chromatin, nuclear membrane irregularities, and monocytoid features and transformed cells with prolymphocytic features including intermediate to large size, more abundant cytoplasm, and prominent nucleoli (a, b). Lymphoma cells expressed CD20 (c), were negative for CD3 (d), a subset expressed dim CD5 (e), and cyclin D1 expression was diffuse and strong (f). (a and b) Hematoxylin and eosin staining, (a) 100 times magnification, (b) 500 times magnification, (c, d, and f) 200 times magnification, (e) 400 times magnification, and inset in (f) 1000 times magnification.

LEF1, and SOX11 (Figures 1(c)–1(f)). EBER staining by *in situ* hybridization was negative. The KI67 proliferation index was estimated at 40%, and it highlighted the large transformed cells in particular. Based on these findings, the possibility of mantle cell lymphoma (MCL) was considered.

The previous material (splenectomy and bone marrow biopsy from 10 years before) was then reviewed at our institution, and the original interpretation of SMZL was indeed confirmed. In the splenic resection, the lymphoma cells were present in a micronodular pattern within white pulp, invaded red pulp, and were composed of small-sized lymphoma cells with monocytoid morphologic features, negative for CD5 and cyclin D1 (Figure 2). Staging bone marrow biopsy performed at the time of initial splenectomy showed extensive involvement by low-grade lymphoma with an interstitial nodular and focally intrasinuoidal pattern (Figure 2). Lymphoid cells in the aspirate smear were small and did not have features of large-cell or prolymphocytic transformation. Karyotype and FISH studies performed in the bone marrow were negative for t (11; 14)(*CCND1-IgH*).

Given the confirmation of the initially diagnosed SMZL, we performed FISH for t(11; 14)(*CCND1-IgH*) using *IgH* and *CCND1* dual-labeled probes in the lymph node sample both at our institution as well as at an external reference lab, and both were negative for *CCND1-IgH* rearrangement

(Figure 3(a)). An additional FISH test using a *CCND1* break apart probe was also performed and failed to detect rearrangements involving *CCND1*. Additional copies of *CCND1* were not present.

To assess the clonal relationship between the splenic and nodal neoplasms, PCR analysis for *IgH* rearrangement was performed in both samples. The same monoclonal *IgH* peaks (framework region (FR) 1: splenectomy: 342.24, lymph node: 342.38; FR2: splenectomy: 277.71, 285.58; lymph node: 277.69 and 285.36; FR3: splenectomy: 146.14, lymph node: 146.3, Figures 3(b) and 3(c)) were identified in the original and current samples, supporting that the two lymphomas were clonally related. Next-generation sequencing (NGS) using the FoundationOne Heme comprehensive genomic profiling assay (Foundation Medicine, https://www.foundationmedicine.com/genomic-testing/foundation-one-heme) identified genomic alterations of *NOTCH2*, *BRCA2*, and *SRSF2* but was negative for rearrangements involving *CCND1* in both samples from the two different time points, further supporting that the lymphomas were clonally related and that despite the acquired strong expression of cyclin D1, the neoplasm lacked *CCND1* gene rearrangement or mutation.

Taken together, these findings indicate that the lymphoma with prolymphocytic transformation involving the lymph node represented disease progression of the patient's original SMZL. The prolymphocytic histologic

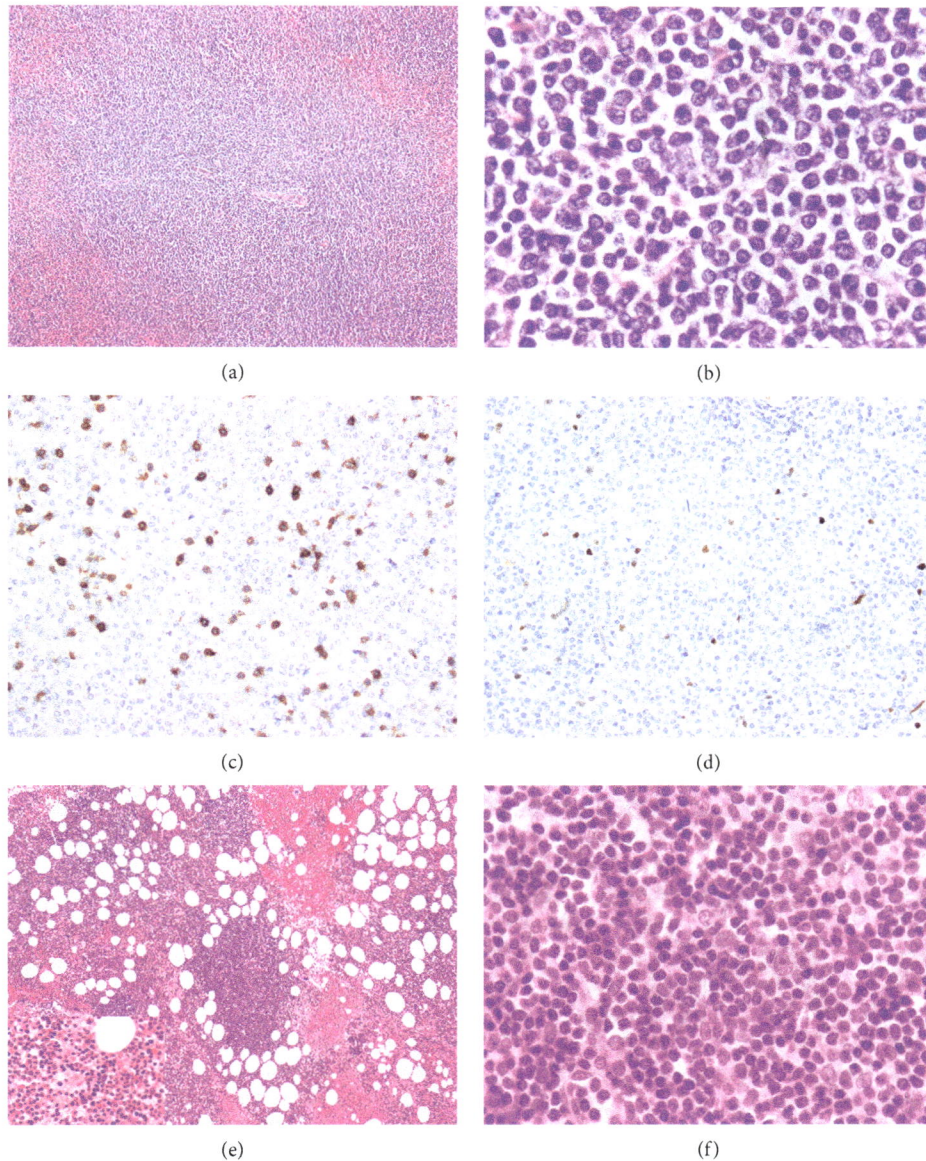

FIGURE 2: Case 1: splenic marginal zone lymphoma and staging bone marrow biopsy. Lymphoma cells are seen in a micronodular distribution expanding splenic white pulp and infiltrating adjacent red pulp (a) and are small with monocytoid morphologic features and minimal cytologic atypia (b). Tumor cells expressed CD20 (not shown) and were negative for CD5 and cyclin D1 (c and d). Bone marrow staging biopsy showed extensive involvement by lymphoma present predominantly in an interstitial nodular distribution with a focal sinusoidal pattern of involvement (inset in (e) showing focal sinusoidal distribution). Lymphoma cells were small in size and prolymphocytic or large cell transformation was not seen (f). (a, b, e, and f) Hematoxylin and eosin stain, (a and e) 100 times magnification, (b and f) 500 times magnification; CD5 (c) and cyclin D1 (d) immunohistochemistry stains shown at 400 and 200 times magnification, respectively.

transformation was defined in this case by the presence of sheets of intermediate to large-sized lymphoma cells with prolymphocytic morphologic features and was associated with acquired partial CD5 and diffuse cyclin D1 expression in the absence of acquired t(11; 14) (*CCND1-IgH*).

2.2. Case 2

2.2.1. Clinical History. This patient was a 53-year-old male without relevant past medical history who presented with one week of intermittent fevers, night sweats, weight loss, early satiety, cough, and exertional shortness of breath. Physical examination revealed diffuse small lymphadenopathy and massive splenomegaly. Imaging studies confirmed massive splenomegaly with the spleen measuring 31 cm in craniocaudal dimension with diffuse hypermetabolic activity, SUV 5.6, in keeping with lymphomatous involvement. There were also numerous subcapsular wedge-shaped areas of photopenia and hypodensities measuring up to 3.5 cm, which were suspected to be splenic infarcts (Figure 4).

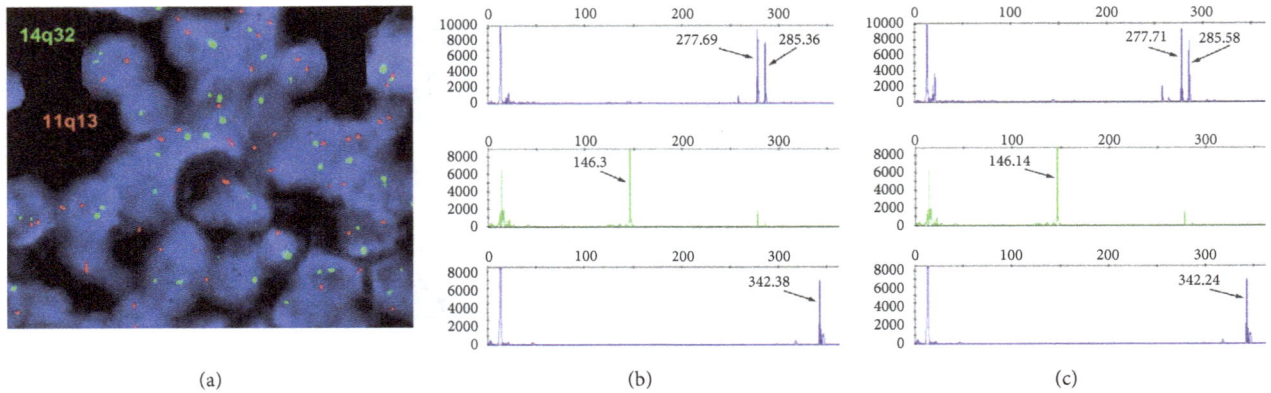

(a)   (b)   (c)

FIGURE 3: Case 1: FISH studies for *IgH-CCND1* fusion were negative (a). This assay was repeated in a reference lab and was again negative. PCR analysis was performed in the original splenic marginal zone lymphoma (b), and in the relapsed lymphoma (lymph node, and clonal PCR amplification products (c) were compared. Amplification products of the same size in base pairs in the initial and relapsed lymphomas were present, supporting that the tumors were clonally related.

2.2.2. Histopathologic, Immunophenotypic, and Molecular Findings. Laboratory analysis showed an elevated LDH of 421 U/L (normal range: 132–225 U/L), leukocytosis (white blood count: 210×10^9 cells/L), anemia, and thrombocytopenia. Peripheral blood smear confirmed lymphocytosis with many circulating lymphoma cells being small to intermediate in size with mature nuclear chromatin (Figure 5(a)). Approximately 50% of circulating lymphoma cells were large with abundant cytoplasm, more open and vesicular nuclear chromatin and prominent nucleoli, consistent with prolymphocytes (Figure 5(b)). Cells with villous or circumferential cytoplasmic projections were not seen. Flow cytometry immunophenotyping in peripheral blood showed that lymphoma cells were positive for CD20, CD19, CD79a, CD22, and CD23 with lambda surface light chain restriction and negative for TdT, CD34, CD10, and CD5. Initial diagnostic considerations included prolymphocytic transformation of atypical CD5 negative CLL, B-prolymphocytic leukemia (B-PLL), and leukemic MCL, noting that the immunophenotypic expression patterns of B-PLL and SMZL can be indistinguishable.

Bone marrow core biopsy showed diffuse infiltration by intermediate-sized cytologically atypical lymphoma cells, and aspirate smear showed that most lymphoma cells had prolymphocytic morphologic features in the bone marrow (Figures 5(c)–5(e)). An intrasinusoidal pattern of involvement was difficult to appreciate due to the extensive degree of marrow involvement. Immunohistochemistry in the bone marrow core biopsy showed lymphoma cells were diffusely and strongly positive for cyclin D1 (Figure 5(f)) and negative for CD5, LEF1, and SOX11. Chromosome analysis in bone marrow aspirate showed a normal karyotype 46, XY in 20 metaphases. FISH studies for t(11; 14) (*CCND1-IgH*) in the peripheral blood and bone marrow aspirate were negative but were positive for deletion 7q (33% of cells), deletion 17p (97% of cells), and deletion 13q (18% of cells). Next-generation sequencing using the FoundationOne Heme comprehensive genomic profiling assay identified a genomic alteration of *TP53* and was

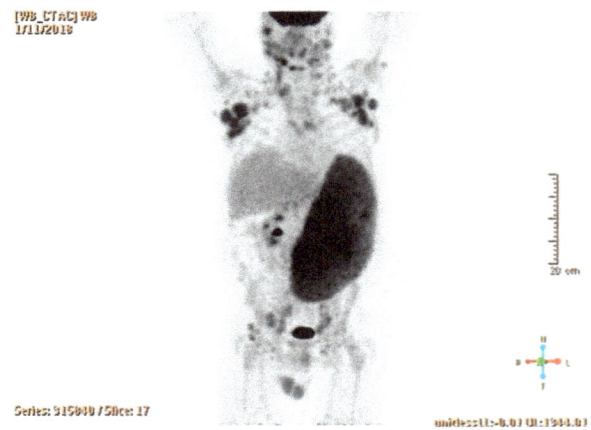

FIGURE 4: Case 2: PET imaging study confirmed massive splenomegaly, spleen measuring 31 cm in craniocaudal dimension, and with diffusely hypermetabolic activity, SUV 5.6, considered to be in keeping with lymphomatous involvement. There were also numerous subcapsular wedge-shaped areas of photopenia and hypodensities measuring up to 3.5 cm, which were suspected to be splenic infarcts.

negative for rearrangements or mutations involving *CCND1* and other tested genomic alterations. Extra copies of *CCND1* were not detected.

Based on the absence of t(11; 14)(*CCND1-IgH*) as detected by FISH, karyotype, and NGS, a diagnosis of MCL was excluded despite diffuse cyclin D1 expression. The presence of massive splenomegaly, the lymphoma cell morphology and immunophenotype, and presence of deletion 7q, support that this lymphoma is best classified as SMZL with prolymphocytic transformation and diffuse cyclin D1 expression. However, extreme leukocytosis, presenting with B symptoms and diffuse lymphadenopathy, as seen in this case, is unusual for SMZL; thus, we cannot exclude that this lymphoma is a B-PLL with diffuse cyclin D1 expression. The presence of deletions 13q and 17p, although not specific, are recurrent abnormalities seen in

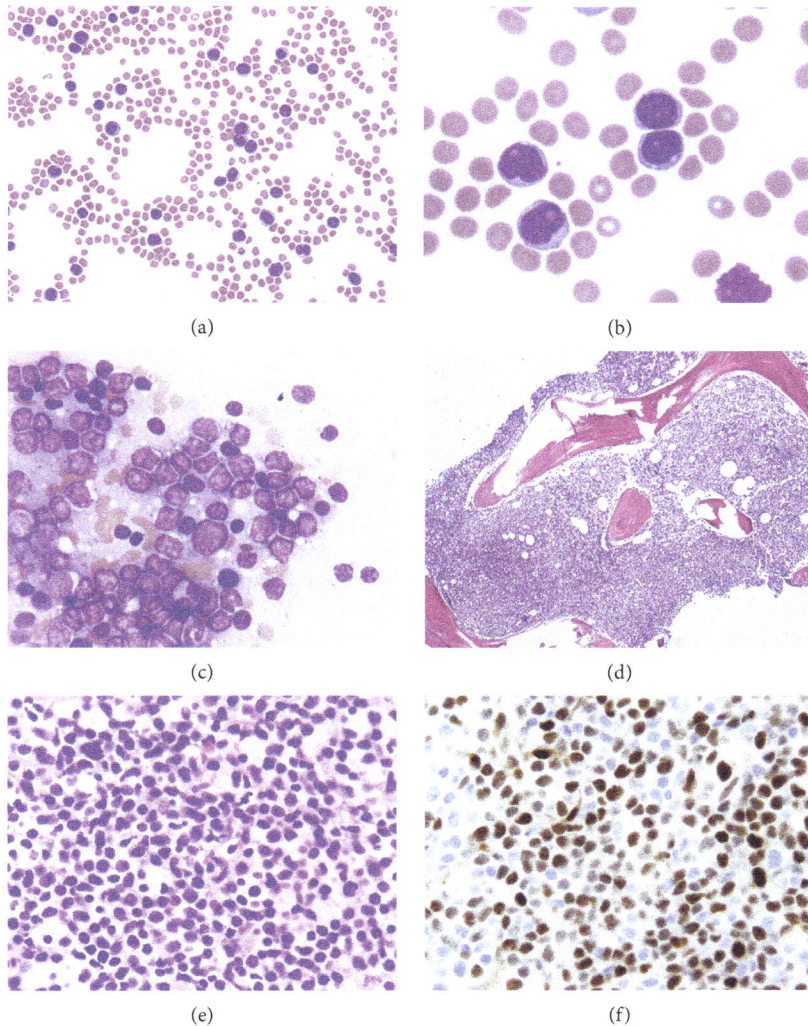

FIGURE 5: Case 2: peripheral blood and bone marrow biopsy. Wright Giemsa-stained peripheral blood smear shows lymphocytosis with many of the circulating lymphoma cells being small in size with round nuclear contours and minimal cytoplasm (a) 500x magnification. Approximately 50% of circulating lymphoma cells had more abundant cytoplasm and prominent nucleoli, consistent with prolymphocytic morphologic features (b) 1000x magnification. Bone marrow aspirate smear shows extensive involvement by lymphoma with a predominance of cells having prolymphocytic features (c 1000x magnification). Hematoxylin and eosin-stained slides of bone marrow core biopsy show extensive marrow involvement by lymphoma ((d) 200x and (e) 500x magnification) with lymphoma cells being diffusely positive for cyclin D1 protein (f) 500x magnification.

approximately 27% and 50% of B-PLL, respectively, and may support this classification [1].

Because this patient did not have splenectomy, we also cannot completely exclude the possibility of splenic diffuse red pulp small B-cell lymphoma, although *CCND3* mutations, which are recurrent in that lymphoma, were not identified, and the presentation was more aggressive than typically reported in diffuse red pulp small B-cell lymphoma.

3. Discussion

We present two chronic B-cell leukemias with splenic involvement, both with increased prolymphocytes and showing misleading diffuse cyclin D1 protein expression. Further confounding the interpretations was that both

leukemias were associated with aggressive clinical features and diffuse lymphadenopathy, clinically simulating MCL.

It is concerning that each of these cases would have been classified as MCL had the patients not had clinical scenarios drawing attention to the possibility of misleading cyclin D1 protein expression. Because FISH is not routinely performed in clinical cases to confirm MCL if diffuse cyclin D1 protein expression is present, it is possible that rare cases are misclassified.

Regarding the first case presented, we were able to identify that this was not an MCL because we were aware that the patient had a history of SMZL in which FISH studies were negative for t(11; 14)(q13; q32). FISH and NGS studies pursued in the relapsed, transformed lymphoma confirmed the lack of t(11; 14)(q13; q31) and variant translocations despite the acquired diffuse cyclin D1 protein expression. Supporting the classification of SMZL expressing cyclin D1 in this case was the initially indolent clinical presentation with splenomegaly and marrow involvement, initial lack of CD5 and cyclin D1 protein expression, lack of CCND1-IgH, and identification of NOTCH2 mutation. Of note, we are able to conclude in this case that the expression of CD5 and cyclin D1 were acquired at or before the time of prolymphocytic transformation, but after initial presentation, given that the previous SMZL (CD5 negative and cyclin D1 negative) and current transformed SMZL (CD5 positive and cyclin D1 positive) were clonally related.

While not absolutely specific and also reported in diffuse large B-cell lymphomas and rarely in other low-grade B-cell lymphomas, activating NOTCH2 genomic alterations are particularly frequent and recurrent in SMZL where they are observed in ~20–25% of patients, establishing this gene mutation as one of the most frequent in SMZL [11, 12]. Due to the relative specificity of activating NOTCH2 mutations, this abnormality informs the diagnosis of SMZL and distinguishes it from histopathologic mimics [11]. The prognostic significance of this mutation in the context of SMZL is controversial, but most studies associate this abnormality with poorer overall survival [4, 11, 13]. Analysis of NOTCH2 mutations in SMZLs has shown a relationship with other alterations involved in lymphoma pathogenesis including deletion of 7q31, over-representation of IgHV1-2 usage, and higher promoter methylation status and correlates with poor outcome and histologic transformation [4, 13].

In addition to NOTCH2 mutation, BRCA2 mutation was also identified in case 1. BRCA2 is a tumor suppressor gene whose protein regulates response to DNA damage and whose mutation causes the inability to repair DNA damage, thereby promoting tumorigenesis [14].

While BRCA2 mutations are reported in DLBCL, we are not aware that this mutation has been reported specifically in SMZL [15]. Similarly, SRSF2 mutation, also identified in this case, is widely reported in myeloid neoplasms, but we are not aware of its significance in MZL [16].

The second case presented is another example of a diffuse cyclin D1 positive B-cell lymphoma presenting initially in the leukemic phase and with increased prolymphocytes (50%), diffuse lymphadenopathy, massive splenomegaly, and aggressive clinical features. Despite diffuse cyclin D1 protein expression, FISH, karyotype and NGS did not identify alterations of CCND1. Deletions of 7q, 17p, and 13q were identified, and TP53 mutation was detected by NGS. While not diagnostically specific, deletion 13q is reported in B-PLL, and 17p deletions and TP53 mutations are particularly frequent in B-PLL (~50% of cases). Given these genetic abnormalities and the clinical presentation, we cannot exclude that this lymphoma is a B-PLL presenting initially with diffuse cyclin D1 protein expression.

However, also present in this case was a 7q deletion, which, although also not specific, is reported in and supports the classification of this lymphoma as SMZL with leukemic prolymphocytic transformation. In fact, similar cases of SMZL with the overt leukemic phase including increased peripheral blood prolymphocytes (>55%), markedly elevated leukocyte count ($>130 \times 10^9$/L), and massive splenectomy are previously reported [9]. Similar to our case, these previously reported SMZL with prolymphocytic transformation presented with a prolymphocytic leukemia-like clinical picture, and the resected spleens showed SMZL with increased nucleoliated cells consistent with prolymphocytes. Deletion 7q was identified in these previously reported cases, supporting the diagnosis of SMZL with prolymphocytic transformation, overt leukocytosis, and a clinical picture mimicking B-PLL.

While SMZL lacks recurrent chromosomal translocations that are typical of other lymphomas, including other MZLs, deletion 7q, the most frequent copy number alteration, is identified in 30% of SMZL, and its presence supports the classification of this lymphoma type [17]. Although deletion 7q is not entirely specific for SMZL, it is seen only rarely in other small and leukemic B-cell lymphomas including chronic lymphocytic leukemia, hairy cell leukemia, and MCL. This deletion is not reported as a recurrent abnormality in B-PLL. In the context of SMZL, deletion 7q is associated with poor clinical outcomes [4, 13].

The target genes lost in the 7q deletion responsible for development of a subset of SMZL have not been clearly identified. Studies aimed at elucidating the oncogenic nature of the 7q deletion have shown that the deleted region in some cases is a 2.8 Mb region at 7q32 [17].

Recurrent breakpoints in this region have not been identified [17]. Loss of the sonic hedgehog gene (SHH) at 7q36.2 and protection of telomere 1 gene (POT1) at 7q31.32 have been reported in array-based comparative genomic hybridization studies aimed at characterization of the deletion 7q abnormality of SMZL [8]. It has been postulated that loss of POT1 in particular may contribute to lymphomagenesis and create an environment of DNA instability, correlating with the poor prognostic significance of this deletion [8].

Unlike previously reported SMZL (with or without prolymphocytic transformation), our report describes diffuse cyclin D1 protein expression in SMZL, which has not been reported previously to our knowledge [18]. This is an important finding given that cyclin D1 protein expression is routinely used in clinical practice to identify leukemias/lymphomas as MCL. In our two cases, the diffuse expression of cyclin D1 was associated with the presence of a prolymphocytic transformation although both small and large (prolymphocytic) cells expressed cyclin D1.

We were able to identify one case report describing cyclin D1 positive marginal zone lymphoma of mediastinum; however, the provided image in this report shows only weak and focal nuclear positivity for cyclin D1 and is not the staining pattern or intensity expected for MCL [19]. Previous reports of SMZL in prolymphocytic transformation in particular have shown all cases to be negative for cyclin D1 protein [9].

CCND1 is an oncogene that promotes progression of the cell cycle at the level of the G1 checkpoint, where its protein binds to CDK4 and CDK6 creating complexes that phosphorylate retinoblastoma protein, inactivating its suppressor effect [20]. Cyclin D1 overexpression in the context of lymphomagenesis is most frequently due to a translocation that juxtaposes the 11q13 band containing *cyclin D1* with the constitutively active *IgH* locus on chromosome 14. In the context of B-cell lymphomas, the presence of this translocation and the resulting diffuse overexpression of cyclin D1 protein, detected by immunophenotyping, have come to define MCL. However, expression of *CCND1* can be modulated at the transcriptional level by other mechanisms including being promoted by transcription factors such as STAT3, independent of the t(11; 14)(q13; q32) translocation [21].

In the cases reported here, cyclin D1 protein expression was upregulated independent of chromosomal translocation or additional *CCND1* copies, neither of which were not detectable by a variety of means. The mechanism of protein overexpression in the cases we present is unclear at this time but is not unique to the lymphomas we report given that overexpression of cyclin D1 is known to occur in other nontranslocated lymphomas including diffuse large B-cell lymphoma and within proliferation centers of CLL/SLL. It is intriguing that cyclin D1 overexpression in our report was associated with prolymphocytic transformation, as is the precedent for this occurrence within prolymphocytes of CLL/SLL and in a subset of diffuse large B-cell lymphoma.

Given our experience of diffuse cyclin D1 expression in SMZL coupled with the fact that FISH studies are not performed in the majority of lymphomas classified as MCL, we suggest the possibility that a subset of splenic and/or leukemic lymphomas classified as MCL based on cyclin D1 expression may in fact be SMZL expressing cyclin D1. This may particularly be the case when increased large cells or prolymphocytic cells are present. Given that diffuse cyclin D1 positive SMZL is not previously reported, the incidence of this finding and its clinical significance are unknown and certainly need to be investigated. The association of prolymphocytic transformation and acquired cyclin D1 protein expression likewise deserves additional investigation. Finally, the cases presented also raise the question of whether FISH studies should be performed in cases of cyclin D1 positive B-cell lymphomas in order to confirm the diagnosis of MCL. We are not doing this in our practice despite acknowledgement of the cases presented.

Conflicts of Interest

The authors declare that they have no conflicts of interest.

References

[1] S. H. Swerdlow, E. Campo, N. L. Harris et al., *WHO Classification of Tumours of Haematopoietic and Lymphoid Tissues*, IARC, Lyon, France, 4th edition, 2017.

[2] C. Kalpadakis, G. A. Pangalis, S. Sachanas et al., "New insights into monoclonal B-cell lymphocytosis," *BioMed Research International*, vol. 2014, Article ID 258917, 11 pages, 2014.

[3] J. M. Hernandez, J. L. Garcia, N. C. Gutierrez et al., "Novel genomic imbalances in B-cell splenic marginal zone lymphomas revealed by comparative genomic hybridization and cytogenetics," *American Journal of Pathology*, vol. 158, no. 5, pp. 1843–1850, 2001.

[4] A. Rinaldi, M. Milan, E. Chigrinova et al., "Genome-wide DNA profiling of marginal zone lymphomas identifies subtype-specific lesions with an impact on the clinical outcome," *Blood*, vol. 117, no. 5, pp. 1595–1604, 2011.

[5] F. I. Camacho, M. Mollejo, M. S. Mateo et al., "Progression to large B-cell lymphoma in splenic marginal zone lymphoma: a description of a series of 12 cases," *American Journal of Surgical Pathology*, vol. 25, no. 10, pp. 1268–1276, 2001.

[6] A. Conconi, S. Franceschetti, K. Aprile von Hohenstaufen et al., "Histologic transformation in marginal zone lymphomas," *Annals of Oncology*, vol. 26, no. 11, pp. 2329–2335, 2015.

[7] J. Lenglet, C. Traullé, N. Mounier et al., "Long-term follow-up analysis of 100 patients with splenic marginal zone lymphoma treated with splenectomy as first-line treatment," *Leukemia & Lymphoma*, vol. 55, no. 8, pp. 1854–1860, 2014.

[8] F. Vega, J. H. Cho-Vega, P. A. Lennon et al., "Splenic marginal zone lymphomas are characterized by loss of interstitial regions of chromosome 7q, 7q31.32 and 7q36.2 that include the protection of telomere 1 (POT1) and sonic hedgehog (SHH) genes," *British Journal of Haematology*, vol. 142, no. 2, pp. 216–226, 2008.

[9] D. Hoehn, R. N. Miranda, R. Kanagal-Shamanna, P. Lin, and L. J. Medeiros, "Splenic B-cell lymphomas with more than 55% prolymphocytes in blood: evidence for prolymphocytoid transformation," *Human Pathology*, vol. 43, no. 11, pp. 1828–1838, 2012.

[10] L. Arcaini, D. Rossi, and M. Paulli, "Splenic marginal zone lymphoma: from genetics to management," *Blood*, vol. 127, no. 17, pp. 2072–2081, 2016.

[11] M. K. Angelopoulou, C. Kalpadakis, G. S. Pangalis, M. C. Kyrtsonis, and T. P. Vassilakopoulous, "Nodal marginal zone lymphoma," *Leukemia & Lymphoma*, vol. 55, no. 6, pp. 1204–1250, 2014.

[12] M. J. Kiel, T. Velusamy, B. L. Betz et al., "Whole-genome sequencing identifies recurrent somatic NOTCH2 mutations in splenic marginal zone lymphoma," *Journal of Experimental Medicine*, vol. 209, no. 9, pp. 1553–1565, 2012.

[13] A. J. Arribas, A. Rinaldi, A. A. Mensah et al., "DNA methylation profiling identifies two splenic marginal zone lymphoma subgroups with different clinical and genetic features," *Blood*, vol. 125, no. 12, pp. 1922–1931, 2015.

[14] H. Yang, P. D. Jeffrey, J. Miller et al., "BRCA2 function in DNA binding and recombination from a BRCA2-DSS1-ssDNA structure," *Science*, vol. 297, no. 5588, pp. 1837–1848, 2002.

[15] W. K. Holloman, "Unraveling the mechanism of BRCA2 in homologous recombination," *Nat Struct Mol Biol*, vol. 18, no. 7, pp. 748–754, 2011.

[16] E. Kim, J. O. Ilagan, Y. Liang et al., "SRSF2 mutations contribute to myelodysplasia by mutant- specific effects on exon recognition," *Cancer Cell*, vol. 27, no. 5, pp. 617–630, 2015.

[17] A. J. Watkins, R. A. Hamoudi, N. Zeng et al., "An integrated genomic and expression analysis of 7q deletion in splenic marginal zone lymphoma," *PLoS One*, vol. 7, no. 9, Article ID e44997, 2012.

[18] M. Kojima, E. Sato, K. Oshimi et al., "Characteristics of CD5-positive splenic marginal zone lymphoma with leukemic manifestation ; clinical, flow cytometry, and histopathological findings of 11 cases," *Journal of Clinical and Experimental Hematopathology*, vol. 50, no. 2, pp. 107–112, 2010.

[19] G. Rymkiewicz, K. Ptaszyński, J. Walewski et al., "Unusual cyclin D1 positive marginal zone lymphoma of mediastinum," *Medical Oncology*, vol. 23, no. 3, pp. 423–428, 2006.

[20] M. E. Ewen, H. K. Sluss, C. J. Sherr et al., "Functional interactions of the retinoblastoma protein with mammalian D-type cyclins," *Cell*, vol. 73, pp. 487–497, 1993.

[21] Y. Xu, Y. Shi, Q. Yuan et al., "Epstein-Barr Virus encoded LMP1 regulated cyclin D1 promoter activity by nuclear EGFR and STAT3 in CNE1 cells," *Journal of Experimental and Clinical Cancer Research*, vol. 32, no. 1, p. 90, 2013.

17

Is There a Role for Biweekly Romiplostim in the Management of Chronic Immune Thrombocytopenia (ITP)?

Jasjit Kaur Rooprai [ID][1] **and Karima Khamisa**[2]

[1]*Faculty of Medicine, University of Ottawa, Ottawa, Ontario, Canada*
[2]*Division of Hematology, Department of Medicine, The Ottawa Hospital, Ottawa, Ontario, Canada*

Correspondence should be addressed to Jasjit Kaur Rooprai; jsing077@uottawa.ca

Academic Editor: Tomás J. González-López

Romiplostim is a peptibody, which stimulates platelet production by a mechanism similar to that of endogenous thrombopoietin. It has an established indication as second-line therapy in patients with chronic immune thrombocytopenia (ITP). The agent is typically administered weekly; however, there are instances where a biweekly (i.e., alternate week) dosing may be feasible in a select group of patients. We conducted a retrospective case review to evaluate the efficacy and safety of biweekly administration of romiplostim in maintaining a platelet count of $>30 \times 10^9$/L in three patients with chronic ITP. Treatment was started with a weekly injection (1 μg/kg) with a dose escalation to achieve a platelet count $>30 \times 10^9$/L. Once stable on weekly romiplostim, these patients received biweekly administration. No bleeding complications were noted during biweekly dosing for these patients. The current findings suggest that lengthening the dose interval of romiplostim is feasible in select patients with chronic ITP to maintain stable platelet counts. Additional studies are therefore warranted to further evaluate biweekly dosing for romiplostim to increase convenience and decrease costs for patients with chronic ITP.

1. Introduction

Chronic idiopathic immune thrombocytopenia (ITP) is an autoimmune bleeding disorder characterized by low platelet counts often below 100×10^9/L for at least 12 months' duration [1]. Recent literature suggests that the pathogenesis of immune thrombocytopenia (ITP) is caused due to both autoantibody-mediated platelet destruction and suboptimal platelet production [2–6]. Most traditional ITP therapies have focused on either inducing short-term increases in platelet counts (via intravenous immunoglobulins (IVIg), steroids, and intravenous anti-D) or long-term maintenance of platelet counts using rituximab and splenectomy [4]. These treatments were effective in many patients but failed to achieve or maintain a durable response in certain patients and were associated with adverse effects [4]. In the past decade, thrombopoietin receptor agonists (TRAs) have been

shown to induce increases in platelet counts in both healthy adults and patients with ITP, with an acceptable safety profile [4–7].

Romiplostim is a thrombopoiesis-stimulating protein, referred to as a peptibody, which stimulates platelet production by a mechanism similar to that of endogenous TPO [8]. Currently, both the American Society of Hematology ITP management guidelines and the International Consensus Report guidelines recommend the use of TRAs for adults with ITP that persists following splenectomy or in patients who are not candidates for splenectomy and for whom at least one other treatment has failed [9]. In addition, the 2015 assessment report released by the European Medicines Agency (EMA) on romiplostim concluded that TRAs can be considered as second-line treatment in non-splenectomized patients [10]. Current evidence on the use of romiplostim in adults with ITP has demonstrated rapid and sustained platelet increases while reducing the use of concomitant medications and the incidence of bleeding [9]. Currently, it is dosed weekly to maintain platelet counts >30 $\times 10^9$/L (in International terms >30,000/μL). Usual starting dose is 1 μg/kg weekly, though some centers have been able to safely start patients on 2-3 μg/kg per week. Vials of romiplostim are only available in 250 μg and 500 μg sizes; titration by weight often involves discarding portions of these vials to meet exact dosing.

We report three cases of patients with chronic ITP who have maintained stable platelet counts >30 $\times 10^9$/L on biweekly dosing of romiplostim. The treatment of these three patients was started with a weekly injection, and the dose was escalated until a titrated dose was achieved that maintained platelet count >30 $\times 10^9$/L. Patients were then switched to a biweekly schedule and were given a rescue dose (and steroids/IVIg) if platelet counts fell to below < 30 $\times 10^9$/L. The characteristics and outcomes of these patients are presented.

2. Methods

2.1. Study Design. This was a retrospective case series analysis of three patients with chronic ITP who were seen at the Ottawa Hospital (Ontario, Canada). These patients were subsequently followed in a community hematology clinic. Data were collected from electronic medical records for patients with chronic ITP, with treatment refractory disease and receiving romiplostim as a part of their therapy. Demographic and disease characteristics, including time of ITP diagnosis, previous ITP treatments, and concomitant ITP treatments, were recorded. This study was approved by the OHSN-REB (Ottawa Health Science Network Research Ethics Board), and written consent was provided by patients.

2.2. Definitions. Guidelines established by the American Society of Hematology (ASH) define a clinical response as a sustained platelet count ≥30 $\times 10^9$/L and a complete response with a platelet count ≥100 $\times 10^9$/L [1]. Further, it defines refractory ITP as severe ITP that persists after splenectomy or patients who respond temporarily to corticosteroid therapy or IVIg [1].

2.3. Case Presentations. We describe three cases of patients who were able to safely maintain their platelet counts on biweekly romiplostim (Table 1).

2.3.1. Case 1. A 62-year-old female diagnosed with ITP after presenting with persistent epistaxis, thrombocytopenia, and wet purpura at age 51; she was known to have a prior history of warm autoimmune hemolytic anemia (although this was stable). She was considered to have Evan's syndrome after her ITP diagnosis. Her other comorbidities included diabetes mellitus (type II) and developmental delay. Over the next 3 years, she had frequent relapses of her ITP requiring hospitalization for epistaxis. She underwent splenectomy within the first 3 months of her ITP diagnosis, and

TABLE 1: Baseline demographic and clinical characteristics.

Characteristic	Case #1	Case #2	Case #3
Age of ITP diagnosis	57	63	46
Gender	Female	Female	Female
Weight	60 kg	120 kg	80 kg
ITP etiology	Primary	Primary	Primary
Number of prior ITP therapies	4	2	2
Prior therapies for ITP			
Prednisone (maintenance)	10 mg	No	No
IVIg (# of doses)	16 doses	4 doses	21 doses
Rituximab	8 doses	4 doses	No
Splenectomy	Yes	No	Yes
Vincristine	Yes	No	No
Eltrombopag	Yes	No	No
Dexamethasone	Yes	No	No

eventually received eight courses of rituximab, multiple courses of IVIg and prednisone, and finally was started on romiplostim three years after her splenectomy. She maintained a stable platelet count on romiplostim 500 μg weekly for 53 weeks. Due to platelet counts remaining in the 200–600 $\times 10^9$/L range, she was switched to biweekly dosing of romiplostim 250 μg and was able to maintain stable platelet counts for 11 consecutive weeks (Figure 1). She experienced a mild respiratory infection after the 11th week mark which caused her platelet counts to fall. She received dexamethasone and IVIg as a rescue medication and eventually modified her romiplostim dosing schedule to alternate week dosing of romiplostim 250 μg and 500 μg. While on biweekly romiplostim, she experienced no bleeding complications. However, given her cognitive issues, she felt weekly dosing a preferable option. Presently, her platelets remain in the 200 to 300 $\times 10^9$/L range while on weekly doses of romiplostim, (presently at 230 μg a week).

2.3.2. Case 2. A 65-year-old female was diagnosed with chronic severe thrombocytopenia at the age of 59. She had a number of comorbidities including diabetes mellitus (type II, poorly tolerant of steroids), chronic iron deficiency, obesity, and nonalcoholic steatohepatitis. She was initially put on intermittent IVIg therapy, with platelet levels increasing from 20–30 $\times 10^9$/L to over 200 $\times 10^9$/L. The patient was not a candidate for splenectomy. The patient was started on romiplostim therapy at an initial dose of 100 μg weekly and was able to maintain stable platelet counts for 38 weeks. Due to cost and convenience, a trial of biweekly dosing of romiplostim was initiated. The patient was able to maintain stable platelet counts for 131 consecutive weeks; however, due to a lapse in private medication coverage, the patient discontinued romiplostim altogether (Figure 2). Six weeks after her last romiplostim dose, she was given 4 doses of rituximab to maintain her platelet counts >30 $\times 10^9$/L. Currently, she is on no treatment for ITP and is in partial remission, maintaining platelet counts in the range of 37–69 $\times 10^9$/L. While on biweekly romiplostim, she experienced no bleeding complications.

2.3.3. Case 3. A 52-year-old female was diagnosed with chronic refractory ITP at the age of 46. She had a number of

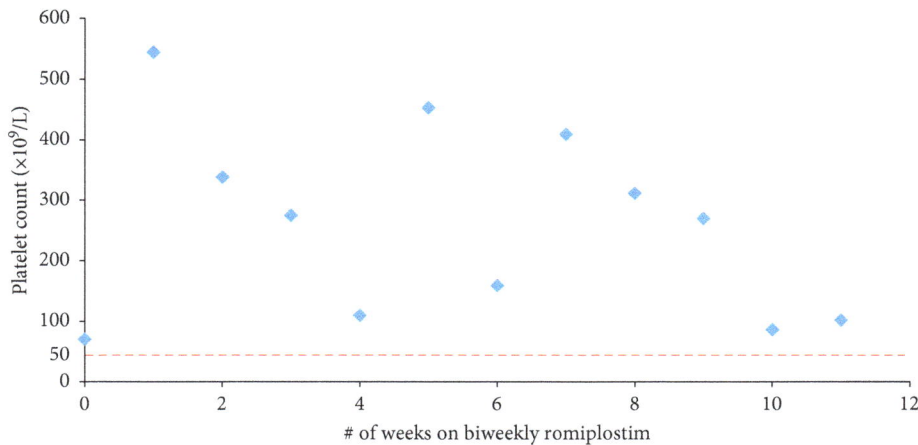

FIGURE 1: Case 1: biweekly romiplostim.

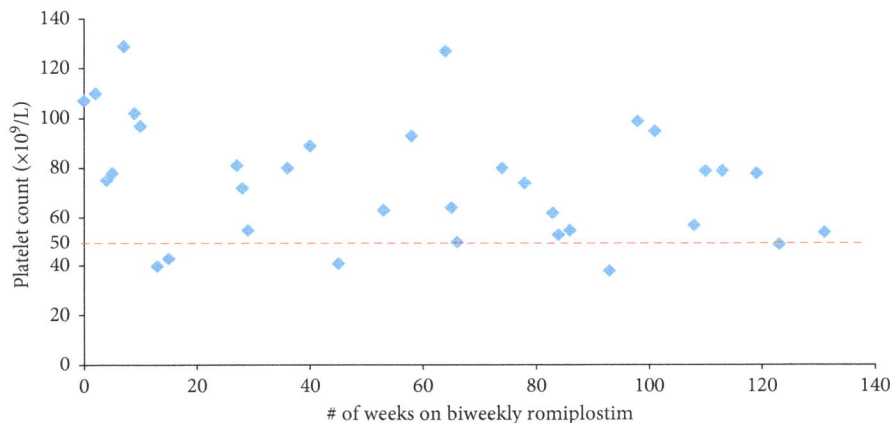

FIGURE 2: Case 2: biweekly romiplostim.

comorbidities including osteoporosis and type I diabetes mellitus. She was initially able to maintain a stable platelet count on prednisone 50–70 mg therapy for 2 years; however, due to her diabetes, she was weaned off prednisone. She underwent a splenectomy three years after her initial presentation; however, her platelet count remained under 10×10^9/L one-week postprocedure. She received multiple doses of IVIg and low dose prednisone to maintain her platelet count above 30×10^9/L. Romiplostim was initiated 13 months postsplenectomy. She was started on weekly romiplostim $75 \mu g$ therapy. She maintained stable platelet counts on weekly romiplostim dosing for 94 weeks before being switched to biweekly romiplostim $75 \mu g$ therapy and was able to maintain stable platelet counts for 20 weeks (Figure 3). She had extremely high platelet counts on biweekly romiplostim ($400–700 \times 10^9$/L range) allowing a trial of triweekly romiplostim dosing to be introduced. On q3weekly dosing, she was still able to maintain high platelet counts for 12 weeks (Figure 4), and thus, romiplostim therapy was discontinued altogether while monitoring the patient closely. The patient maintained a durable remission three years after her last dose of romiplostim. Like the other

two patients, she experienced no bleeding complications while on biweekly dosing of the drug.

3. Discussion

In this paper, we report three cases of adult patients with chronic ITP who were administered biweekly dosing of romiplostim after achieving stable platelet counts (often with platelet counts well above 400×10^9/L). Romiplostim, a TPO-receptor agonist, is a highly effective treatment for patients with chronic ITP following splenectomy or in patients who are not candidates for splenectomy and have failed one other form of treatment. Dosing is typically weekly via subcutaneous injection. Withholding the drug for a week is recommended if a patient's platelet count is above 400×10^9/L [7]. In some instances, withholding weekly dosing of the medication (despite platelet counts over 400×10^9/L) can cause a paradoxical worsening of thrombocytopenia [7]. There is a paucity of the literature regarding the clinical use of biweekly dosing of romiplostim. However, a recent study by Park et al. did address this issue in patients with acute ITP [11]. While platelet counts remained labile in

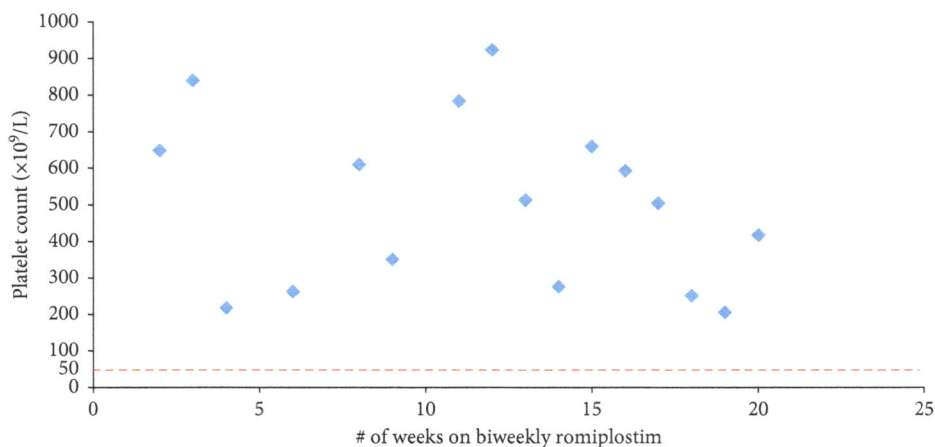

FIGURE 3: Case 3: biweekly romiplostim.

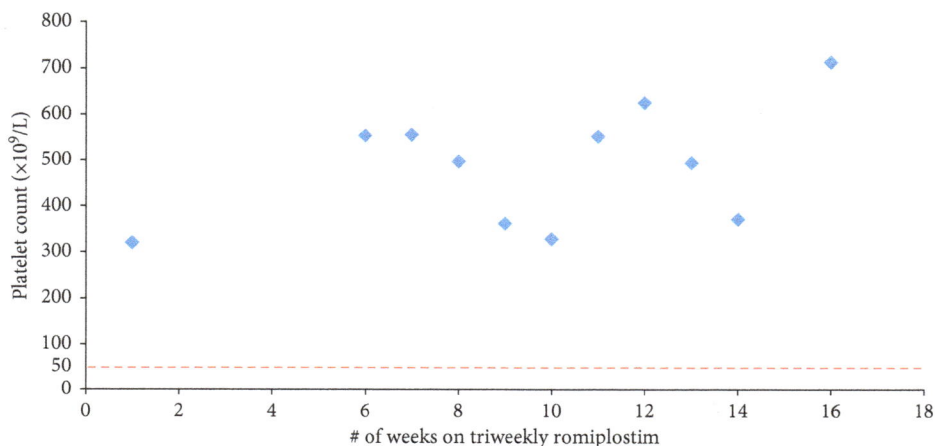

FIGURE 4: Case 3: triweekly romiplostim.

patients on biweekly dosing, no bleeding complications occurred in patients on this dosing schedule.

In this case series, we retrospectively evaluated the efficacy and safety of biweekly romiplostim therapy in three patients with chronic ITP, who had been previously stable on weekly therapy. Despite the differential characteristics of the described patients (Table 1), platelet responses were rapidly observed after romiplostim therapy (1-2 weeks) in all cases. All 3 patients had maintained stable platelet counts on weekly romiplostim for at least 38 weeks prior to being switched to the biweekly dosing schedule. All three patients maintained a platelet count >30 × 10⁹/L while on biweekly romiplostim therapy (Table 2). Park et al. previously reported that a biweekly romiplostim schedule was not effective in producing a stable platelet response in patients with chronic ITP [11]. However, the three patient cases presented in this paper suggest otherwise. Furthermore, Park et al. reported that a rapid drop in platelet count was observed in all cases shortly after switching to a biweekly dosing schedule [11]. However, in the three case studies being reported, no such rapid drop in platelet count was observed. This may be due to a longer duration of stability on

weekly dosing (9 months versus 3 months in the Park study) before transitioning to biweekly dosing.

In another study by Sekeres et al., patients with myelodysplastic syndrome were administered either weekly or biweekly romiplostim [12]. Durable responses were attained in patients administered weekly or biweekly romiplostim, and no differences in adverse outcomes were noted between the two groups. This study also noted that thrombocytopenic patients do not need to achieve normal platelet levels to derive clinical and quality-of-life benefit from this therapeutic intervention [12]. The goal was to achieve platelet levels that obviated the need for transfusions and lowered the risks of spontaneous or traumatic bleeding [12].

Romiplostim is administered by subcutaneous injections in a dose based on a patient's body weight and platelet count. Romiplostim, however, is only available in two doses in prefilled vials, 250 μg and 500 μg, costing approximately $882.50 and $1765 Cdn, respectively [13]. The dose is potentially administered indefinitely for patients with chronic ITP. At the present time, in the Canadian health care system, the yearly medication costs between $45,890 Cdn (for the 250 μg weekly dose) and $91,780 Cdn (500 μg weekly dose).

TABLE 2: Detailed summary of romiplostim dosing schedule.

Parameter	Case #1	Case #2	Case #3
Romiplostim started (postdiagnosis)	3 years (2015)	2 years	3 years
Trial 1			
Dose	500 μg	100 μg	75 μg
Frequency	Weekly	Weekly	Weekly
Duration	53 weeks	38 weeks	94 weeks
Platelet range ($\times 10^9$/L)	31–722	35–221	42–595
Trial 2			
Dose	250 μg	250 μg	75 μg
Frequency	Biweekly	Biweekly	Biweekly
Duration	11 weeks	131 weeks	20 weeks
Platelet range ($\times 10^9$/L)	86–454	40–129	217–922
Trial 3			
Dose	500 μg	—	75 μg
Frequency	Weekly	—	Triweekly
Duration	42 weeks	—	12 weeks
Platelet range ($\times 10^9$/L)	31–1277	—	321–625
Current ITP status	Stable*	Partial remission	Complete remission

*On weekly dosing of romiplostim 230 μg.

However, certain patients, such as those presented in this case series report, can maintain stable platelet counts while on a biweekly dosing of romiplostim. On a biweekly dosing schedule, patients are able to save between $22,945 and $45,890 Cdn annually.

Interestingly, one patient (Case 3) achieved clinical remission after discontinuation of romiplostim. Several other studies have demonstrated sustained remission and a positive safety profile after discontinuing romiplostim, mainly in chronic relapsing or refractory ITP patients [14–17]. The mechanisms and factors of remission in patients with ITP remain unknown, although some studies suggest a restoration of immune tolerance and a decrease of inflammatory state after continuous treatment with TPO-receptor agonists through the stimulation of regulatory B and T lymphocytes [18, 19]. We conclude that if a patient does appear to be entering a remission from ITP while on romiplostim, there may be a role for attempting biweekly dosing as part of a potential tapering strategy.

The half-life of romiplostim is estimated to be from 1 to 34 days, suggesting that lengthening the interval of romiplostim administration to more than a week may be possible in some patients, and should cautiously be evaluated on a case-by-case basis [8, 11, 20, 21]. Early pharmacokinetic mathematical modeling studies further lend support to this possibility; weekly romiplostim dosing has a more predictable platelet count profile, but biweekly dosing can still lead to acceptable platelet counts, above the minimum requirements of 30 × 10^9/L [21]. The maintenance of stable platelet counts after initiating biweekly dosing of romiplostim suggests different physiological responses to romiplostim in ITP patients and highlights the importance of a close follow-up in these patients. Based on our real-life experience, a transition to biweekly romiplostim dosing may be attempted in those who have achieved clinical stability on a weekly dosing regimen for at least six months and have demonstrated platelet counts typically of 400 × 10^9/L or greater while on weekly dosing. This is especially helpful for patients with financial challenges. Finally,

the alternate week dosing may be attempted in those that may be entering a remission from their ITP with eventual goal to stop all therapies.

4. Conclusion

In conclusion, lengthening the dosing frequency of romiplostim to biweekly may have a role to select patients with chronic ITP. Our data suggest that a trial of biweekly dosing may be implemented in patients who have been stable on weekly dosing for at least six months and may be entering clinical remission. All three patients reported in this case series had no adverse bleeding symptoms while on biweekly romiplostim dosing; one patient eventually experienced a sustained remission from her ITP. Although romiplostim is traditionally given on a weekly schedule, based on the present findings, it might be valuable to evaluate the efficacy of biweekly dosing on a case-by-case basis. In clinical practice, required doses and intervals are expected to differ between patients and the minimal effective dose to maintain adequate platelet levels should be determined individually. Further studies are warranted to determine which patients can safely be transitioned to biweekly dosing; this will ultimately reduce the cost of the medication and increase convenience to patients.

Consent

Written informed consent was obtained from the included patients for publication of this case report series.

Conflicts of Interest

J. R. has no conflicts of interest to disclose. K. K. has received Speaker's Fees for Alexion, Amgen, and Novartis.

References

[1] C. Neunert, W. Lim, M. Crowther, A. Cohen, L. Solberg, and M. A. Crowther, "The American Society of Hematology 2011

evidence-based practice guideline for immune thrombocytopenia," *Blood*, vol. 117, no. 16, pp. 4190–4207, 2011.

[2] P. J. Ballem, G. M. Segal, J. R. Stratton, T. Gernsheimer, J. W. Adamson, and S. J. Slichter, "Mechanisms of thrombocytopenia in chronic autoimmune thrombocytopenic purpura. Evidence of both impaired platelet production and increased platelet clearance," *Journal of Clinical Investigation*, vol. 80, no. 1, pp. 33–40, 1987.

[3] D. Nugent, R. McMillan, J. L. Nichol, and S. J. Slichter, "Pathogenesis of chronic immune thrombocytopenia: increased platelet destruction and/or decreased platelet production," *British Journal of Haematology*, vol. 146, no. 6, pp. 585–596, 2009.

[4] D. B. Cines and J. B. Bussel, "How I treat idiopathic thrombocytopenic purpura (ITP)," *Blood*, vol. 106, no. 7, pp. 2244–2251, 2005.

[5] M. Chang, P. E. Nakagawa, S. A. Williams et al., "Immune thrombocytopenic purpura (ITP) plasma and purified ITP monoclonal autoantibodies inhibit megakaryoctopoiesis in vitro," *Blood*, vol. 102, no. 3, pp. 887–895, 2003.

[6] R. McMillan, L. Wang, A. Tomer, J. Nichol, and J. Pistillo, "Suppression of in vitro megakaryocyte production by antiplatelet autoantibodies from adult patients with chronic ITP," *Blood*, vol. 103, no. 4, pp. 1364–1369, 2004.

[7] J. B. Bussel, D. J. Kuter, V. Pullarkat, R. M. Lyons, M. Guo, and J. L. Nichol, "Safety and efficacy of long-term treatment with romiplostim in thrombocytopenic patients with chronic ITP," *Blood*, vol. 113, no. 10, pp. 2161–2171, 2009.

[8] D. Hubulashvili and N. Marzella, "Romiplostim (Nplate), a treatment option for immune (idiopathic) thrombocytopenic purpura," *Pharmacy and Therapeutics*, vol. 34, no. 9, pp. 482–485, 2009.

[9] S. Chalmers and M. D. Tarantino, "Romiplostim as a treatment for immune thrombocytopenia: a review," *Journal of Blood Medicine*, vol. 6, pp. 37–44, 2015.

[10] European Medicines Agency, *Assessment Report: Nplate*, European Medicines Agency, London, UK, 2016.

[11] S. Park, S. S. Yoon, J. H. Lee, J. S. Park, J. H. Jang, and J. W. Lee, "Multicenter, prospective study to evaluate the efficacy of biweekly romiplostim administration in patients with immune thrombocytopenia," *International Journal of Hematology*, vol. 103, no. 1, pp. 44–52, 2016.

[12] M. A. Sekeres, H. Kantarjian, P. Fenaux et al., "Subcutaneous or intravenous administration of romiplostim in thrombocytopenic patients with lower risk myelodysplastic syndromes," *Cancer*, vol. 117, no. 5, pp. 992–1000, 2011.

[13] M. Pettigrew, K. Garces, R. Deuson, J. Kassis, and V. Laroche, "Comparative net cost impact of the utilization of romiplostim and intravenous immunoglobulin for the treatment of patients with immune thrombocytopenia in Quebec, Canada," *Journal of Medical Economics*, vol. 16, no. 2, pp. 318–326, 2013.

[14] M. Mahevas, O. Fain, M. Ebbo et al., "The temporary use of thrombopoietin-receptor agonists may induce a prolonged remission in adult chronic immune thrombocytopenia. Results of a French observational study," *British Journal of Haematology*, vol. 165, no. 6, pp. 865–869, 2014.

[15] L. Cervinek, J. Mayer, and M. Doubek, "Sustained remission of chronic immune thrombocytopenia after discontinuation of treatment with thrombopoietin-receptor agonists in adults," *International Journal of Hematology*, vol. 102, no. 1, pp. 7–11, 2015.

[16] C. Santoro, F. De Angelis, E. Baldacci et al., "Thrombopoietin receptor agonists in primary immune thrombocytopenia: evaluation of efficacy (response and sustained response off treatment) and safety in a single center population," *Haematologica*, vol. 99, no. 1, p. 205, 2014.

[17] M.-E. Mingot-Castellano, C. Grande-García, D. Valcárcel-Ferreiras, C. Conill-Cortés, and L. de Olivar-Oliver, "Sustained remission in patients with primary immune thrombocytopenia after romiplostim tapering and discontinuation: a case series in real life management in Spain," *Case Reports in Hematology*, vol. 2017, Article ID 4109605, 8 pages, 2017.

[18] W. Bao, J. B. Bussel, S. Heck et al., "Improved regulatory T-cell activity in patients with chronic immune thrombocytopenia treated with thrombopoietic agents," *Blood*, vol. 116, no. 22, pp. 4639–4645, 2010.

[19] H. Zhong, W. Bao, X. Li et al., "CD16 + monocytes control T-cell subset development in immune thrombocytopenia," *Blood*, vol. 120, no. 16, pp. 3326–3335, 2012.

[20] R. K. DasGupta, L. Levine, T. Wiczer, and S. Cataland, "Initial romiplostim dosing and time to platelet response in patients with treatment refractory immune thrombocytopenia," *Journal of Oncology Pharmacy Practice*, 2018.

[21] C.-H. Tsai, J. Bussel, A. Imahiyerobo, S. I. Sandler, and B. A. Ogunnaike, "Platelet count control in immune thrombocytopenic purpura patient: optimum romiplostim dose profile," *IFAC Proceedings Volumes*, vol. 47, no. 3, pp. 11800–11805, 2014.

18

De Novo Psoriasis Vulgaris Diagnosed after Nivolumab Treatment for Refractory Hodgkin's Lymphoma, Completely Resolved after Autologous Hematopoietic Stem Cell Transplantation

Panayotis Kaloyannidis[ID],[1] **Eshrak Al Shaibani,**[1] **Miral Mashhour,**[2] **Mohammed Gamil,**[3] **Ioannis Apostolidis,**[1] **Hani Al Hashmi,**[1] and **Khalid Ahmed Al Anazi**[ID][1]

[1]*Adults Hematology and Stem Cell Transplantation Department, King Fahad Specialist Hospital, Dammam, Saudi Arabia*
[2]*Department of Pathology and Laboratory Medicine, King Fahad Specialist Hospital, Dammam, Saudi Arabia*
[3]*Dermatology Department, King Fahad Specialist Hospital, Dammam, Saudi Arabia*

Correspondence should be addressed to Panayotis Kaloyannidis; pkaloyannidis@yahoo.gr

Academic Editor: Masayuki Nagasawa

The programmed cell death protein-1 (PD-1) inhibitor nivolumab has been recently approved as an effective and safe treatment for patients with refractory/relapsed Hodgkin's lymphomas. Dermatological adverse events, mainly skin rash, have been reported in 1–5% of patients. We describe a case of de novo psoriasis vulgaris (PsV), diagnosed after nivolumab treatment for refractory Hodgkin's lymphoma. After administration of 6 cycles, skin lesions appeared in the right tibia, forearms, and dorsum of hands, and biopsy confirmed the diagnosis of PsV. The lesions completely resolved after autologous stem cell transplantation (ASCT) which was performed in the context of the treatment for the primary disease. PsV is an inflammatory skin disease, and it is considered to be mediated through cytotoxic T-cells. PD-1 blockage may lead to expansion of such T-cells, resulting thus in PsV appearance. The early published studies showed that nivolumab represents a safe treatment approach. PsV occurrence has not been reported so far in patients treated with nivolumab for hematological diseases, and it seems that long-term follow-up is necessary to fully clarify the entirety of PD-1 inhibitors' skin adverse events. Additionally, this clinical observation provides an evidence for a potential exploitation of ASCT in refractory and severe forms of PsV.

1. Introduction

The blockade of immunosuppressive pathways, also known as "immune checkpoints," represents an innovative treatment approach for patients with refractory solid and hematological malignancies [1–4]. Nivolumab (Opdivo, Bristol-Myers Squibb Company), a monoclonal antibody against programmed cell death protein-1 (PD-1), has shown extremely promising results with durable disease responses, and in May 2016, it was approved by the U.S. Food and Drug Administration for the treatment of refractory Hodgkin's lymphoma patients [5]. Given the mechanism of action that triggers T-cell activation, nivolumab may induce specific adverse events (AEs), including immune-related cutaneous toxicities. In the published clinical trials, the cutaneous complications among patients with hematological diseases are reported to be nonspecific, such as macular papular rash and pruritus, which usually are readily manageable [2–6].

We herein describe a rare dermatologic AE psoriasis vulgaris (PsV) that appeared in a patient who was treated with nivolumab for refractory classical Hodgkin's lymphoma (cHL).

2. Case Report

A 53-year-old man who was firstly treated for diffuse large B-cell lymphoma (DLBCL) presented 45 months after induction remission treatment with abdominal and inguinal lymph node (L/N) enlargement. An excisional L/N biopsy confirmed the histological type of mixed cellularity cHL; malignant cells were positive for CD30, CD15, and PAX5 and negative for CD20, CD10, CD3, BCL-2, and EMA antigens. ESHAP (etoposide, cisplatin, methylprednisolone, and cytarabine) was given as salvage treatment, and after 2 cycles, he achieved very good partial remission. Since the treatment plan was to proceed with high-dose chemotherapy and rescue with autologous stem cells transplantation (ASCT), he received an additional 3rd cycle of ESHAP for further disease control and autologous stem cell collection. After the 3rd cycle of salvage chemotherapy, the disease further responded and the stem cells collection was successful. However, he developed acute kidney injury, and the ASCT postponed till renal function recovery; the patient, based on his previous medical history (DLBCL and cHL diagnoses), received a combination of rituximab plus brentuximab vedotin as bridge treatment to ASCT. Four months later, the renal function became normal, but evaluation with PET-CT (after six cycles of combination treatment) confirmed disease progression. Subsequently, nivolumab at the dose of $3 \, mg/m^2$ every two weeks was given as a new salvage therapy. The medication was well tolerated, and no renal or any other organ function impairment was noticed. However, after the sixth infusion of nivolumab, he presented with raised nonitchy, erythematous scaly papules with silver-white coating and some annular plaques with collarettes of scales of different sizes involving the anterolateral aspects of shins and dorsa of hands, distal forearms, and both tibias (Figure 1(a)). The Köbner phenomenon was not noticed. The clinical differential diagnosis included (1) PsV, (2) erythema annulare, or (3) tinea circinata. To confirm the diagnosis, a 5 mm punch skin biopsy was obtained from the right tibia. The epidermis findings revealed hyperkeratosis and irregular acanthosis with regular elongation of rete ridges and suprapapillary thinning (Figures 1(c) and 1(d)). The upper dermis showed mild perivascular lymphocytic infiltration (Figure 1(d)). There were no evidence of Munro microabscesses and no evidence of granuloma or other specific inflammation. Although the histological findings were not the typical one, the diagnosis of PsV was made based on the clinicopathological findings and the exclusion of the other aforementioned dermatological diseases.

The patient initially received only topical treatment with steroids, and the skin lesions partially improved. He next underwent ASCT, with a conditioning regimen consisted of single-agent chemotherapy of melphalan $200 \, mg/m^2$. The skin lesions gradually improved, and 3 months after ASCT, they almost disappeared. Currently, one year after ASCT, the patient was alive in complete metabolic remission regarding his primary disease and without any evidence of residual skin lesions (Figure 1(b)).

3. Discussion

Nivolumab, although it belongs to the "monoclonal antibodies family" agents, unlikely to other monoclonal antibodies, directly triggers the T-cell activation and therefore is associated with a specific toxicity profile and adverse events that are mostly of immune origin.

In a series of patients treated with nivolumab for solid malignant diseases or lymphomas, cutaneous reactions were not uncommon and mainly concerned skin rash, pruritus, and vitiligo [2–7]. Although the exacerbation of previously diagnosed PsV is a well-described phenomenon after PD-1 inhibitor treatment, the *de novo* appearance of PsV is uncommon, and only few sporadic cases have been described so far, all of them in patients with nonhematological cancers [8–12]. Among patients with cHL who were treated with nivolumab, although skin reactions have been noticed, drug-induced psoriasis never has been reported, at least to our best knowledge [2–8, 13].

PsV is a chronic inflammatory skin disease with a complex autoimmune etiology, and it is considered to be mediated by cytotoxic T-cells and more specifically by T-cells polarized to a Th1 and Th17 fate [14]. PD-1 inhibitors have been demonstrated to augment Th1 and Th17 cell activities, and by these immunological consequences, nivolumab has been potentially implicated in either PsV new occurrence or PsV reactivation [15]. We assume that in our heavily pretreated patient, the exposure to nivolumab (even for short tem period), was quite enough to trigger residual T cells which subsequently targeted antigens on the dermis/epidermis cells resulting thus in PsV appearance.

The treatment of PsV still remains challenging, and several topical and systemic treatments (including monoclonal antibodies and immunomodulating factors) have been used and proposed so far [16, 17].

Regarding the correlation of PD-1 inhibitors treatment and PsV, Bonigen et al. published recently a review study, the largest so far, of 21 patients with reactivated or newly diagnosed PsV after PD-1 inhibitors treatment . All patients had diagnosis exclusively of solid tumor (melanoma or lung cancer). Fourteen out of 21 had been previously treated with nivolumab, and 12 of them showed improvement after local (7 patients) or systemic (5 patients) treatment. However, it is not reported whether complete resolution of PsV occurred in any patient [8].

In our case, the skin lesions mildly improved after local steroids treatment and finally resolved almost completely within 3 months after ASCT. It is well known that the symptoms of several autoimmune diseases, including psoriasis disease, can be controlled and minimized after high-dose chemotherapy followed by allogeneic or autologous stem cells rescue [18]. However, the experience of ASCT in psoriasis with only skin involvement, especially in PsV form, is extremely limited, and only sporadic cases have been reported [19–22]. We speculate that, in our case, the conditioning regimen consisted of $200 \, mg/m^2$ melphalan followed by autologous stem cell infusion facilitated the process of the complete PsV resolution.

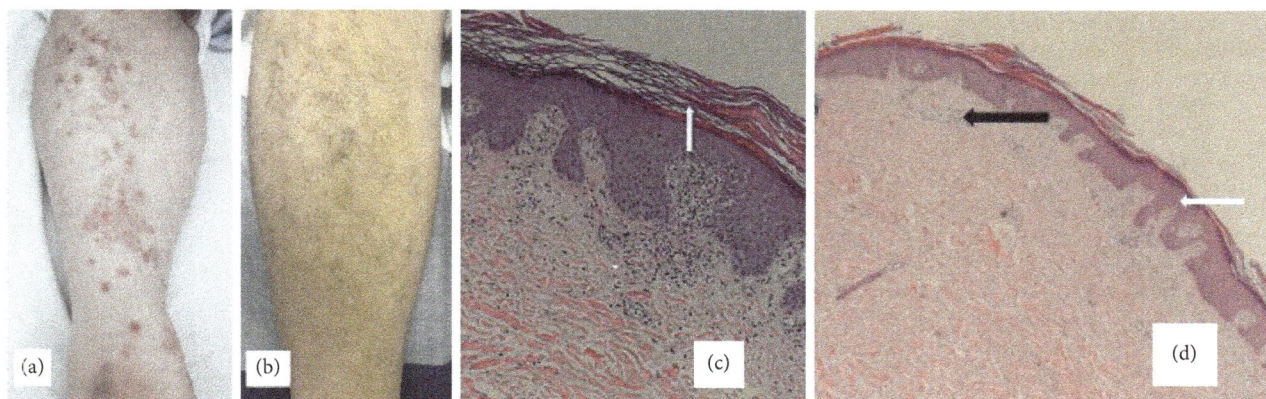

FIGURE 1: Skin lesions and skin biopsy with hematoxylin-eosin stain. (a) After 6 cycles of nivolumab and before ASCT: scaly erythematous annular plaque on the right tibia. (b) Twelve months after ASCT: skin lesions completely disappeared. (c) Skin biopsy: epidermis lesions showing hyperkeratosis. (d) Skin biopsy: lesions showing acanthosis (white arrow) and perivascular infiltration of mononuclear cells indicating chronic inflammation (black arrow).

PD-1 inhibitors have been only recently introduced in physicians' "pharmaceutical quiver" for the treatment of advanced hematological diseases. Although the early published studies showed only mild and easily manageable immune skin reactions, it seems that long-term follow-up is necessary to clarify the entirety of PD-1 inhibitors' skin adverse events. On the contrary, given its mechanism of action and its current low toxicity profile, ASCT could be studied in clinical trials as a potential therapeutic approach for patients with a severe and refractory form of PsV.

Conflicts of Interest

The authors declare that there are no conflicts of interest.

References

[1] J. Sunshine and J. M. Taube, "PD-1/PD-L1 inhibitors," *Current Opinion in Pharmacology*, vol. 23, pp. 32–38, 2015.

[2] A. M. Lesokhin, S. M. Ansell, P. Armand et al., "Nivolumab in patients with relapsed or refractory hematologic malignancy: preliminary results of a phase Ib study," *Journal of Clinical Oncology*, vol. 34, no. 23, pp. 2698–2704, 2016.

[3] P. Armand, A. Engert, A. Younes et al., "Nivolumab for relapsed/refractory classic Hodgkin lymphoma after failure of autologous hematopoietic cell transplantation: extended follow-up of the multicohort single-arm phase II checkmate 205 trial," *Journal of Clinical Oncology*, vol. 36, no. 14, pp. 1428–1439, 2018.

[4] A. Younes, A. Santoro, M. Shipp et al., "Nivolumab for classical Hodgkin's lymphoma after failure of both autologous stem-cell transplantation and brentuximab vedotin: a multicentre, multicohort, single-arm phase 2 trial," *Lancet Oncology*, vol. 17, no. 9, pp. 1283–1294, 2016.

[5] Y. L. Kasamon, R. A. de Claro, Y. Wang et al., "FDA approval summary: nivolumab for the treatment of relapsed or progressive classical Hodgkin lymphoma," *Oncologist*, vol. 22, no. 5, pp. 585–591, 2017.

[6] V. Kumar, N. Chaudhary, M. Garg, C. S. Floudas, P. Soni, and A. B. Chandra, "Current diagnosis and management of immune related adverse events (irAEs) induced by immune checkpoint inhibitor therapy," *Frontiers in Pharmacology*, vol. 8, p. 49, 2017.

[7] V. Sibaud, N. Meyer, L. Lamant et al., "Dermatologic complications of anti-PD-1/PD-1 immune checkpoint antibodies," *Current Opinion in Oncology*, vol. 28, no. 4, pp. 254–263, 2016.

[8] J. Bonigen, C. Raynaud-Donzel, J. Hureaux et al., "Anti-PD1-induced psoriasis: a study of 21 patients," *Journal of European Academy of Dermatology and Venereology*, vol. 31, no. 5, pp. e254–e257, 2017.

[9] N. Matsumara, M. Ohtsuka, N. Kikuchi, and T. Yamamoto, "Exacerbation of psoriasis during nivolumab therapy for metastatic melanoma," *Acta Dermato Venereologica*, vol. 96, no. 2, pp. 259-260, 2016.

[10] Y. Kato, A. Otsuka, Y. Miyachi, and K. Kabashima, "Exacerbation of psoriasis vulgaris during nivolumab for oral mucosal melanoma," *Journal of the European Academy of Dermatology and Venereology*, vol. 30, no. 10, pp. e89–e91, 2016.

[11] M. Ohtsuka, T. Miura, T. Mori, M. Ishikawa, and T. Yamamoto, "Occurrence of psoriasiform eruption during nivolumab therapy for primary oral mucosal melanoma," *JAMA Dermatology*, vol. 151, no. 7, pp. 797–799, 2015.

[12] S. Murata, S. Kaneko, Y. Harada, N. Aoi, and E. Morita, "Case of de novo psoriasis possibly triggered by nivolumab," *Journal of Dermatology*, vol. 44, no. 1, pp. 99-100, 2017.

[13] J. D. Ransohoff and B. Y. Kwong, "Cutaneus adverse events of targeted therapies for hematolymphoid malignancies," *Clinical Lymphoma Myeloma and Leukemia*, vol. 17, no. 12, pp. 834–851, 2017.

[14] C. W. Lynde, Y. Poulin, R. Vender, M. Bourcier, and S. Khalil, "Interleukin 17A: toward a new understanding of psoriasis pathogenesis," *Journal of American Academy of Dermatology*, vol. 71, no. 1, pp. 141–150, 2014.

[15] J. Dulos, G. J. Carven, S. J. van Boxtel et al., "PD-1 blockade augments Th1 and Th17 and suppresses Th2 responses in peripheral blood from patients with prostate and advanced melanoma cancer," *Journal of Immunotherapy*, vol. 35, no. 2, pp. 169–178, 2012.

[16] A. Nast, L. Amelunxen, M. Augustin et al., "S3 Guideline for the treatment of psoriasis vulgaris,update-short version part 1-systemic treatment," *Journal der Deutschen Dermatologischen Gesellschaft*, vol. 16, no. 5, pp. 645–669, 2018.

[17] A. Nast, L. Amelunxen, M. Augustin et al., "S3 Guideline for the treatment of psoriasis vulgaris, update-Short version part 2-Special patient populations and treatment situations," *Journal der Deutschen Dermatologischen Gesellschaft*, vol. 16, pp. 806–813, 2018.

[18] J. A. Snowden, M. Badoglio, M. Labopin et al., "Evolution, trends, outcomes, and economics of hematopoietic stem cell transplantation in severe autoimmune diseases," *Blood Advances*, vol. 1, no. 27, pp. 2742–2755, 2017.

[19] B. H. Kaffenberger, H. K. Wong, W. Jarjour, and L. A. Andritsos, "Remission of psoriasis after allogeneic, but not autologous, hematopoietic stem-cell transplantation," *Journal of American Academy of Dermatology*, vol. 68, no. 3, pp. 489–492, 2013.

[20] A. Azevedo, C. Gonçalves, M. Selores et al., "Remission of psoriasis after autologous stem cell transplantation-until when?," *European Journal of Dermatology*, vol. 27, no. 1, pp. 74-75, 2017.

[21] K. Held, R. Rahmetulla, T. W. Loew, and M. A. Radhi, "Complete resolution of guttate psoriasis following autologous SCT for Ewing's sarcoma in a pediatric patient," *Bone Marrow Transplant*, vol. 47, no. 12, pp. 1585-1586, 2012.

[22] F. Braiteh, S. R. Hymes, S. A. Giralt, and R. Jones, "Complete remission of psoriasis after autologous hematopoietic stem-cell transplantation for multiple myeloma," *Journal of Clinical Oncology*, vol. 26, no. 27, pp. 4511–4513, 2008.

19

Rare Coexistence of Acute Monoblastic Leukemia with Chronic Lymphocytic Leukemia

Vikrant Singh Bhar ⓘ,[1] Vasudha Gupta,[1] Mahak Sharma,[2] Rishi Dhawan,[3] Shilpi Modi,[4] and Mona Vijyaran[5]

[1]Associate Consultant, Department of Haematopathology, Artemis Hospitals, Gurgaon, India
[2]Senior Resident, Department of Haematopathology, Artemis Hospitals, Gurgaon, India
[3]Assistant Professor, Department of Hematology, AIIMS, New Delhi, India
[4]Associate Consultant, Department of Histopathology, Artemis Hospitals, Gurgaon, India
[5]Associate Consultant, Department of Hematooncology, Artemis Hospitals, Gurgaon, India

Correspondence should be addressed to Vikrant Singh Bhar; vikrantbhar86@gmail.com

Academic Editor: Alessandro Gozzetti

Acute monoblastic leukemia (AMoL) is a rare hematopoietic neoplasm, and simultaneous occurrence of acute monoblastic leukemia with chronic lymphocytic leukemia is very rare and only a few cases have been reported in the literature. We here report a rare case of dual hematological malignancy in an 85-year-old male. The peripheral blood and bone marrow examination revealed dual population of atypical cells, comprising large cells with opened-up chromatin having monocytic appearance and small mature-appearing lymphocytes. Flowcytometric immunophenotyping confirmed the monocytic lineage of cells, whereas small lymphocytes showed the immunophenotype consistent with chronic lymphocytic leukemia (CLL). The final diagnosis was made as acute monoblastic leukemia with associated CLL. This is a rare case scenario, and this highlights the importance of careful morphological examination and flowcytometric immunophenotyping in the exact characterization of hematopoietic malignancies.

1. Introduction

Dual hematological malignancy occurring simultaneously in a patient is a rare phenomenon. There are many case reports in literature describing dual coexistence of CLL with other hematological disorders. Brouet et al. reported eleven cases of CLL with coexistent multiple myeloma. Six of these cases expressed different immunoglobulins, suggesting biclonal nature of the disease [1]. Similar cases of dual coexistence of CLL with multiple myeloma have been reported in the past [2]. Coexistence of CLL with acute myeloid leukemia is even rarer, and only a few case reports have been reported so far. Carulli et al. have reported a case of acute myeloid leukemia with monoblastic features associated with CLL [3]. Gottardi et al. reported a similar case of acute myeloid leukemia with maturation and CLL. Authors also did clonal studies and showed that both diseases represent two different clones [4]. Lai et al. reported five cases of untreated CLL with acute myelogenous leukemia and myelodysplastic syndrome [5].

Apart from de-novo occurrence of concomitant CLL and acute myeloid leukemia, patients with CLL can rarely show transformation to acute myeloid leukemia (AML). Hatoum et al. in their review of literature found only 6 cases of CLL transforming to AML [6]. We here report such a rare case of dual hematological disorder, acute monoblastic leukemia with chronic lymphocytic leukemia confirmed by flowcytometric immunophenotyping.

2. Case Report

We here report a case of an 85-year-old male who was apparently well 15 days back, when he started developing swelling of bilateral feet. The patient also complained of decreased urine output with poor urinary stream. The patient has a history of breathlessness, more so on exertion. The patient is an ex-smoker and has a history of loss of appetite and loss of weight since 1-2 months. Also, there is a history of anemia in the past with a recorded haemoglobin

TABLE 1: Findings of bone marrow aspirates.

Blast (%)	Promonocyte (%)	Metamyelocyte (%)	Lymphocyte (%)	Monocytes (%)	Erythroid precursor (%)
54	02	01	40	01	02

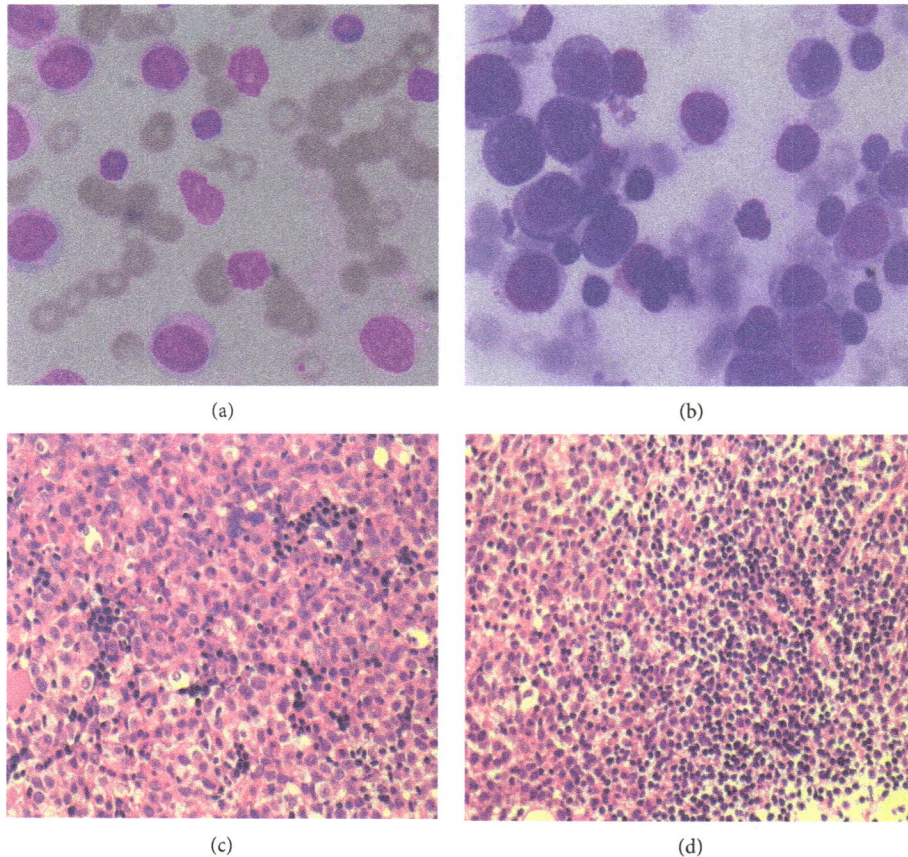

FIGURE 1: (a, b) Peripheral blood film and bone marrow aspirate showing dual population (×40, May Grunwald Giemsa). (c, d) Bone biopsy with sheets of immature cells with interstitial infiltration and nodular aggregates of lymphocytes, respectively (×40, H&E).

(Hb) level of 78 g/l. The patient's clinical examination showed multiple, nontender firm lymph nodes in the right upper jugular, middle jugular, right and left submandibular, and multiple right-sided axillary lymph nodes. His complete blood count parameters were as follows: Hb, 58 g/l; platelet count, 63×10^9/l; and total leukocyte count (TLC), 230×10^9/l. Differential counts on peripheral blood smear (PBS) were as follows: blasts, 30%; promonocytes, 5%; monocytes, 5%; neutrophils, 3%; and lymphocytes, 57%. Lymphocytes appeared mature with many smudge cells. Clinical and laboratory features of the patient were consistent with tumor lysis syndrome (TLS). Laboratory parameters supporting TLS were as follows: uric acid, 11.5 mg/dl; calcium, 7.7 mg/dl; phosphorus, 4.8 mg/dl; potassium, 4.2 meq/L;and serum creatinine, 2.42 mg/dl.

Bone marrow examination showed markedly hypercellular smears with reduced megakaryocytes and erythropoiesis. Bone marrow differential counts are summarized in Table 1. Bone marrow biopsy was markedly hypercellular

TABLE 2: Immunophenotyping results of large cells (Population 1) and small cells (Population 2).

Population 1: CD45 positive with moderate side scatter	
Positive markers	CD33, CD64, CD14(Only in minor subset with bright CD45), HLA-DR, dim CD13
Negative markers	CD19, CD3, CD5, CD10, cyCD79a, CD22, MPO, CD34, TdT, CD117
Population 2: CD45 positive with low side scatter	
Positive markers	CD19, cyCD79a, dim CD20, CD5, CD23, CD200, dim kappa
Negative markers	CD3, myeloid and monocytic markers, CD22, FMC7, CD10, immaturity markers, lambda

with sheets of immature cells with abundant cytoplasm (monocytic look) replacing normal hematopoietic elements. In addition, there were interstitial increase and intertrabecular small to large collections of mature lymphocytes. Representative pictures of peripheral blood and bone marrow findings are compiled in Figure 1.

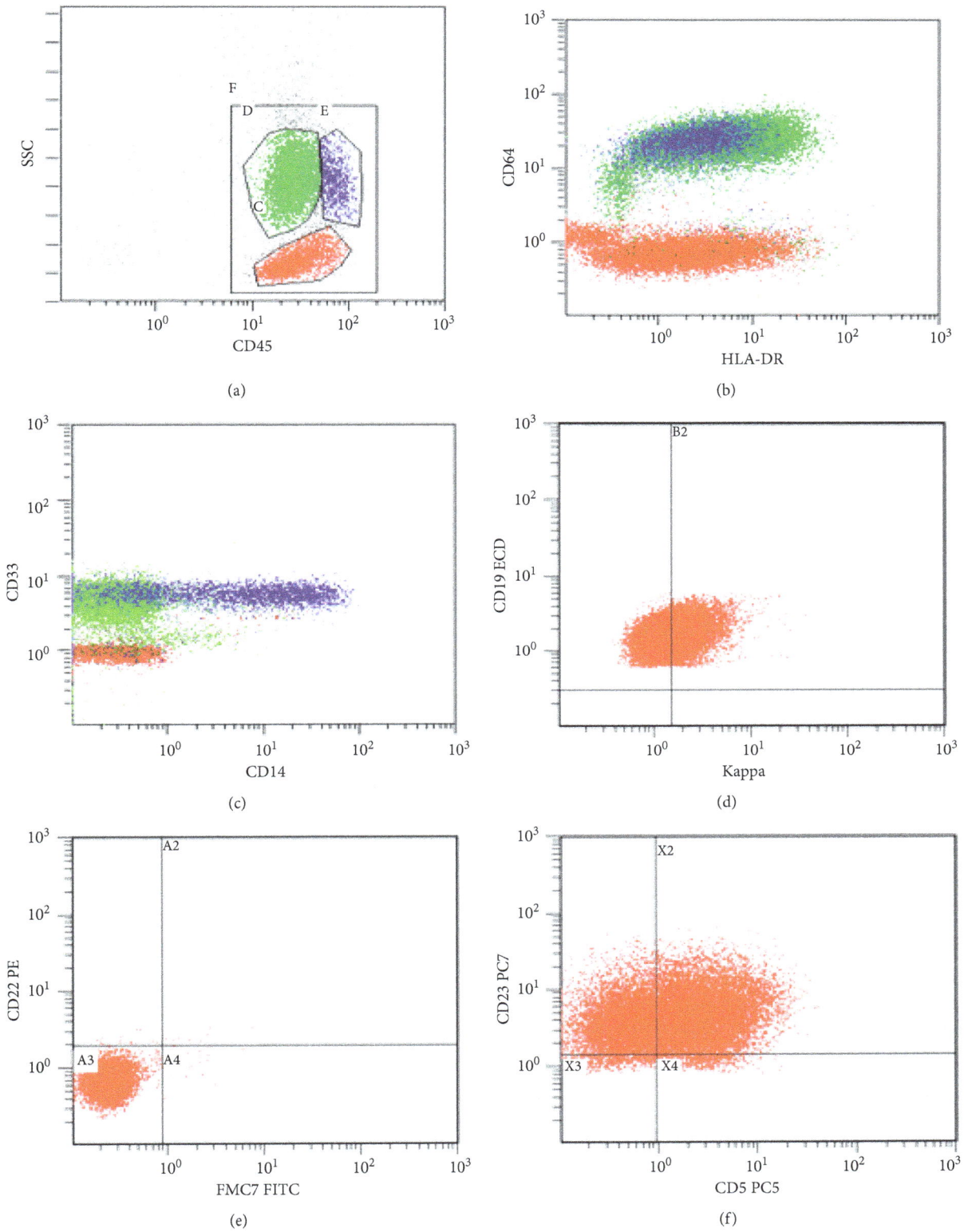

(a)

(b)

(c)

(d)

(e)

(f)

FIGURE 2: (a) CD45 versus side scatter (SSC) dot plot showing three distinct populations. Lymphocytes: CD45 positive and low side scatter (red color). Monocytic precursors and monocytes: CD45 positive and moderate side scatter (green and blue color, respectively). (b, c) Population in green and blue color was positive for CD64, CD33, and HLA-DR. More mature cells were also positive for CD14. (d–f) Lymphocytes were predominantly B cells and showed dual positivity for CD5 and CD23 with dim kappa and negative FMC7 and CD22.

PBS and bone marrow aspirate lymphocytosis made us to suspect a dual disorder, and we put a combined flowcytometry panel for acute leukemia and chronic lymphoproliferative disorder. Gating was done on CD45 versus the side scatter plot. The gating plot revealed two different populations, CD45 positive with moderate side scatter (Population 1-monoblasts) and CD45 positive with low side scatter (Population 2-lymphocytes). Population 1 showed monocytic markers with negative MPO, B-lineage, and T-lineage markers. Population 2 was positive for CD19 and showed dual positivity for CD5 and CD23. Overall immunophenotyping features were consistent with acute leukemia with monocytic differentiation and chronic lymphocytic leukemia. Immunophenotyping features are compiled in Table 2 and Figure 2.

The patient was explained about treatment options and prognosis, and he refused to undergo any further investigations and therapy.

3. Discussion

The B-cell non-Hodgkin lymphoma (B-cell NHL) makes up to 80–85% of all NHLs in India. Diffuse large B-cell lymphoma (DLBCL) is the commonest type of B-cell NHL. The prevalence of CLL of all NHL cases in India has been reported to be around 4-5% as compared to the much higher prevalence of CLL from Western countries [7].

This is a rare case of simultaneous presentation of untreated CLL with acute myeloid leukemia with monoblastic differentiation. Similar rare case reports of dual hematological malignancy have been reported in the past. In these case reports, CLL is a common partner with the second disease being plasma cell neoplasm, acute myeloid leukemia, or myelodysplastic syndrome [1–5]. The mean age of patients was 73.8 and 67.2 years in the case series reported by Brouet et al. [1] and Lai et al. [5]. Our patient was 85 years old indicating the fact that chances of having dual malignancy are higher in elderly patients as chances of acquiring plasma cells neoplasms, CLL increases, and other hematological malignancies increases with age. The peripheral smear of the patient showed distinct double population of small mature-appearing lymphocytes and large immature cells with monocytic morphological features. In addition, smudge cells were seen. Bone marrow examination also showed blasts with the second population of small lymphocytes. The review by Kotchetkov et al. at their center of 3,036 patients revealed 41 cases of synchronous dual hematological malignancy (SDHM). The authors divided SDHM cases in three groups based on the type of combination. The myeloid/lymphoid group revealed monoclonal gammopathy of unknown significance (MGUS) as the most common hematological malignancy occurring with myeloid neoplasms. This study did not find combination of CLL with AMoL [8]. The present case here represents a rare myeloid/lymphoid type of SDHM. This case highlighted the importance of careful morphological examination and deciding immunophenotyping panels as guided by morphological findings. Similarly, a close careful follow-up of the cases on therapy might help in picking up cases of CLL transforming to AML as has been rarely reported in the literature [6]. The systemic approach not only helps in exact

characterization of the disease but also saves time, labour, and reagents. Flowcytometry immunophenotyping is indispensable for exact typing and confirmation of the disease. So, a high index of suspicion, careful morphological examination, and flowcytometric immunophenotyping are required to diagnose rare case presentations.

Conflicts of Interest

The authors have declared that they have no conflicts of interest.

Acknowledgments

We are highly thankful to Mr. Gaurav Pandya and Mr. Rakesh for providing technical support for immunophenotyping.

References

[1] J. C. Brouet, J. P. Fermand, G. Laurent et al., "The association of chronic lymphocytic leukaemia and multiple myeloma: a study of eleven patients," British Journal of Haematology, vol. 59, no. 1, pp. 55–66, 1985.

[2] K. D. Hoffman and R. A. Rudders, "Multiple myeloma and chronic lymphocytic leukemia in a single individual," Archives of Internal Medicine, vol. 137, no. 2, pp. 232–235, 1977.

[3] G. Carulli, A. Marini, E. Baccelli, P. Lambelet, T. Lari, and A. Azzarà, "Association of B-chronic lymphocytic leukemia and acute myeloid leukemia," Journal of Experimental and Clinical Cancer Research, vol. 26, no. 3, pp. 421–424, 2007.

[4] M. Gottardi, V. Gattei, M. Degan et al., "Concomitant chronic lymphocytic leukemia and acute myeloid leukemia: evidence of simultaneous expansion of two independent clones," Leukemia and Lymphoma, vol. 47, no. 5, pp. 885–889, 2006.

[5] R. Lai, D. A. Arber, R. K. Brynes, O. Chan, and K. L. Chang, "Untreated chronic lymphocytic leukemia concurrent with or followed by acute myelogenous leukemia or myelodysplastic syndrome. a report of five cases and review of the literature," American Journal of Clinical Pathology, vol. 111, no. 3, pp. 373–378, 1999.

[6] H. A. Hatoum, R. A. Mahfouz, Z. K. Otrock, A. R. Hudaib, A. T. Taher, and A. I. Shamseddine, "Acute myeloid leukemia with T-cell receptor gamma gene rearrangement occurring in a patient with chronic lymphocytic leukemia: a case report," American Journal of Hematology, vol. 82, no. 1, pp. 69–72, 2007.

[7] R. Nair, N. Arora, and M. K. Mallath, "Epidemiology of non-hodgkin's lymphoma in India," Oncology, vol. 91, no. 1, pp. 18–25, 2016.

[8] R. Kotchetkov, E. Ellison, B. Pressnail, and D. Nay, "Characterization and management of synchronous dual hematological malignancies," Blood, vol. 128, no. 22, p. 5975, 2016.

20

Dural Plasmacytoma with Meningeal Myelomatosis in a Patient with Multiple Myeloma

Nieves Gascón, Héctor Pérez-Montero ⓘ, Sandra Guardado, Rafael D'Ambrosi, María Ángeles Cabeza, and José Fermín Pérez-Regadera

Radiation Oncology Department, Hospital Universitario 12 de Octubre, Madrid, Spain

Correspondence should be addressed to Héctor Pérez-Montero; hectorperezmontero@gmail.com

Academic Editor: Yusuke Shiozawa

Here, we describe the case of a 66-year-old male diagnosed with multiple myeloma who presented with generalized tonic-clonic seizures. Magnetic resonance imaging demonstrated a right solid extra-axial parieto-occipital lesion with typical characteristics of meningeal myelomatosis. Biopsy was performed, which diagnosed a dural plasmacytoma. Because of this, we started concomitant therapy with radiotherapy and lenalidomide, but the patient has a poor response to treatment and died few weeks after its initiation. Myelomatous involvement of the dura mater is a rare occurrence, given that only few cases were reported in the English literature. This presentation confers an ominous prognosis and must be a suspect diagnosis in patients diagnosed with multiple myeloma presenting neurological symptoms.

1. Introduction

Plasma cell tumors are characterized by proliferation of monoclonal plasma cells. They may appear as single lesions (solitary plasmacytoma) or multiple ones (multiple myeloma). Plasmacytomas usually develop in the bone, although they may also do so in soft tissues (called extramedullary plasmacytoma). Extramedullary plasmacytomas can arise without evidence of multiple myeloma or also in patients with multiple myeloma at any time during the course of the disease [1].

Extramedullary plasmacytoma appears most frequently in head and neck locations [2], although cases have also been reported in the upper aerodigestive tract, gastrointestinal tract, urinary bladder, central nervous system, thyroids, breast, testicles, parotid gland, lymph nodes, and skin. They represent approximately 3% of plasma cell tumors, with median age at diagnosis being 55–60. Around 2/3 of the patients are male [3, 4]. Clinical presentation depends on lesion location, direct involvement of structures or organs, or their compression [5]. Extramedullary plasmacytomas with an intracranial location can develop from the cranium,

meninges, or parenchyma. Meningeal involvement is a rare presentation with an ominous prognosis for patients [6].

We present a rare case of a patient with multiple myeloma that developed a secondary cranial plasmacytoma with meningeal involvement in the form of myelomatosis.

2. Case Study

A 66-year-old male patient presented with a history of liver transplant in 1993 due to severe acute hepatic insufficiency. Six months after transplant, he developed acute rejection with Epstein–Barr virus (EBV) viremia, requiring aggressive immunosuppression with cyclosporine and corticosteroids.

In 2009, due to generalized musculoskeletal pain not responding to analgesics, he was diagnosed with stage IIA multiple myeloma. He initiated treatment with bortezomib-dexamethasone receiving 5 cycles, after which he achieved complete remission (with disappearance of monoclonal spike in blood and urine, negative electrophoresis, and negative immunofixation).

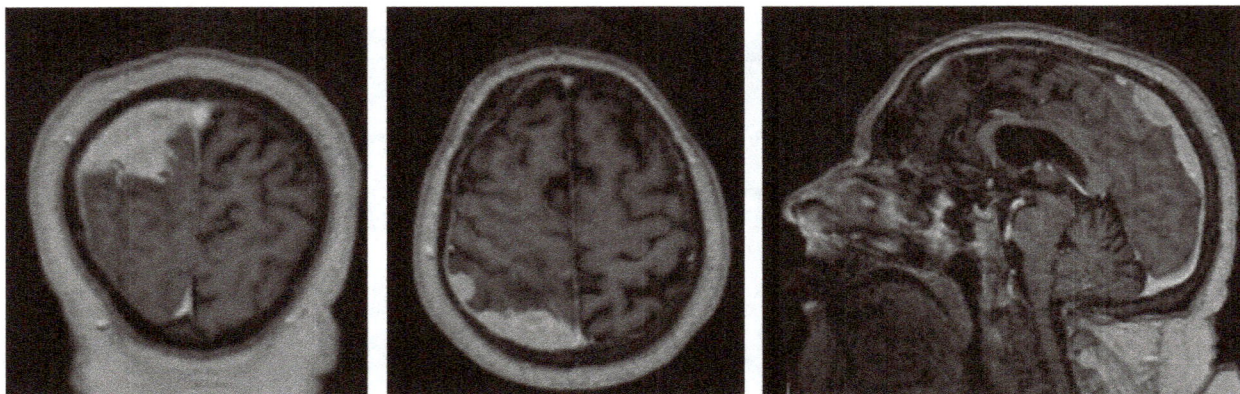

FIGURE 1: MRI showing right solid extra-axial parieto-occipital lesion with typical characteristics of meningeal myelomatosis. The tumor adapts to the underlying brain surface, is intensely enhanced with contrast, and shows adjacent pachymeningeal enhancement with focal spread through leptomeninges towards sulci in the proximal convexity, associated with vasogenic edema but not causing intracranial herniation.

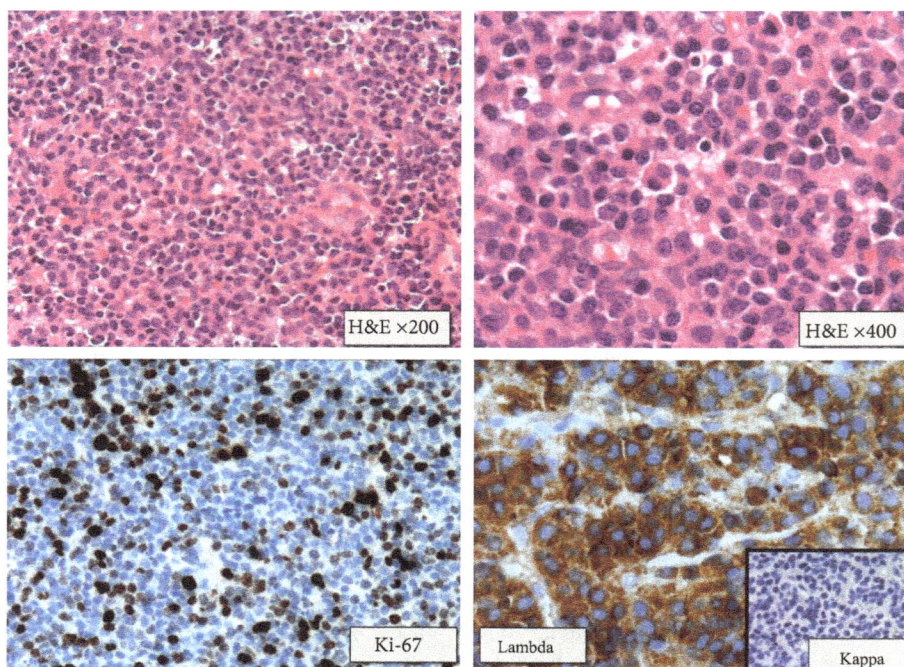

FIGURE 2: Pathological study: tumor proliferation of diffuse growth plasma cells made up of atypical plasma cells. The tumor immunophenotype shows lambda light chain restriction. The rest of the markers analyzed were negative (EMA, CD56, CD117, CD20, CD79a, and CD3). The Ki-67 proliferative index was approximately 30–40%.

In January 2013, he presented with new-onset pain in the left hip, for which a pelvic MRI was conducted which showed a lesion in the left greater trochanter compatible with a multiple myeloma secondary lesion. Treatment with bortezomib-dexamethasone was resumed with very poor tolerance leading to severe hydroelectrolytic disorders, altered bowel function, and pneumonia. At that moment, treatment was interrupted for this reason and only monthly zoledronic acid was maintained.

In May 2014, he presented with reappearance of IgA monoclonal spike, and therefore treatment with bortezomib-dexamethasone was reinitiated with excellent tolerance and

significant diminishment of pain in the left femur. He completed 4 cycles and then had bortezomib-dexamethasone every 2 months and concomitant zoledronic acid monthly.

On November 8, 2015, he was admitted to the Neurosurgery Unit due to generalized tonic-clonic seizures accompanied by sialorrhea, gaze deviation, and disorientation, with subsequent postcritical period and without sphincter relaxation. A cranial MRI was performed to investigate these symptoms. This study revealed a right solid extra-axial parieto-occipital lesion with typical characteristics of meningeal myelomatosis. The tumor adapted to the underlying brain surface showing adjacent pachymeningeal enhancement with focal spread through leptomeninges (Figure 1). A biopsy of the cranial lesion was conducted on November 12, 2015, with pathological diagnosis of plasmacytoma (Figure 2). Given the existence of meningeal myelomatosis, a spine MRI was requested that ruled out spread to this level.

Finally, it was decided to administer radiotherapy on the right parieto-occipital meningeal lesion, prescribing a total initial dose of 40 Gy with a fractionation of 2 Gy per day. Radiotherapy was administered concurrently with lenalidomide (15 mg a day) and dexamethasone (20 mg a week).

At the time 16 Gy had been received, the patient was hospitalized due to progressive deterioration of his general condition together with cognitive impairment, diminished mobility, urinary incontinence, and grade 4 thrombocytopenia. During admission, the patient deteriorated progressively with the increase of these symptoms and the appearance of clinical signs of intracranial hypertension. Given this situation and in agreement with the Hematology Service, we decided to interrupt active treatment and request evaluation from the Palliative Care Service.

3. Discussion

There are very few cases described in literature of intracranial involvement of plasmacytoma and multiple myeloma. Dural involvement without spreading from the bone and meningeal spreading of the disease are even rarer scenarios [1, 7, 8]. There is theory that this meningeal involvement may be present from the start of the disease, increasing its presence during development of this pathology. This is based on the fact that most treatments for myeloma do not cross the blood-brain barrier [9–11].

Our case is a patient diagnosed with multiple myeloma who subsequently developed a secondary dural plasmacytoma; this is usually a benign scenario with relative good prognosis. Nevertheless, this case further developed meningeal myelomatosis, which changed the course of the disease giving it an ominous prognosis.

The main diagnosis of dural plasmacytoma should be based on clinical suspicion, which shall depend on the region where the lesion is located and its extension. Clinical presentation of plasmacytomas in the dura mater is usually related to space occupation such as headache, seizures, or focal neurological deficit [1, 5, 7, 12–15]. Diagnosis should be conducted with imaging tests: in a CT scan, it is possible to confirm signal iso- or hyperintensity. An MRI shows T1 signal iso- or hyperintensity and marked T2 signal hypointensity. This presentation mimics the image of a meningioma, which is the main differential diagnosis together with metastases and lymphoma [10–12, 15]. Therefore, a histological study is essential to confirm the diagnosis. Tumor proliferation of diffuse growth atypical plasma cells with lambda chain positivity is characteristic [1, 15].

Apart from extramedullary plasmacytoma, our patient had underlying liver transplantation and long-standing immunosuppression. An increased risk of transplantation-related malignancies has been described in patients in this situation [16–19], the most common being nonmelanoma skin cancers and non-Hodgkin's lymphoma. Despite its rarity, transplant patients carry a higher risk of multiple myeloma as well. Transplant-associated non-Hodgkin's lymphomas are also commonly associated with EBV infection in extranodal sites [16]. In addition, an association between cyclosporine treatment and the development of malignancy is widely known [16, 17]. Otherwise, prognosis of transplant-related neoplasms in comparison to standard malignancies has not been well studied [18, 19].

Due to its rarity, the definitive treatment for these patients is not well known. Given its high radiosensitivity, reasonable options include radiotherapy given with curative intent, or surgical resection of the plasmacytoma, as thorough as possible, followed by adjuvant radiotherapy. The optimal doses of radiotherapy are controversial due to the scarcity of publications, but authors seem to agree that, in the absence of surgery, the minimum advisable is a total dose of 40–50 Gy given with conventional fractionation [1, 12–15].

In our case, the surgical option was discarded due to the extensive dural affectation and to the medical history of the patient, fundamentally the state of immunosuppression presented. As this was ruled out, we had to explore other therapeutic options, and together with Hematology Service, we decided to provide combined treatment with radiotherapy and lenalidomide. We based this decision on current literature supporting this drug to manage intracranial involvement of these lesions [20]. We decided to prescribe 40 Gy due to the fragile status of the patient and the use of concomitant lenalidomide. Unfortunately, during its administration, the patient presented with severe deterioration of his general condition and treatment had to be interrupted. As in previous literature, describing median survival of 6 weeks [8, 21], the meningeal involvement gave the patient an ill-fated prognosis in spite of the local and systemic treatments.

This ominous outcome in the short term may be due mainly to the massive dural involvement that affected a large part of the central nervous system. Additionally, the patient had undergone a transplant with its associated complications and had suffered a long illness receiving numerous lines of chemotherapy. This background had deteriorated its baseline situation, preventing surgical treatment and decreasing tolerance to the aggressive treatments carried out in this case. This poor tolerance caused severe clinical deterioration during admission showing intracranial hypertension symptoms and a worsening of meningeal symptoms. This deterioration precluded further active treatment.

Although dural involvement of a multiple myeloma is a very infrequent situation, it should be suspected in patients with this disease that present neurological symptoms. It is essential to conduct an imaging test, preferably an MRI to reach the diagnosis. Treatment for these patients has not been clearly defined to date. Meningeal involvement gives it an ill-fated prognosis.

Conflicts of Interest

The authors declare that they have no conflicts of interest.

References

[1] A. Cerase, A. Tarantino, A. Gozzetti et al., "Intracranial involvement in plasmacytomas and multiple myeloma: a pictorial essay," *Neuroradiology*, vol. 50, no. 8, pp. 665–674, 2008.

[2] K. M. Creach, R. L. Foote, M. A. Neben-Wittich, and R. A. Kyle, "Radiotherapy for extramedullary plasmacytoma of the head and neck," *International Journal of Radiation Oncology∗Biology∗Physics*, vol. 73, no. 3, pp. 789–794, 2009.

[3] G. M. Dores, O. Landgren, K. A. McGlynn, R. E. Curtis, M. S. Linet, and S. S. Devesa, "Plasmacytoma of bone, extramedullary plasmacytoma, and multiple myeloma: incidence and survival in the United States, 1992–2004," *British Journal of Haematology*, vol. 144, no. 1, pp. 86–94, 2009.

[4] D. A. Frassica, F. J. Frassica, M. F. Schray, F. H. Sim, and R. A. Kyle, "Solitary plasmacytoma of bone: Mayo Clinic experience," *International Journal of Radiation Oncology∗Biology∗Physics*, vol. 16, no. 1, pp. 43–48, 1989.

[5] S. Kilciksiz, O. Karakoyun-Celik, F. Y. Agaoglu, and A. Haydaroglu, "A review for solitary plasmacytoma of bone and extramedullary plasmacytoma," *The Scientific World Journal*, vol. 2012, Article ID 895765, 6 pages, 2012.

[6] M. C. Chamberlain and M. Glantz, "Myelomatous meningitis," *Cancer*, vol. 112, no. 7, pp. 1562–1567, 2008.

[7] T. H. Schwartz, R. Rhiew, S. R. Isaacson, A. Orazi, and J. N. Bruce, "Association between intracranial plasmacytoma and multiple myeloma: clinicopathological outcome study," *Neurosurgery*, vol. 49, no. 5, pp. 1039–1044, 2001.

[8] J. Bladé and L. Rosiñol, "Complications of multiple myeloma," *Hematology/Oncology Clinics of North America*, vol. 21, no. 6, pp. 1231–1246, 2007.

[9] K. Laribi, C. Mellerio, A. Baugier et al., "Meningeal involvement in multiple myeloma," *Clinical Case Reports*, vol. 3, no. 2, pp. 84–87, 2015.

[10] K. Hirata, T. Takahashi, K. Tanaka et al., "Leptomeningeal myelomatosis in well-controlled multiple myeloma," *Leukemia*, vol. 10, pp. 1672-1673, 1996.

[11] R. L. Sham, P. D. Phatak, P. A. Kouides, J. A. Janas, and V. J. Marder, "Hematologic neoplasia and the central nervous system," *American Journal of Hematology*, vol. 62, no. 4, pp. 234–238, 1999.

[12] M. Manabe, H. Kanashima, Y. Yoshii et al., "Extramedullary plasmacytoma of the dura mimicking meningioma," *International Journal of Hematology*, vol. 91, no. 5, pp. 731-732, 2010.

[13] N. Azarpira, P. Noshadi, S. Pakbaz, S. Torabineghad, M. Rakei, and A. Safai, "Dural plasmacytoma mimicking meningioma," *Turkish Neurosurgery*, vol. 24, no. 3, pp. 403–405, 2014.

[14] A. E. Hasturk, M. Basmaci, F. Erten, N. Cesur, E. R. Yilmaz, and H. Kertmen, "Solitary dural plasmacytoma mimicking meningioma and invading calvarium," *Journal of Craniofacial Surgery*, vol. 24, no. 2, pp. e175–e177, 2013.

[15] R. P. Khalili, M. Mokhtari, S. A. Fard, A. Neshat, and R. Norouzi, "Solitary dural plasmacytoma with parenchymal invasion," *Asian Journal of Neurosurgery*, vol. 10, no. 2, pp. 102–104, 2015.

[16] T. R. Pacheco, L. Hinther, and J. Fitzpatrick, "Extramedullary plasmacytoma in cardiac transplant recipients," *Journal of the American Academy of Dermatology*, vol. 49, no. 5, pp. S255–S258, 2003.

[17] R. Dempewolf and J. H. Lee, "Extramedullary plasmacytoma presenting as a nasal mass in an immunosuppressed patient: treatment after failed primary radiotherapy," *Ear Nose and Throat Journal*, vol. 87, no. 4, pp. 223–225, 2008.

[18] A. C. Wilberger and R. A. Prayson, "Intracranial involvement of posttransplant lymphoproliferative disorder multiple myeloma," *Journal of Clinical Neuroscience*, vol. 22, no. 11, pp. 1850-1851, 2015.

[19] T. Aoki, M. Kasai, Y. Harada et al., "Stable renal engraftment in a patient following successful tandem autologous/reduced-intensity conditioning allogeneic transplantation for treatment of multiple myeloma with del(17p) that developed as a post-transplantation lymphoproliferative disease following renal transplantation," *International Journal of Hematology*, vol. 98, no. 1, pp. 129–134, 2013.

[20] C. E. Devoe, J. Y. Li, and A. M. Demopoulos, "The successful treatment of a recurrent intracranial, dural-based plasmacytoma with lenalidomide," *Journal of Neuro-Oncology*, vol. 119, no. 1, pp. 217–220, 2014.

[21] S. L. Petersen, A. Wagner, and P. Gimsing, "Cerebral and meningeal multiple myeloma after autologous stem cell transplantation: a case report and review of the literature," *American Journal of Hematology*, vol. 62, no. 4, pp. 228–233, 1999.

21

High-Grade B-Cell Neoplasm with Surface Light Chain Restriction and Tdt Coexpression Evolved in a *MYC*-Rearranged Diffuse Large B-Cell Lymphoma: A Dilemma in Classification

Dina Sameh Soliman,[1,2] **Ahmad Al-Sabbagh,**[1] **Feryal Ibrahim,**[1]
Ruba Y. Taha,[3] **Zafar Nawaz,**[1] **Sarah Elkourashy,**[3] **Abdulrazzaq Haider,**[1]
Susanna Akiki,[1] **and Mohamed Yassin**[3]

[1]*Department of Laboratory Medicine and Pathology, National Center for Cancer Care and Research, Hamad Medical Corporation, Doha, Qatar*
[2]*Department of Clinical Pathology, National Cancer Institute, Cairo University, Cairo, Egypt*
[3]*Department of Hematology and Medical Oncology, National Center for Cancer Care and Research, Hamad Medical Corporation, Doha, Qatar*

Correspondence should be addressed to Dina Sameh Soliman; DSoliman@hamad.qa

Academic Editor: Tatsuharu Ohno

According to World Health Organization (WHO) classification (2008), B-cell neoplasms are classified into precursor B-cell or a mature B-cell phenotype and this classification was also kept in the latest WHO revision (2016). We are reporting a male patient in his fifties, with tonsillar swelling diagnosed as diffuse large B-cell lymphoma (DLBCL), germinal center. He received 6 cycles of RCHOP and showed complete metabolic response. Two months later, he presented with severe CNS symptoms. Flow cytometry on bone marrow (BM) showed infiltration by CD10-positive Kappa-restricted B-cells with loss of CD20 and CD19, and downregulation of CD79b. Moreover, the malignant population showed Tdt expression. BM Cytogenetics revealed t(8;14)(q24;q32) within a complex karyotype. Retrospectively, MYC and Tdt immunostains performed on original diagnostic tissue and came negative for Tdt and positive for MYC. It has been rarely reported that mature B-cell neoplasms present with features of immaturity; however the significance of Tdt acquisition during disease course was not addressed before. What is unique in this case is that the emerging disease has acquired an immaturity marker while retaining some features of the original mature clone. No definitive WHO category would adopt high-grade neoplasms that exhibit significant overlapping features between mature and immature phenotypes.

1. Introduction

The accurate classification of lymphoid neoplasms is vital for determining subsequent therapy and requires a multiparametric approach blending clinical, morphologic, immunophenotypic, and cytogenetic/molecular data to formulate a final diagnosis. Diffuse large B-cell lymphoma (DLBCL) is a diverse disease that had been subdivided into biologically heterogeneous subgroups based on morphological, molecular, and immunophenotypic diversity.

In the diagnostic evaluation of B-cell neoplasms, flow cytometric and immunohistochemical immunophenotyping

have a critical role in the differentiation of a precursor B-cell phenotype from a mature B-cell phenotype [1]. The most common types of mature B-cell neoplasms are DLBCL and follicular lymphoma (FL) (excluding Hodgkin's lymphoma and plasma cell myeloma) [2]. Tdt and CD34 are considered as surrogate immaturity markers while surface light chain restriction generally indicates a mature phenotype. Burkitt lymphoma (BL) is an aggressive B-cell neoplasm. Most of BL cases (90%) harbor the characteristic *MYC* translocation t(8;14)(q24;q32) which juxtaposes the *MYC* (previously known as *cMYC*) gene normally located at 8q24 with the *IG* heavy-chain locus, as well as the so-called

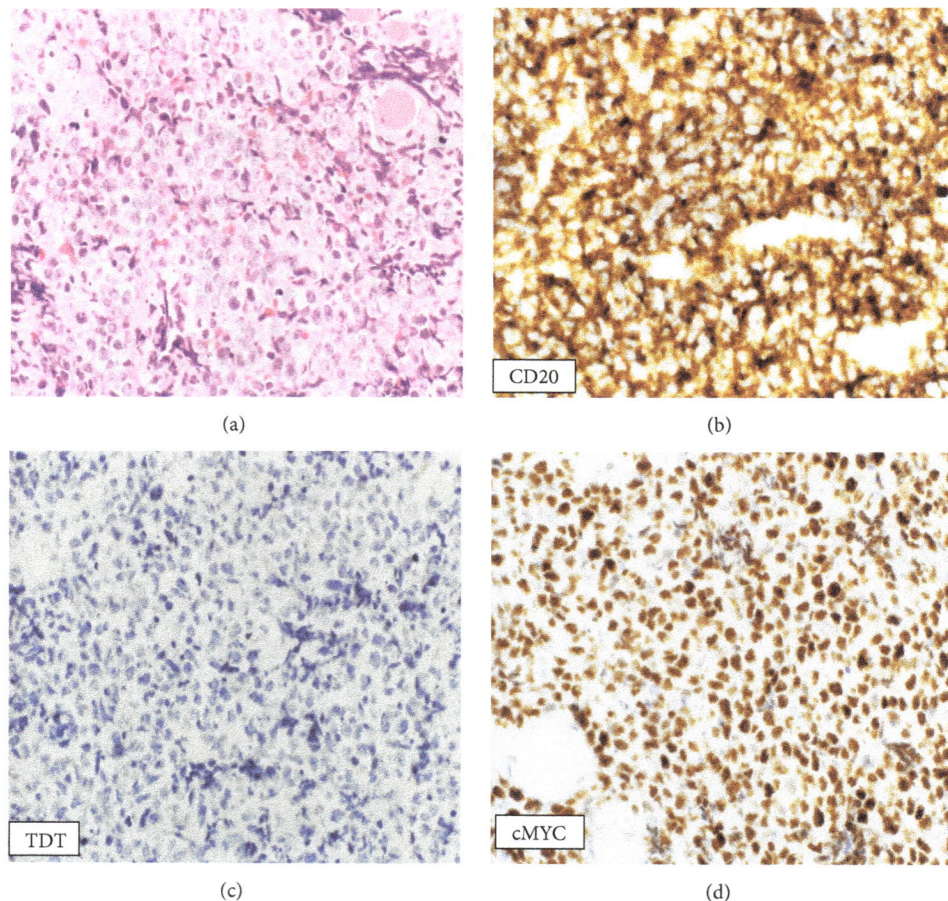

FIGURE 1: Tosillar tissue: H&E sections showing large to medium sized lymphoid cells with round to oval vesicular nuclei (a). The malignant cells are positive for CD20 immunostain (b). Immunohistochemistry (40x): Retrospectively performed on original diagnostic tonsillar tissue. Negative for TDT (c) and positive for MYC immunostains (d).

variant translocations, t(2;8)(p12;q24) and t(8;22)(q24;q11), involving the *IG* light chain genes; these are considered genetic hallmarks of BL. *MYC* rearrangements can also be found in DLBCL [3] and even in precursor B-lymphoblastic leukaemia/lymphoma (B-ALL/LBL) [4]. B-ALL is a neoplasm of B-lymphoblasts that are characteristically negative for surface immunoglobulins and express immaturity markers and markers related to the degree of B-cell differentiation. Few cases of B-ALL/LBL with surface light chain restriction have been previously reported [5].

Herein, we report unique case of an aggressive *MYC*-rearranged high-grade B-cell neoplasm with monotypic surface light chain and Tdt coexpression along with loss of pan B-cell antigens (CD19, CD20) evolved in a patient with two-month history of diffuse large B-cell lymphoma, germinal center (GC) origin.

2. Case Report

Our patient is a male in his fifties with type II diabetes, dyslipidemia, and chronic hepatitis C who presented in 2016 with a two-month history of odynophagia and neck swelling with no B-symptoms. On physical examination, a left para-tonsillar swelling was noted. Further, computerized tomography (CT) imaging showed a large soft tissue mass extending from the left tonsillar fossa and inferiorly to the left parapharyngeal wall. Magnetic resonance imaging (MRI) redemonstrated the pharyngeal mass but also bilateral cervical lymphadenopathy. The patient subsequently underwent a pan-endoscopy and excisional biopsy of the pharyngeal mass. Morphologic and immunohistochemical studies revealed a final diagnosis of DLBCL, germinal center (GC) subtype. Histopathological examination showed medium sized to large lymphoid cells with round to oval vesicular nuclei containing single to multiple nuclei (Figure 1(a)). The malignant lymphoid cells were positive for CD20 (Figure 1(b)), CD79a, PAX-5, BCL-2, BCL-6, and CD10. *cMYC* immunostain was not performed at time of diagnosis. Laboratory investigations including complete blood counts (CBC), electrolytes, and renal and liver function tests were unremarkable except for a thrombocytopenia of $102 \times 10^3/\mu L$ (150–400) and slightly elevated Lactate dehydrogenase (LDH) (274.0 U/L; *n*: 135–225).

Bone marrow examination (BM) was performed as a part of staging work-up and showed small atypical CD20-positive

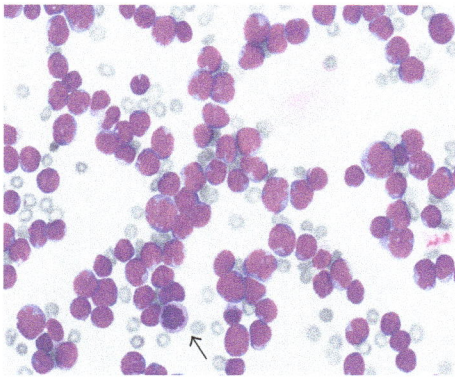

FIGURE 2: CSF cytospin preparation smear (50x) shows infiltration with many malignant lymphoid cells, some of which are larger with irregular nuclear contours, less clumped nuclear chromatin, and prominent nucleoli with few mitotic figures (black arrow) (Wright stain, ×500).

lymphoid aggregates; however BM involvement could not be confidently concluded due to suboptimal specimen quality. CSF cytologies were negative for lymphomatous involvement. The patient was diagnosed as oropharyngeal DLBCL, unconfirmed stage I, International Prognostic Index (IPI) 1-2, and he subsequently received treatment with RCHOP for 21 days and CNS prophylaxis with intrathecal (IT) methotrexate. The patient completed 6 cycles of therapy, with uncomplicated course. Mid-treatment and end of treatment Positron Emission topography (PET/CT) showed complete metabolic response.

Two months later, the patient presented with subacute onset bilateral upper limb weakness, which progressed to dense right-sided upper limb weakness, complete left sided facial weakness, and blurred vision (bilateral 6th nerve palsies). He also had a decreased level of consciousness and intermittent tonic-clonic seizures, no headache, neck stiffness, or vomiting. CT and MRI scans of the brain were unremarkable.

CBC showed thrombocytopenia ($94 \times 10^3/\mu L$); with mild leukopenia ($3.6 \times 10^3/\mu L$; 4–10). LDH was elevated at 257.0.

PET/CT imaging was unremarkable except for mild subfrontal increase uptake (possibly leptomeningeal involvement).

A lumbar puncture showed marked lymphocytic pleocytosis (WBC: 651/ul; n: 0–5) and CSF cytology showed many malignant lymphoid cells, compatible with relapsed lymphoma (Figure 2).

Restaging BM showed infiltration by abnormal medium to large-sized lymphoid cells (~40%) with slightly irregular nuclear contours, dispersed nuclear chromatin, few nucleoli, and basophilic cytoplasm (Figure 3(a)). Few cells also showed prominent cytoplasmic vacuolation. The BM biopsy was hypocellular (20–30%) with interstitial infiltration by many malignant lymphoid cells (Figure 3(b)). By immunohistochemistry (IHC), the lymphoid cells were positive for PAX-5, BCL-2 (more than 50%), cMYC, and Tdt immunostains (Figures 4(a)–4(d)) with high mitotic index reflected by strong KI-67 positivity (Figure 4(e)). The neoplastic cells

were negative for CD20 (Figure 4(f)), CD5, BCL6, CD23, MUM-1, and Cyclin D1. Flow cytometry (FCM) of the BM aspirate (Figure 5) revealed a population of kappa-restricted monotypic B-cells (~15%), expressing CD45, CD10, and CD38 (bright) and showed surface kappa light chain restriction. The monotypic B-cells are negative for CD5 and showed downregulation of pan B markers (partial expression of CD79 (dim), loss of CD19 and CD20). Moreover, the malignant population showed partial dim expression of Tdt (Figure 5(g)). FCM on CSF showed infiltration with malignant cells with the same phenotype.

Conventional cytogenetics studies revealed a complex karyotype: (48,XY,+X,t(8;14)(q24;q32),+12,13,der(14)t(1;14)(q21;p11.2),+der(?)t(1;?)(q21;?)[8]/50,idem,+der(?)t(1;?),+mar[2]/46, XY[22]) and subsequent FISH analysis confirmed the MYC/IGH, t(8;14) rearrangement in 41% of cells analyzed (Figure 6(b)). There was no evidence of BCL-6 or BCL-2 gene rearrangement.

Retrospectively, MYC and Tdt immunostains performed on original diagnostic tissue and came positive for MYC and confirmed negativity for Tdt (Figures 1(c) and 1(d)).

Screening of the original diagnostic tonsillar tissue for double hit gene rearrangement IGH/BCL2, MYC/IGH by FISH analysis was also performed at this stage and revealed positivity for MYC/IGH (Figure 6(a)) and negativity for BCL-2 gene rearrangement. Unfortunately, additional molecular studies were not available in our centre.

A final diagnosis of MYC-rearranged high-grade B-cell neoplasm stage IV (leptomeningeal and bone marrow involvement), IPI 4, with Tdt expression, likely representing early relapse/transformation of previous MYC-rearranged DLBCL was agreed upon at a multidisciplinary meeting.

The patient received triple intrathecal (Methotrexate/Cytarabine/Hydrocortisone) chemotherapy twice weekly till clearance of CSF from malignant cells. Concurrently, he started on high-dose methotrexate therapy alternating with high-dose Cytarabine (total of four cycles). Mid-treatment BM examination showed no evidence of disease. The therapy was complicated with decompensated liver failure manifested with hyperbilirubinemia, encephalopathy, and multiple sepsis with Pseudomonas aeruginosa and accordingly the patient was not a candidate for consolidation with high-dose therapy and SCT.

The patient was maintained throughout the treatment on extensive physiotherapy program. After recovery from last cycle of chemotherapy, he started to walk independently. Unfortunately, the patient relapsed again within few weeks where circulating malignant cells ~10% were detected in peripheral smear (Figure 7(a)), for which flow cytometry was performed and revealed a population of monotypic B-cells ~10% expressing CD45, CD10, CD20, and CD38, with kappa light chain restriction, loss of CD19, and acquisition of CD5 expression (Figure 7(b)). Shortly after, the patient passed away and this was four months after his first relapse.

3. Discussion

According to World Health Organization (WHO) classification system for Hematopoietic and Lymphoid

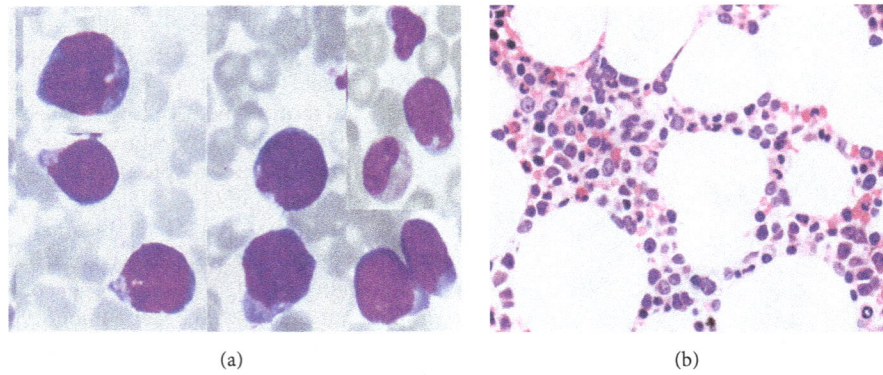

(a)

(b)

FIGURE 3: BM aspirate smear shows numerous abnormal medium to large-sized lymphoid cells. The cells showed slightly irregular nuclear contours, dispersed nuclear chromatin, and basophilic cytoplasm (Wright stain, 1,000x) (a). BMB biopsy (H&E 50x): interstitial infiltration with malignant lymphoid cells (b).

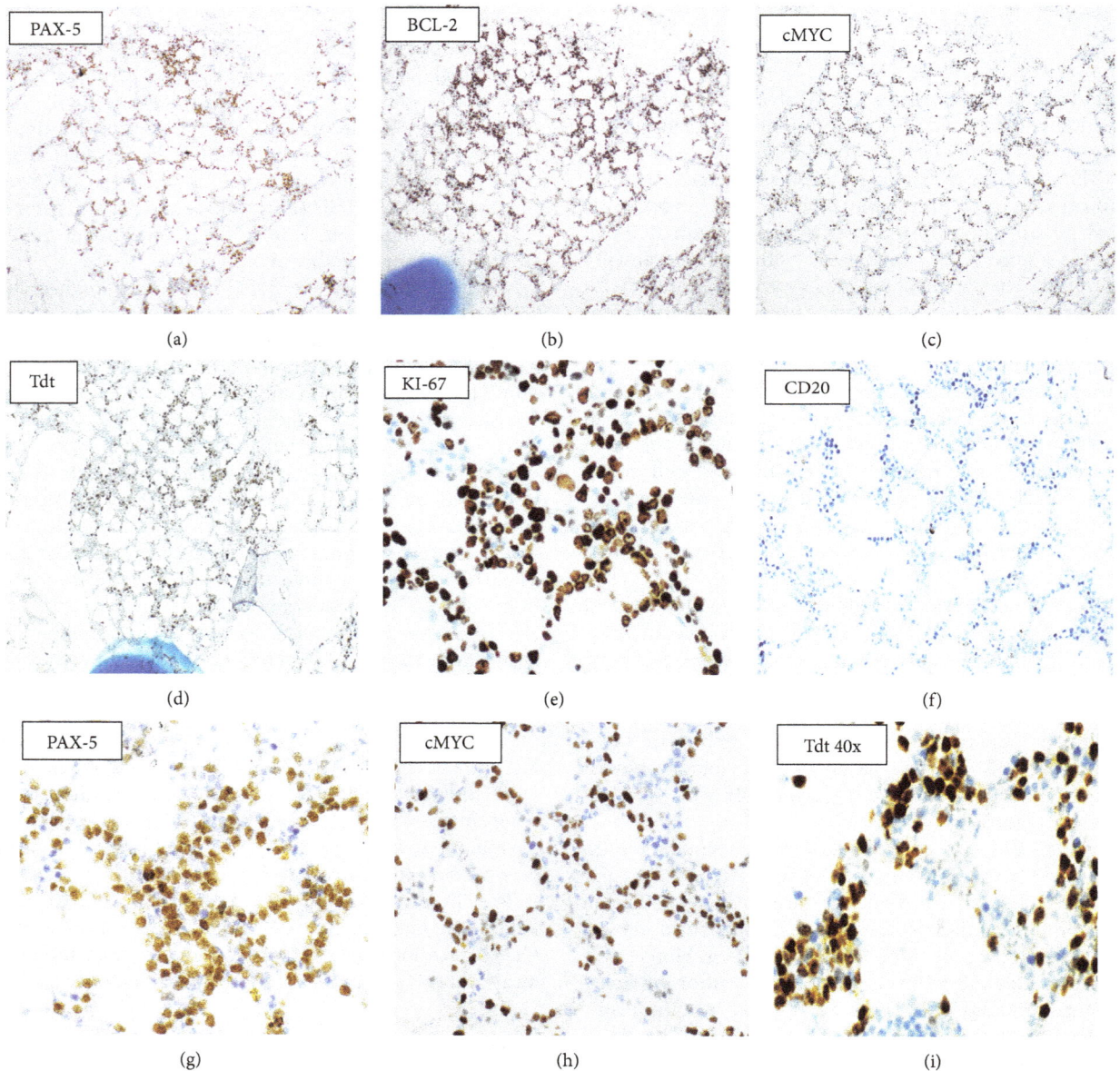

(a)   (b)   (c)

(d)   (e)   (f)

(g)   (h)   (i)

FIGURE 4: Immunohistochemistry performed on bone marrow biopsy (first relapse). The abnormal lymphoid cells are positive for PAX-5, BCL-2, *cMYC*, and TDT (a–d). KI-67 shows high proliferative index (e). The neoplastic cells are negative for CD20 (f). PAX-5 50x (g), cMYC 40x, and Tdt 40x (i).

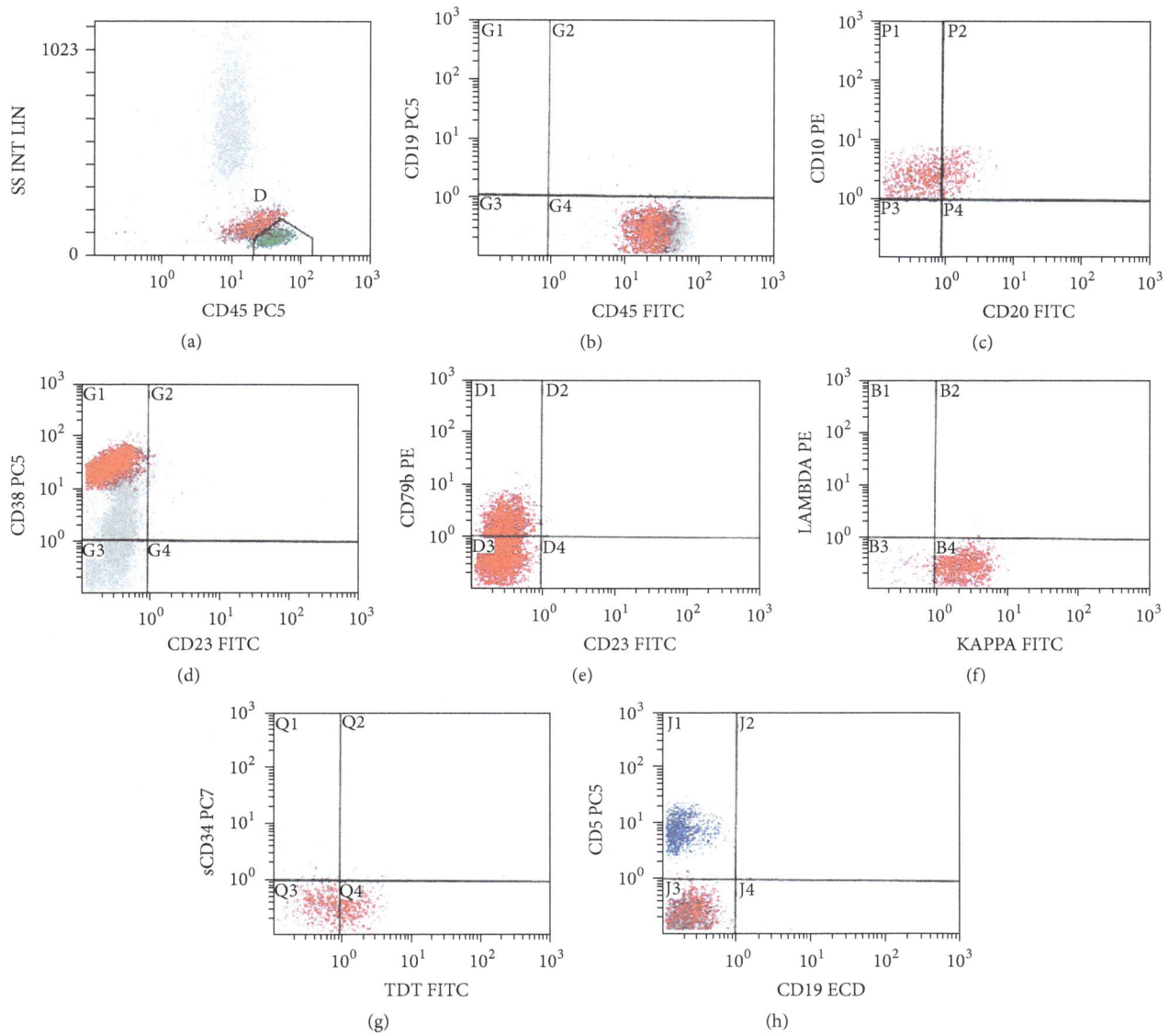

FIGURE 5: Flow cytometry on bone marrow aspirate: a population of monotypic B-cells, expressing CD45, CD10, CD38, and surface kappa light chain restriction. The monotypic B-cells are negative for CD 5 with downregulation of pan B markers (partial CD79 (dim), loss of CD19 and CD20).

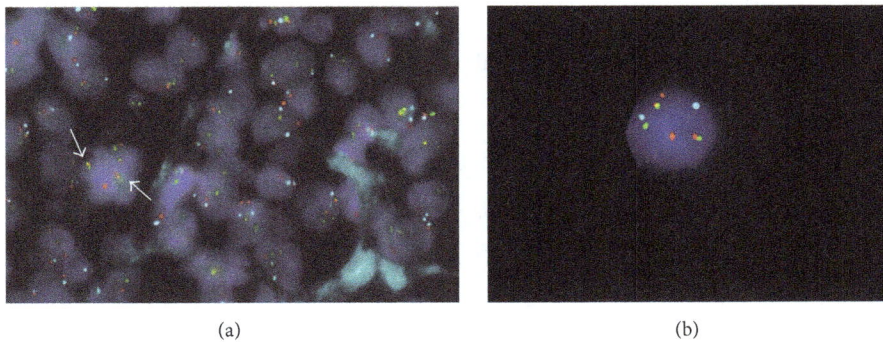

FIGURE 6: CEP8/MYC/IGH probes on tonsils (a) and bone marrow biopsy (b). The FISH analysis was performed using probes from Vysis; MYC-Orange spectrum, CEP8-Aqua spectrum, and IGH-Green spectrum. White arrows indicate the fusion signal a result of MYC/IGH translocation.

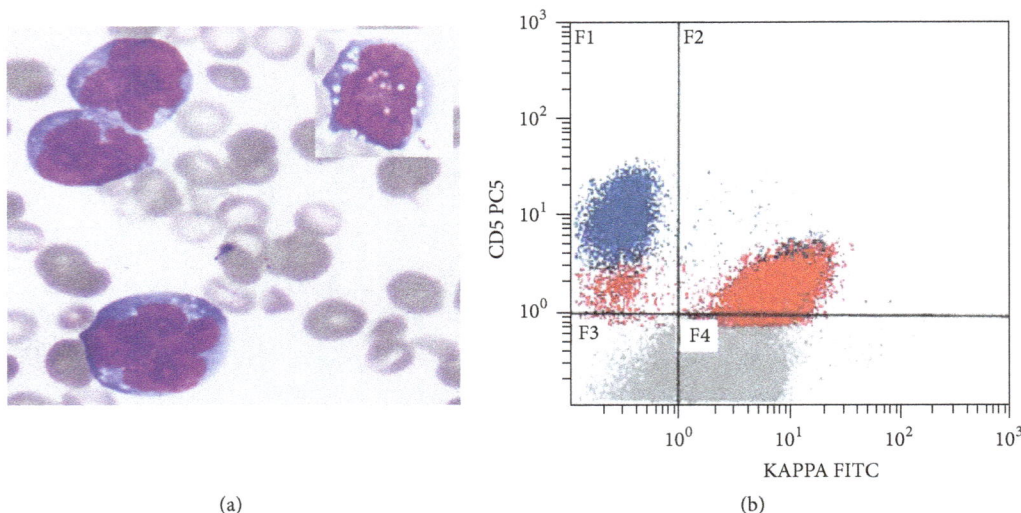

(a)   (b)

FIGURE 7: Peripheral smear at time of second relapse: Neoplastic cells show more pronounced nuclear irregularities with variable cytoplasmic vacuolation (a). Wright stain, 1,000x magnification. Flow cytometry on peripheral blood showed malignant cells with CD5 acquisition (b).

neoplasms (2008) [6], neoplasms of the B-lymphoid cell lineage can be broadly classified into those having a precursor B-cell or a mature B-cell phenotype and this is also kept in the latest WHO 2016 update in which Tdt expression was considered exclusive for precursor B-cell neoplasms [7]. MYC gene is rearranged in 5% to 15% of DLBCL, NOS, and is frequently associated with BCL2 or, to a lesser extent, BCL6 translocation, in the so-called "double hit" (DH) or "triple-hit" lymphomas that are included in the updated revision of WHO classification within the new category of high-grade B-cell lymphoma (HGBL), with rearrangements of MYC and BCL2 and/or BCL6 [7, 8]. MYC protein expression is detected in a much higher proportion of DLBCL (30%–50%) and is associated with concomitant expression of BCL2 in 20% to 35% of cases [9]. Most of these tumors do not carry MYC/BCL2 chromosomal rearrangements and have been labelled as "double-expressor lymphoma (DE)." There is some controversy about the prognosis of DE lymphomas, however; several studies showed that this category has an inferior outcome compared to other DLBCL, NOS, but they are not as aggressive as the HGBL with rearrangements of MYC and BCL2 and/or BCL6 [10, 11].

Back to our case, which demonstrated quite unusual morphologic, immunophenotypic, and cytogenetics combination, it was rather challenging to classify the disease according to WHO, to ascertain the cell of origin or to link it to original disease (at presentation).

Given the prior history of recently diagnosed DLBCL (GC), the most relevant diagnosis was relapsing DLBCL. However, in view of the aggressive presentation with systemic involvement and the marked immunophenotypic aberrancies (including Tdt expression), a simple diagnosis of relapsed DLBCL could not be committed.

An alternative scenario was to consider the latter presentation as a different emerging immature clone unrelated to original disease. This proposition was supported by the purely extranodal involvement (BM and CSF), aggressive behavior, and immunophenotypic differences especially the acquisition of Tdt, the hallmark of cell immaturity. For the latter reason, B-lymphoblastic leukaemia/lymphoma (B-ALL) was considered in the differential diagnosis.

Despite the unequivocal expression of Tdt (by IHC and FCM) and the well documented expression of surface immunoglobulin in cases of B-lymphoblastic lymphoma [3], in addition to the fact that classic MYC translocation can be detected in about 7% of B-ALL/LBL cases [12] and its presence by no means excludes a diagnosis of B-ALL/LBL, however, there was a more convincing evidence that we are dealing with a mature B-cell neoplasm that acquired Tdt expression as an immunophenotypic drift or as a manifestation of higher grade transformation/clonal evolution rather than a novel immature clone. This was supported by lack of any additional morphologic or immunophenotypic features that are supportive of immaturity; as the malignant cells were not really having blastoid morphology, with bright CD45 expression, negative CD34, and positive surface immunoglobulin with kappa light chain restriction. In addition, loss of CD20 could not be considered as supportive evidence of immaturity as this could be simply related to Rituximab treatment rather than de novo, especially that the cells had regained CD20 expression in second relapse. All the aforementioned features made the diagnosis of denovo B-ALL less likely.

Regain of CD20 within relatively short time from Rituximab therapy and the acquisition of CD5 later in the course of the disease would suggest a malignant clone with high genomic instability evidenced by the complex karyotype detected.

Putting together the morphologic, immunophenotypic, and cytogenetic findings as well as the prior history of recently diagnosed DLBCL with triple BCL-2, BCL-6, and cMYC protein expression (on the original diagnostic tissue), the diagnostic category of "B-cell lymphoma unclassifiable, with features intermediate between DLBCL and BL (BCLU)" (WHO 2008) was proposed.

According to the revised WHO (2016) [7], it was again difficult to confidently categorize this disease; however the three most relevant categories are as follows:

> Diffuse large B-cell lymphoma, NOS, with coexpression of MYC and BCL2 protein.
>
> Or high-grade B-cell lymphoma, with MYC and BCL2 and/or BCL6 rearrangements*: includes all "double-/triple-hit" lymphomas other than FL or lymphoblastic lymphomas.
>
> Or high-grade B-cell lymphoma, NOS*: for cases intermediate between DLBCL and BL, but lack a MYC and BCL2 and/or BCL6 rearrangement.

In the case reported here, the first presentation (but not at relapse) would probably fit into the first category with coexpression of MYC and BCL2 protein (double-expressor lymphoma). The absence of solid evidence of BCL2/BCL-6 gene rearrangements by FISH or standard cytogenetics together with detection of classic MYC translocation and coexpression of surface immunoglobulin and Tdt: the latter presentation would not fit into any of the previously listed categories as all should be negative for Tdt.

Even though no definite final classification could be confidently made, we considered the case as high-grade B-cell neoplasm probably representing a clonal evolution/transformation/dedifferentiation from MYC-R DLBCL with acquired Tdt expression.

MYC-R DLBCL have a higher rate of CNS involvement at presentation and posttreatment [13, 14]. Furthermore, a recent study [15] demonstrated that coexpression of MYC and BCL2 by IHC in DLBCL predicted risk of CNS relapse independent of other established variables. However, thus far there are no unique clinical or pathologic features that can identify MYC-R lymphomas in practice. However, a recent study [16] showed that bright CD38 expression and dim CD45 expression are unique to MYC-R and not non-MYC-R DLBCL.

The loss of pan-B-cell markers in our case was also rather peculiar. The vast majority of de novo cases of mature B-cell lymphoma express CD20 and/or CD19 although any one of these pan-B-cell markers may be rarely lost [17, 18]. The most common clinical scenario where CD20 loss is seen in mature B-cell lymphomas is in the relapse/recurrence setting post-Rituximab therapy months or even years after therapy [19]. While CD20 loss can possibly be explained by Rituximab effect, concurrent absence of CD19 and CD20 and downregulation of CD79 are extremely rare in mature B-cell neoplasms neither at initial diagnosis nor at relapse. CD19-cre/Pax5fl/- mice, which lose Pax5 in CD19 positive cells, die within 8 months of birth from aggressive lymphomas that express B220 and Ig μ but lack CD19 and other B-cell markers [20].

Rare cases of DHL presenting with Tdt expression have been reported, most with the morphology and immunophenotype of B-LBL, arising from or presenting simultaneously with FL [21–23]. Loghavi et al., 2015 [24], have reported five

cases of Tdt-positive B-cell neoplasms with BCL2 rearrangements and MYC rearrangements; four of these had high-grade blastoid neoplasms at presentation while the fifth case was transformed from preceding follicular lymphoma. All these reported tumors were positive for CD10, CD19, and Tdt and negative or only dimly positive for CD20 and importantly negative for surface immunoglobulins.

Blastic transformation of FL to BL is a rare event but has been documented for more than 25 years [25]. DHL arising from or presenting concurrently with FL has also been rarely reported [14, 21, 24–26]. On the other hand, transformation of DLBCL (GC) into B-LBL is a very rare event. The mechanism of transformation of FL is not well understood and different models had been proposed.

A mechanism of "dedifferentiation" of lymphoma cells into more immature stages as a result of secondary genetic events has been suggested in our case. Although no molecular studies were performed as this test is not available in our institution, the immunophenotypic and genetic similarities between the original neoplasm and the second presentation (including mature phenotype, CD10 positivity, BCL-2 expression, and cMYC gene rearrangement) have suggested that the two neoplasms probably had originated from a common B-cell clone or the second presentation has emerged from clonal evolution of its former DLBCL and "dedifferentiated" into more immature stage. Another possibility is that there was an additional minor undetected clone at time of presentation.

It has been rarely reported that MYC-rearranged B-lymphomas can present with features suggestive of immaturity, including Tdt expression. However, the significance of Tdt acquisition during disease course/relapse was not clearly addressed before. What is unique in this case is that the emerging disease has acquired an immaturity marker (Tdt) while keeping some immunophenotypic and cytogenetics features of the original mature clone.

4. Conclusion

In conclusion, in this case, the changes in the biological characteristics of tumor cells postchemotherapy and acquisition of immunophenotypic aberrancies including Tdt expression had led to early relapse with aggressive clinical presentation and fatal outcome. The importance of early recognition of MYC expression (which might have modified the treatment protocol) is questionable. An extensive literature review did not identify a similar case of a B-cell neoplasm with such unusual immunophenotypic aberrancies (particularly Tdt expression) that likely clonally evolved from MYC-R DLBCL. Reporting this case with such peculiar immunophenotypic features would probably spotlight cases of Tdt-positive mature B-cell neoplasms. Although these cases were rarely reported, there is no definitive WHO category that can adopt such high-grade neoplasms with significant overlapping features between mature and immature phenotypes.

As Tdt is a hall mark of immaturity and considered as a differentiating marker between mature and immature B-cell neoplasms (WHO 2016), we recommend including Tdt in the routine immunophenotyping panel in cases of aggressive mature B-cell neoplasms particularly DH and DE DLBCL to recognize those aggressive neoplasms which lack solid clinicopathological characterization in the literature, to draw more attention to the effect of Tdt expression on treatment response and disease outcome. It is also of interest to identify the probable molecular mechanisms implemented in disease pathogenesis and exploring the role of "dedifferentiation" which has not been previously discussed in context of DLBCL transformation.

Conflicts of Interest

The authors declare that there are no conflicts of interest regarding the publication of this paper.

Acknowledgments

The authors gratefully acknowledge the contributions of all the staff of the flow cytometry and cytogenetics laboratories at the National Center for Cancer Care and Research in specimen processing and data collection. The authors also gratefully acknowledge the contribution of Dr. Vignesh Shanmugam.

References

[1] C. D. Jennings and K. A. Foon, "Recent advances in flow cytometry: application to the diagnosis of hematologic malignancy," *Blood*, vol. 90, no. 8, pp. 2863–2892, 1997.

[2] Anon, "A clinical evaluation of the International Lymphoma Study Group clas- sification of non-Hodgkins lymphoma. The Non-Hodgkins Lymphoma Classification Project," *Blood*, vol. 89, pp. 3909–3918, 1997.

[3] M. Hummel, S. Bentink, H. Berger et al., "A biologic definition of Burkitt's lymphoma from transcriptional and genomic profiling," *The New England Journal of Medicine*, vol. 354, no. 23, pp. 2419–2430, 2006.

[4] A. V. Moorman, L. Chilton, J. Wilkinson, H. M. Ensor, N. Bown, and S. J. Proctor, "A population-based cytogenetic study of adults with acute lymphoblastic leukemia," *Blood*, vol. 115, pp. 206–214, 2010.

[5] R. Kansal, G. Deeb, M. Barcos et al., "Precursor B lymphoblastic leukemia with surface light chain immunoglobulin restriction: a report of 15 patients," *American Journal of Clinical Pathology*, vol. 121, no. 4, pp. 512–525, 2004.

[6] S. H. Swerdlow, E. Campo, N. L. Harris et al., *WHO Classification of Tumours of Haematopoietic and Lymphoid Tissues*, 4 edition, 2008.

[7] S. H. Swerdlow, E. Campo, S. A. Pileri et al., "The 2016 revision to the World Health Organization classification of myeloid neoplasms and acute leukemia," *Blood*, vol. 127, no. 20, pp. 2375–2390, 2016.

[8] S. H. Swerdlow, "Diagnosis of 'double hit' diffuse large B-cell lymphoma and B-cell lymphoma, unclassifiable, with features intermediate between DLBCL and Burkitt lymphoma: When and how, FISH versus IHC," *Hematology*, vol. 2014, no. 1, pp. 90–99, 2014.

[9] K. Karube and E. Campo, "MYC Alterations in Diffuse Large B-Cell Lymphomas," *Seminars in Hematology*, vol. 52, no. 2, pp. 97–106, 2015.

[10] Johnson N. A., Slack G. W., Savage K. J. et al., "Concurrent expression of MYC and BCL2 in diffuse large B-cell lymphoma treated with rituximab plus cyclophosphamide, doxorubicin, vincristine, and prednisone," *Journal of Clinical Oncology*, vol. 30, no. 28, pp. 3452–3459, 2012.

[11] T. J. Molina, D. Canioni, C. Copie-Bergman et al., "Young patients with non–germinal center B-cell–like diffuse large B-cell lymphoma benefit from intensified chemotherapy with ACVBP plus rituximab compared with CHOP plus rituximab: analysis of data from the Groupe d'Etudes des Lymphomes de l'Adulte/Lymphoma Study Association phase III trial LNH 03-2B," *Journal of Clinical Oncology*, vol. 32, no. 35, pp. 3996–4003, 2014.

[12] A. V. Moorman, L. Chilton, J. Wilkinson, H. M. Ensor, N. Bown, and S. J. Proctor, "A population-based cytogenetic study of adults with acute lymphoblastic leukemia," *Blood*, vol. 115, pp. 206–214, 2010.

[13] S. Li, P. Lin, L. E. Fayad et al., "B-cell lymphomas with MYC/8q24 rearrangements and IGH@BCL2/t(14;18) (q32;q21): an aggressive disease with heterogeneous histology, germinal center B-cell immunophenotype and poor outcome," *Modern Pathology*, vol. 25, no. 1, pp. 145–156, 2012.

[14] M. Snuderl, O. K. Kolman, Y.-B. Chen et al., "B-cell lymphomas with concurrent IGH-BCL2 and MYC Rearrangements are aggressive neoplasms with clinical and pathologic features distinct from burkitt lymphoma and diffuse Large B-cell lymphoma," *American Journal of Surgical Pathology*, vol. 34, no. 3, pp. 327–340, 2010.

[15] K. J. Savage, G. W. Slack, A. Mottok et al., "Impact of dual expression of MYC and BCL2 by immunohistochemistry on the risk of CNS relapse in DLBCL," *Blood*, vol. 127, no. 18, pp. 2182–2188, 2016.

[16] H. Horn, A. M. Staiger, M. Vöhringer et al., "Diffuse Large B-cell Lymphomas of Immunoblastic Type Are a Major Reservoir for MYC-IGH Translocations," *The American Journal of Surgical Pathology*, vol. 39, no. 1, pp. 61–66, 2015.

[17] M. Kimura, M. Yamaguchi, S. Nakamura et al., "Clinicopathologic significance of loss of CD19 expression in diffuse large B-cell lymphoma," *International Journal of Hematology*, vol. 85, no. 1, pp. 41–48, 2007.

[18] P. G. Chu, S. Loera, Q. Huang, and L. M. Weiss, "Lineage Determination of CD20- B-Cell Neoplasms: an Immunohistochemical Study," *American Journal of Clinical Pathology*, vol. 126, no. 4, pp. 534–544, 2006.

[19] J. Hiraga, A. Tomita, T. Sugimoto et al., "Down-regulation of CD20 expression in B-cell lymphoma cells after treatment with rituximab-containing combination chemotherapies: Its prevalence and clinical significance," *Blood*, vol. 113, no. 20, pp. 4885–4893, 2009.

[20] C. Cobaleda, W. Jochum, and M. Busslinger, "Conversion of mature B cells into T cells by dedifferentiation to uncommitted progenitors," *Nature*, vol. 449, no. 7161, pp. 473–477, 2007.

[21] L. Moench, Z. Sachs, G. Aasen, M. Dolan, V. Dayton, and E. L. Courville, "Double- and triple-hit lymphomas can present with features suggestive of immaturity, including TdT expression, and create diagnostic challenges," *Leukemia and Lymphoma*, vol. 57, no. 11, pp. 2626–2635, 2016.

[22] D. De Jong, B. M. H. Voetdijk, G. C. Beverstock, G. J. B. Van Ommen, R. Willemze, and P. M. Kluin, "Activation of the c-myc oncogene in a precursor-B-cell blast crisis of follicular lymphoma, presenting as composite lymphoma," *New England Journal of Medicine*, vol. 318, no. 21, pp. 1373–1378, 1988.

[23] A. M. Harrington, H. Olteanu, S. H. Kroft, and C. Eshoa, "The unique immunophenotype of double-hit lymphomas," *American Journal of Clinical Pathology*, vol. 135, no. 4, pp. 649-650, 2011.

[24] S. Loghavi, J. L. Kutok, and J. L. Jorgensen, "B-acute lymphoblastic leukemia/lymphoblastic lymphoma," *American Journal of Clinical Pathology*, vol. 144, no. 3, pp. 393–410, 2015.

[25] S. Li, V. L. Weiss, X. J. Wang et al., "High-grade B-cell lymphoma with MYC rearrangement and without BCL2 and BCL6 rearrangements is associated with high P53 expression and a poor prognosis," *American Journal of Surgical Pathology*, vol. 40, no. 2, pp. 253–261, 2016.

[26] K. H. Young, Q. Xie, G. Zhou et al., "Transformation of follicular lymphoma to precursor B-cell lymphoblastic lymphoma with c-myc gene rearrangement as a critical event," *American Journal of Clinical Pathology*, vol. 129, no. 1, pp. 157–166, 2008.

22

Extensive Bone Marrow Necrosis: Initial Presentation in Sickle Cell Anemia

Sameera A. Alsafwani,[1] Abdulwahed Al-Saeed,[2] and Rehab Bukhamsin[3]

[1]*Qatif Central Hospital (QCH), Qatif, Saudi Arabia*
[2]*Dammam Medical Complex (DMC), Dammam, Saudi Arabia*
[3]*Dammam Regional Laboratory and Blood Bank (DRL), Dammam, Saudi Arabia*

Correspondence should be addressed to Sameera A. Alsafwani; sameeraalsafwani@gmail.com

Academic Editor: Akimichi Ohsaka

Bone marrow necrosis (BMN) is a rare clinical entity that was first described in an autopsy of a sickle cell disease (SCD) patient and is defined as ill-defined necrotic cells in an amorphous eosinophilic background with preservation of cortical bone. The pathophysiology of BMN is not well known; however, occlusion of the bone marrow microcirculation with subsequent hypoxia and cell injury has been thought to be common underlying features. Malignancy has been identified to be the primary cause in 90% of the cases whereas SCD was found in only 2%. In this report we present an unusual case of SCD with late onset of the disease whose initial presentation was extensive BMN. The patient was not known previously to have SCD, when suddenly she presented with severe cytopenias and marked elevation in serum lactate dehydrogenase (LDH). Bone marrow examination was done to exclude bone marrow infiltration, and BMN with dilated marrow sinuses full of irreversibly sickled cells were the unexpected findings. Patients with a mild SCD phenotype are at high risk of BMN. Thus, a high index of suspicion must be borne in mind, particularly in an area of high SCD prevalence, to recognize and prevent this catastrophic complication.

1. Introduction

Bone marrow necrosis (BMN) is rarely encountered in clinical practice. It was first described in an autopsy of a sickle cell disease (SCD) patient by Wade and Stevenson [1]. BMN refers to necrosis of myeloid tissue and medullary stroma in large areas of the haemopoietic bone marrow that results in an amorphous eosinophilic background, ill-defined necrotic cells with preservation of the cortical bone [2]. The bone marrow trephine shows disruption of normal marrow architecture with loss of fat spaces but generally with preservation of the specular architecture [3]. The incidence of BMN varies among different reports, ranging from 0.3 to 37% [3]. Malignancy has been identified to be the primary cause of BMN in more than 90% of the cases [4]. Other nonmalignant causes include hemoglobinopathies, infections, drugs, anorexia nervosa, hemolytic uremic syndrome (HUS), antiphospholipid syndrome, and disseminated intravascular coagulopathy (DIC) [3, 5, 6]. SCD was found to be the primary cause in only 2% of the cases [4]. Although the pathophysiology of BMN is not well defined, occlusion of the bone marrow microcirculation is assumed to be the initiating factor [7]. Occlusion of the microcirculation could be caused by variable factors such as tumor cell emboli, fibrin thrombi, toxic effect of drugs, radiation, bacterial infection, or cytokines [2, 8, 9]. Patients with extensive BMN usually present with fever, bone pain, and fatigue and have pancytopenia with a leucoerythroblastic picture in the peripheral blood film (PBF) and, characteristically, a striking number of nucleated red blood cells (NRBCs) [10]. Elevated serum lactate dehydrogenase (LDH), alanine transferase (ALT), alkaline phosphates (ALP), and uric acid levels are also common features [4]. Examination of bone marrow biopsy is a prerequisite for the accurate diagnosis of BMN. We report an unusual case of a 26-year-old Saudi female whose bone marrow was referred for evaluation due to her clinical presentation with generalized body aches, jaundice, hepatosplenomegaly with anemia, and thrombocytopenia.

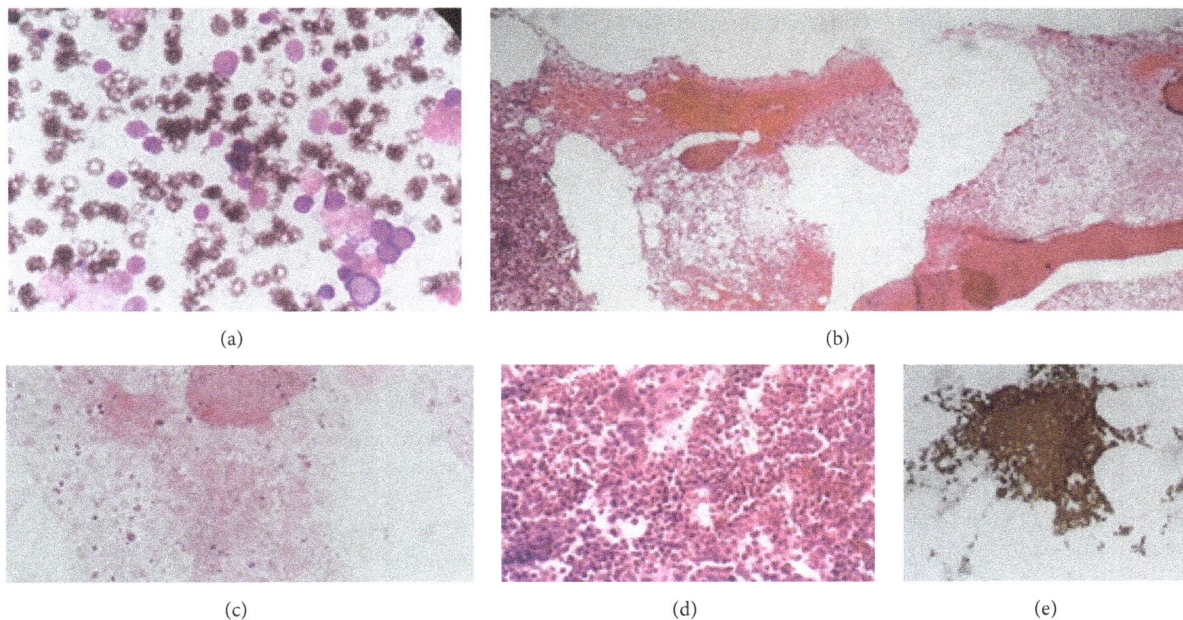

FIGURE 1: (a) Bone marrow aspirate showing an amorphous necrotic material (Giemsa stain ×100). (b) Extensive BMN in the trephine biopsy (H&E ×4). (c) Dilated sinus full of sickle cells in a background of ill-defined eosinophilic material (H&E ×40). (d) Intact area with erythroid hyperplasia (H&E ×40). (e) Spectrin stain showing the extent of erythroid hyperplasia (IHC, spectrin ×10).

2. Case Presentation

A 26-year-old Saudi female with known diabetes mellitus (DM) type-1 was admitted with jaundice, generalized body aches, and abdominal distention. She gave a history of chest infection that has been treated with antibiotics three days prior to her presentation. The family denied any previous hospitalizations or similar episodes in the past. Her mother and father are second-degree relatives with a history of sickle cell trait (SCT) in the father and DM type-1 in her identical twin sister. On examination the patient was conscious, alert, jaundiced, and not in distress and looked pale. Her vital signs were normal with clear chest examination and had a normal cardiovascular examination. Abdominal examination showed hepatosplenomegaly with ascites and she had intact central nervous system (CNS) examination. The initial blood count showed severe anemia with hemoglobin (Hb) of 5 g/dL (normal range 12.5–18 g/dL) and thrombocytopenia with platelet count of 5×10^9/L (normal range 150–450 × 10^9/L). Reticulocyte count was 4.2% (normal range 0.5–2.5%). PBF showed polychromasia with a marked leucoerythroblastic picture. Serum LDH was markedly elevated to 3000 U/L (normal range 135–255 U/L) and high total bilirubin 3.1 g/dL (normal range 0–1.2 g/dL), mainly indirect bilirubin. Renal function and other liver enzymes, however, were within the normal range. Computed tomography (CT) scan showed hepatosplenomegaly. Virology screen for corona, H1N1, and parvo virus was negative. During admission, the patient's condition deteriorated with declines in Hb and platelet count and an increase in serum LDH level. The patient was admitted to the intensive care unit (ICU) and bone marrow examination was done to exclude bone marrow infiltration. PBF after transfusion of 10 units of packed red blood cells (PRBC) showed a leucoerythroblastic picture with polychromasia and rare sickle cells. Bone marrow aspirate showed gelatinous basophilic material with distorted morphology. The bone marrow biopsy revealed extensive bone marrow necrosis involving more than half of the one centimeter length biopsy, markedly increased erythropoietic activity in the intact area, and dilated sinusoids which were full of sickled red blood cells (Figure 1). The diagnosis of extensive bone marrow necrosis secondary to sickle cell disease was reported based on these findings. Hb electrophoresis after transfusion showed HbS level of 34%. Family studies were done and revealed that both parents had SCT and her identical twin was found to have SCD with a HbS level of 75%. The patient received supportive therapy and eventually did very well. She subsequently received full vaccinations and began regular follow-up in the hematology clinic. Five months later her Hb electrophoresis showed a HbS level of 80%.

3. Discussion

BMN is infrequently encountered in clinical practice. The incidence of BMN varies from 0.3 to 37% among different reports [11]. Such variability in the results could be attributed to the difference in the type of specimens examined (in vivo or postmortem), pathologist experience, and diagnostic criteria used (the incidence was reduced to 0.3 to 12% when only those biopsies with more than half bone marrow involvement by necrosis were included) [11]. BMN is defined as necrosis of hematopoietic tissue and stroma with preservation of cortical bone [2, 4]. It has been identified with various clinical conditions including malignancy, infection, autoimmune disease, chemotherapy, DIC, anorexia nervosa, antiphospholipid syndrome, and sickle cell disease [3–6, 8–10].

Although the first case of BMN was reported in SCD patient, the association of BMN with SCD was reported in only 2% of the cases [4]. One possible cause of the paucity of this association is that bone marrow examination is not commonly done during sickle cell crisis [12]. Charache and Page stated that one of six patients with SCD has some degree of BMN during painful crisis; usually these patients have full recovery [4]. The largest review on BMN in SCD was done by Tsitsikas et al. who identified 58 cases of BMN with fat embolization syndrome (FES) and 16 cases of BMN without FES. In both groups there were a number of patients who were not known to have SCD prior to the presentation of BMN 19 (33%) and 4 (25%), respectively. It has been found that patients with genotype SS were at low risk for BMN/FES and, paradoxically, those with mild phenotypes were at higher risk of this catastrophic complication [10].

SCD is a relatively common genetic disorder in Saudi Arabia with the highest prevalence noticed in eastern province (approximately 21% for SCT and 2.6% for SCD) [13]. There are two major clinical phenotypes of SCD in Saudis. Patients from the western province have the severe phenotype which is consistent with the Benin haplotype. Acute chest syndrome with recurrence, stroke, dactylitis, lower base line total hemoglobin and hemoglobin F level, and early presentation with painful crisis are common clinical features of SCD in the western province. On the other hand patients with SCD from the eastern province have a more benign phenotype which is consistent with the Arab/Indian haplotype. They have a greater incidence of associated deletional alpha thalassemia, higher total hemoglobin and hemoglobin F levels, persistent splenomegaly, more avascular necrosis of the femoral head, and later disease presentation [14].

In our case, the first clinical disease presentation of SCD was extensive bone marrow necrosis with crisis at age of 26 years. She was not suspected to have the SCD prior to her presentation. She had never complained of bone pain and Hb electrophoresis had never been previously performed. Her identical twin sister as well was not known to have the disease nor did she complain of bone pain prior to the family study. Although the presentation of SCD in the eastern province of Saudi Arabia is relatively late as compared with the western province, presentation at this age (26 years old) in our patient and her identical twin is thought to be extremely uncommon. Also, the initial disease presentation with development of extensive BMN is rarely reported in the literature [15–18]. Having a mild SCD phenotype, the limited family history and lack of neonatal or later screening for hemoglobinopathies all contributed to the late diagnosis of SCD and postponed interventions that could possibly prevent life threatening complications of the disease such as BMN. This case presentation emphasizes the importance of SCD screening and need for follow-up of the patients as catastrophic complications could occur irrespective of the disease phenotype. This is especially important in an area with high SCD prevalence such as the eastern province of Saudi Arabia.

Another unique finding in our case is that she has coexistence of SCD and type-1 DM which is rarely reported as well in the literature [19, 20]. Presence of the high prevalence of both diseases in this part of the world could provide a logical explanation for the coexistence of these disorders in these identical twin sisters.

4. Conclusions

BMN is infrequently encountered in clinical practice and rarely reported in association with SCD. As the initial presentation of SCD, BMN was previously reported only in a few cases in the literature. Patients with a mild SCD phenotype are at high risk of BMN. Thus, a high index of suspicion must be borne in mind to prevent the development of catastrophic complications particularly, in an area with a high prevalence of SCD.

Consent

Written informed consent was obtained from the patient for publication of this case report and any accompanying images.

Conflicts of Interest

The authors declare that they have no conflicts of interest.

Authors' Contributions

Sameera A. Alsafwani, Abdulwahed Al-Saeed, and Rehab Bukhamsin were involved actively in the management of the patient. Sameera A. Alsafwani drafted the manuscript. All the others provided valuable inputs and guidance during the preparation of the manuscript. All authors read and approved the final manuscript.

Acknowledgments

The authors of this article acknowledged the hematopathology consultants in DRL, Mariam Alghazal, Azza Abualam, and Mohamed Khan, for their opinions in writing the bone marrow report.

References

[1] L. J. Wade and L. D. Stevenson, "Necrosis of bone marrow with fat embolism in sickle cell anemia," *American Journal of Pathology*, vol. 17, pp. 47–54, 1941.

[2] D. Maisel, J. Y. Lim, W. J. Pollock, R. Yatani, and P. I. Liu, "Bone marrow necrosis: an entity often overlooked," *Ann Clin Lab Sci*, vol. 18, pp. 109–115, 1988.

[3] S. Paydas, M. Ergin, F. Baslamisli et al., "Bone marrow necrosis: clinicopathologic analysis of 20 cases and review of the literature," *American Journal of Hematology*, vol. 70, no. 4, pp. 300–305, 2002.

[4] A. M. Janssens, F. C. Offner, and W. Z. Van Hove, "Bone marrow necrosis," *Cancer*, vol. 88, no. 8, pp. 1769–1780, 2000.

[5] L. Ding, A. Rawal, S. Luikart, and P. Wadhwa, "Necrosis of uninvolved bone marrow following filgrastim administration in

a patient with Burkitt lymphoma undergoing chemotherapy," *British Journal of Haematology*, vol. 159, no. 1, p. 2, 2012.

[6] K. Foucar, K. Reichard, and D. Czuchlewski, *Bone Marrow Pathology*, ASCP, Chicago, IL, USA, 3rd edition, 2010.

[7] A. Almeida and I. Roberts, "Bone involvement in sickle cell disease," *British Journal of Haematology*, vol. 129, no. 4, pp. 482–490, 2005.

[8] P. Ricci, G. Bandini, M. Baccarani, F. Bazzocchi, G. Martinelli, and S. Tura, "Bone marrow necrosis by diffuse metastatic intravascular obstruction," *Haematologica*, vol. 67, no. 5, pp. 754–759, 1982.

[9] C. Knupp, P. H. Pekala, and P. Cornelius, "Extensive bone marrow necrosis in patients with cancer and tumor necrosis factor activity in plasma," *American Journal of Hematology*, vol. 29, no. 4, pp. 215–221, 1988.

[10] D. A. Tsitsikas, G. Gallinella, S. Patel, H. Seligman, P. Greaves, and R. J. Amos, "Bone marrow necrosis and fat embolism syndrome in sickle cell disease: Increased susceptibility of patients with non-SS genotypes and a possible association with human parvovirus B19 infection," *Blood Reviews*, vol. 28, no. 1, pp. 23–30, 2014.

[11] T. C. S. Cabral, C. M. Fernandes, L. A. C. Lage, M. C. Zerbini, and J. Pereira, "Bone marrow necrosis: literature review," *Jornal Brasileiro de Patologia e Medicina Laboratorial*, vol. 52, no. 3, pp. 182–188, 2016.

[12] P. D. Ziakas and M. Voulgarelis, "Bone marrow necrosis in sickle cell anaemia," *Blood Transfusion*, vol. 8, no. 3, p. 211, 2010.

[13] Z. Naserullah, A. Alshammari, M. Al Abbas et al., "Regional experience with newborn screening for sickle cell disease, other hemoglobinopathies and G6PD deficiency," *Annals of Saudi Medicine*, vol. 23, no. 6, pp. 354–357, 2003.

[14] W. Jastaniah, "Epidemiology of sickle cell disease in Saudi Arabia," *Annals of Saudi Medicine*, vol. 31, no. 3, pp. 289–293, 2011.

[15] M. Shafiq and N. Ali, "Bone marrow necrosis—initial presentation in sickle cell anaemia," *American Journal of Case Reports*, vol. 14, pp. 416–418, 2013.

[16] G. El Hachem and N. Chamseddine, "Bone marrow necrosis: an unusual initial presentation of sickle cell anemia," *Clinical Lymphoma, Myeloma and Leukemia*, vol. 16, pp. S195–S196, 2016.

[17] J. Adamski, C. A. Hanna, V. B. Reddy, S. H. Litovsky, C. A. Evans, and M. B. Marques, "Multiorgan failure and bone marrow necrosis in three adults with sickle cell-β^+-thalassemia," *American Journal of Hematology*, vol. 87, no. 6, pp. 621–624, 2012.

[18] F. Simon, E. Carloz, B. Chaudier, P. Kraemer, P. Colbacchini, and P. Hovette, "Extensive bone marrow necrosis as presenting manifestation of sickle cell disease in Africa," *Medecine tropicale : revue du Corps de sante colonial*, vol. 64, no. 2, pp. 179–182, 2004.

[19] O. O. Jarrett and E. I. Olorundare, "Type 1 diabetes mellitus in a known sickle cell anaemia patient: a rare combination in Nigeria," *African Journal of Medicine and Medical Sciences*, vol. 43, no. 2, pp. 177–181, 2014.

[20] Z. Shoar, G. Rezvani, and F. De Luca, "Type 1 diabetes mellitus in a patient with homozygous sickle cell anemia," *Journal of Pediatric Endocrinology and Metabolism*, vol. 26, no. 11-12, pp. 1205–1207, 2013.

23

Upper Limb Deep Vein Thrombosis in Patient with Hemophilia A and Heterozygosity for Prothrombin G20210A

Fares Darawshy,[1] Yosef Kalish,[2] Issam Hendi,[1] Ayman Abu Rmelieh,[1] and Tawfik Khoury[1]

[1]*Department of Medicine, Hadassah-Hebrew University Medical Center, Jerusalem, Israel*
[2]*Department of Hematology, Hadassah-Hebrew University Medical Center, Jerusalem, Israel*

Correspondence should be addressed to Tawfik Khoury; tawfikkhoury1@hotmail.com

Academic Editor: Simon Davidson

Deep vein thrombosis (DVT) is a rare disease in patients with hemophilia A. We report a case of 22-year-old male with severe hemophilia A who presented to the emergency room with 5-day history of right arm pain that was attributed initially to bleeding event. In the absence of external signs of bleeding or hematoma and normal hemoglobin level, we suspected an underlying DVT. Doppler ultrasonography of the right upper limb revealed thrombosis of the subclavian vein and this was confirmed by CT venography. The d-dimer level was normal and investigations for prothrombotic state revealed heterozygosity for prothrombin G20210A mutation. Treatment with factor VIII and low molecular weight heparin led to successful resolution and marked improvement of his clinical condition.

1. Introduction

Hemophilia A is a hereditary hemorrhagic disease characterized by the deficiency of the coagulation FVIII. Due to the bleeding tendencies in hemophilia A patients, the occurrence of spontaneous venous thromboembolism is a rare and even surprising but has been reported in the literature [1–4]. The mechanism of spontaneous venous thromboembolism in hemophilia A patient is unclear due to limited number of cases and there are no clear guidelines for its treatment.

We report a case of 22-year-old male patient with severe hemophilia A who developed DVT in the right upper arm.

2. Case Presentation

A 22-year-old male diagnosed with severe hemophilia A on F VIII prophylaxis (recombinant F VIII therapy, 3000 units 3 times a week) self-administered into a peripheral vein of the right arm presented to the emergency room for evaluation of right arm and shoulder pain in the past 5 days. On admission, the patient was hemodynamic and respiratory stable. His physical examination was unremarkable except for right arm tenderness without swelling, erythema, or increased vascular markings.

Prothrombotic workups including protein C activity, protein S activity, antithrombin III level, APC resistance, lupus anticoagulant, anticardiolipin antibodies, factor VIII inhibitor screening, and factor V Leiden defect were all negative, except for heterozygous mutation for prothrombin G20210A; the d-dimer level was normal 0.14 mcg/mL (0–0.5) and coagulation tests revealed low FVIII levels. A Doppler ultrasonography (US) of the right upper limb showed an echogenic thrombosis in the right subclavian vein. CT venography confirmed the diagnosis of right subclavian DVT (Figure 1). All imaging studies ruled out thoracic outlet syndrome.

Further investigations were performed to rule out other causes of DVT; inflammatory markers C reactive protein (CRP) and erythrocyte sedimentation rate (ESR) were within normal range (Table 1). HLA-B51 was performed to rule out Bechet disease and was negative.

The patient was treated with low molecular weight heparin (LMWH) enoxaparin 100 mg once daily (1.5 mg/kg),

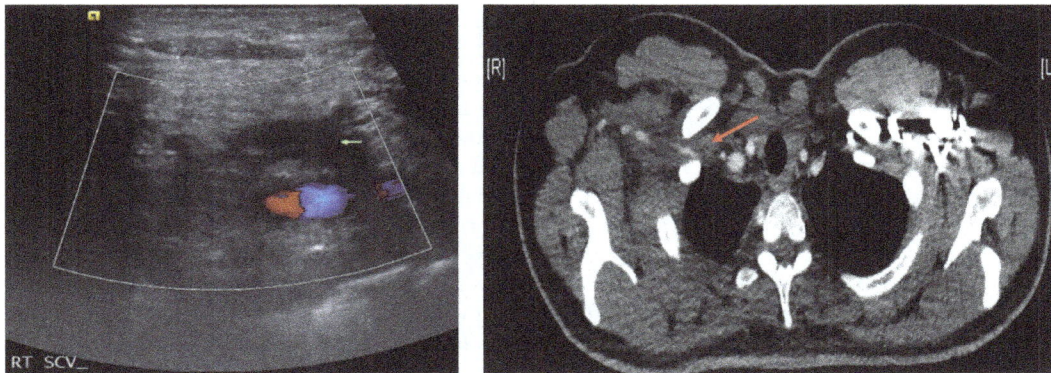

FIGURE 1: Doppler US and CT scan showing DVT in the right subclavian vein. Arrows refer to deep vein thrombosis.

TABLE 1: Laboratory tests results.

Parameter	Result	Normal values
WBC count ($*10^9$/L)	8.4	4–10
Platelets count ($*10^9$/L)	209	140–400
Hemoglobin (Gr%)	15.1	14–18
PT (%)	73.03	60–100
aPTT (s)	54.7	25–49
INR	1.22	1–1.4
D-DIMER (mcg/mL)	0.14	0–0.5
Factor VIII level (%)	17	70–140
Factor VIII inhibitor screening	Negative	
Protein C activity	Normal	70–120
Protein S activity	Normal	70–140
Antithrombin III level	Normal	
APC resistance	Negative	
Lupus anticoagulant	Absent	
Anticardiolipin antibodies	Absent	
Factor V Leiden defect	Absent	
Prothrombin G20210A	Heterozygote	
ESR	28	1–20
CRP (mg%)	1.42	<0.5
ANA	Absent	
C-ANCA (unit/mL)	8	>18
P-ANCA (unit/mL)	1.6	>18
C3 (mg/dL)	138	90–180
C4 (mg/dL)	27	10–40

along with prophylactic FVIII 2000 units per day. This regimen increased FVIII levels up to 49.2% measured 1 hour after FVIII injection and was continued for 2 months.

After two months, the dose of LMWH was reduced to 40 mg and the dose of FVIII was escalated to 3000 units, given three times a week for another 3 months, followed by another six weeks of treatment with 40 mg LMWH and 2000 units of FVIII administered every other day. There was complete resolution of DVT accompanied with significant clinical improvement without recurrence of the thrombosis to date.

3. Discussion

Thrombotic events have been rarely reported among patients with hemophilia [1–3]. Goodnough et al. [5] found no thrombotic complications in 178 patients with hemophilia A over a 30-year follow-up period. The exact pathomechanism and the predisposing factors for the occurrence of venous thrombosis in hemophilic patients are still not well established. Kasper found no evidence of thrombosis in major orthopedic operations in patients with hemophilia A [6]. However, Pruthi et al. reported case report of DVT in hemophilia B patient and factor V Leiden following hip fracture surgery [7]. In another recent study, Buckner et al. reported symptomatic venous thromboembolism incidence of 4.3% in hemophilia patients undergoing major orthopedic surgery [8]. Girolami et al. have reviewed all reported patients with hemophilia A and hemophilia B in the literature and found that the administration of factor VIII inhibitor bypassing activity (FEIBA) or recombinant activated FVII (rFVIIa) in patients with inhibitors and surgery was the most frequent risk factor for thromboembolism development in hemophilia A and B patients, respectively, in addition to variable prothrombotic conditions and administration of prothrombin complex concentrate (PCC) [9]. Stewart et al. reported the occurrence of venous thrombosis in a patient with hemophilia A after a long flight [4]. On the other hand, few previous case reports reported venous thrombosis in hemophilia A with no prothrombotic risk factor identified [2, 3]. Our patient developed right subclavian DVT in the arm used for self-injected FVIII prophylactic therapy and was found to have heterozygous mutation for prothrombin G20210A. There were no other identifiable predisposing risk factors as assessed by an extensive investigation that ruled out inflammatory, mechanical obstructive, and neoplastic causes. Prothrombin is a precursor of the serine protease thrombin and is a key enzyme in the process of hemostasis. Prothrombin heterozygosity is related to a single-nucleotide substitution (G to A) at position 20210 in the $3'$ untranslated region of the gene encoding prothrombin. Its heterozygous state, 20210A, is a risk factor for the development of deep vein thrombosis [10]. Deep vein thrombosis and cerebral vein thrombosis have been reported in association with heterozygous prothrombin mutation [11, 12]. Interestingly, one may postulate that the low FVIII in our patient of 17% is in favor of bleeding tendency; however, the occurrence of DVT in the setting of low systemic level of FVIII may suggest the strong hypercoagulability potential of heterozygous prothrombin G20210A mutation or, on the other hand, might suggest the hypothesis of FVIII administration as a predisposing factor for local thromboembolism development in hemophilia A patients. Another interesting point is that our patient had normal d-dimer level although he had upper extremity DVT. Normal d-dimer level in two patients with pacemaker and upper extremity DVT was previously reported [13]. In a study for evaluating the usefulness of d-dimer in the evaluation of upper extremity DVT [14], the reported sensitivity was 100% but the 95% confidence interval was 78–100. The specificity was 14%, not surprising given the poor specificity of d-dimer in venous thromboembolism. Based on these previous studies, the use of d-dimer in our case to rule out upper extremity DVT is limited and a Doppler US should be the initial test of choice for upper extremity DVT once suspected.

The treatment of spontaneous venous thrombosis in patients with hemophilia A is not well defined, and the recommended treatment of this condition is based on case reports as different regimens have been used for its treatment. Stewart et al. [4] treated their patient with LMWH for 5 days and tinzaparin for 6 weeks. Dargaud et al. used the unfractionated heparin in addition to FVIII replacement therapy for 1 month [2]. Kashyap et al. used LMWH for 9 weeks [3]. Oral anticoagulation was not used, probably since

it increases the risk of bleeding. Bicer et al. [1] treated their patient with LMWH for 2 days followed by warfarin for 6 weeks. No bleeding complications were reported in all cases.

In our case, we treated the patient according to hematological consultation with LMWH on one hand for DVT and with FVIII prophylaxis treating the hemophilia A coagulopathy on the other hand. The regimen was continued for 3 months and then tapered down the administration of LMWH for another six weeks till treatment cessation. This patient was monitored closely and marked clinical and radiological improvement was observed.

In conclusion, spontaneous venous thromboembolism is a very rare and unexpected disease in patients with hemophilia A. Clinicians should be aware about this entity and should consider this differential diagnosis per patient individually especially in the FVIII injected limb. This case shed light on the uncertainty of the mechanism involved in the occurrence of venous thromboembolism in hemophilia A patients especially with low FVIII level. Therefore, further preclinical and clinical trials should be carried out to elucidate the mechanism and treatment of venous thrombosis in patients with hemophilia and to perform larger studies evaluating the exact predictive value of d-dimer in upper limb DVT.

Conflicts of Interest

The authors report no conflicts of interest regarding this manuscript.

Authors' Contributions

Fares Darawshy, Tawfik Khoury, and Yosef Kalish contributed to the concept and design of the study, all authors contributed to the analysis and interpretation of data, Fares Darawshy and Tawfik Khoury contributed to critical writing and revising the intellectual content, and all authors approved the final version to be published.

References

[1] M. Bicer, M. Yanar, and O. Tuydes, "Spontaneous deep vein thrombosis in hemophilia A: a case report," *Cases Journal*, vol. 2, no. 9, Article no. 6390, 2009.

[2] Y. Dargaud, B. B. Cruchaudet, A. Lienhart, B. Coppéré, J. Ninet, and C. Négrier, "Spontaneous proximal deep vein thrombosis in a patient with severe haemophilia A," *Blood Coagulation and Fibrinolysis*, vol. 14, no. 4, pp. 407–409, 2003.

[3] R. Kashyap, L. M. Sharma, S. Gupta, R. Saxena, and D. N. Srivastava, "Deep vein thrombosis in a patient with severe haemophilia A," *Haemophilia*, vol. 12, no. 1, pp. 87–89, 2006.

[4] A. J. Stewart, L. M. Manson, R. Dennis, P. L. Allan, and C. A. Ludlam, "Thrombosis in a duplicated superficial femoral vein in a patient with haemophilia A," *Haemophilia*, vol. 6, no. 1, pp. 47–49, 2000.

[5] L. T. Goodnough, H. Saito, and O. D. Ratnoff, "Thrombosis or myocardial infarction in congenital clotting factor abnormalities and chronic thrombocytopenias: A report of 21 patients and

a review of 50 previously reported cases," *Medicine*, vol. 62, no. 4, pp. 248–255, 1983.

[6] C. K. Kasper, "Postoperative thromboses in hemophilia B," *New England Journal of Medicine*, vol. 289, no. 3, 160 pages, 1973.

[7] R. K. Pruthi, J. A. Heit, M. M. Green et al., "Venous thromboembolism after hip fracture surgery in a patient with haemophilia B and factor V Arg506Gln (factor V Leiden)," *Haemophilia*, vol. 6, no. 6, pp. 631–634, 2000.

[8] T. W. Buckner, A. D. Leavitt, M. Ragni et al., "Prospective, multicenter study of postoperative deep-vein thrombosis in patients with haemophilia undergoing major orthopaedic surgery," *Thrombosis and Haemostasis*, vol. 116, no. 1, pp. 42–49, 2016.

[9] A. Girolami, R. Scandellari, E. Zanon, R. Sartori, and B. Girolami, "Non-catheter associated venous thrombosis in hemophilia A and B. A critical review of all reported cases," *Journal of Thrombosis and Thrombolysis*, vol. 21, no. 3, pp. 279–284, 2006.

[10] M. W. Kellett, P. J. Martin, T. P. Enevoldson, C. Brammer, and C. M. Toh, "Cerebral venous sinus thrombosis associated with 20210A mutation of the prothrombin gene," *Journal of Neurology Neurosurgery and Psychiatry*, vol. 65, no. 4, pp. 611-612, 1998.

[11] V. Biousse, J. Conard, C. Brouzes, M. H. Horellou, and A. Ameri, "Frequency of the 20210 G–>A mutation in the 3'-untranslated region of the prothrombin gene in 35 cases of cerebral venous thrombosis," *Stroke*, vol. 29, pp. 1398–1400, 1998.

[12] O. Hudaoglu, S. Kurul, U. Yis, E. Dirik, H. Cakmakci, and S. Men, "Basilar artery thrombosis in a child heterozygous for prothrombin gene G20210A mutation," in *Journal of Child Neurology*, vol. 22, pp. 329–331, 22, 2007.

[13] C. Byrne, J. Abdulla, and J. K. Christensen, "Normal D-dimer in two patients with pacemaker and deep venous thrombosis in an upper extremity," in *Ugeskr Laeger*, vol. 177, pp. 12-13, 2015.

[14] T. Merminod, S. Pellicciotta, and H. Bounameaux, "Limited usefulness of D-dimer in suspected deep vein thrombosis of the upper extremities," *Blood Coagulation and Fibrinolysis*, vol. 17, no. 3, pp. 225-226, 2006.

24

A Case of Levamisole-Induced Agranulocytosis

Thamer Kassim ⓘ,[1] **Lakshmi Chintalacheruvu,**[1] **Osman Bhatty** ⓘ,[1] **Mohammad Selim** ⓘ,[1] **Osama Diab,**[1] **Ali Nayfeh** ⓘ,[1] **Jayadev Manikkam Umakanthan,**[2] and **Maryam Gbadamosi-Akindele** ⓘ[1]

[1]Department of Internal Medicine, Creighton University, Omaha, NE, USA
[2]University of Nebraska Medical Center, Omaha, NE, USA

Correspondence should be addressed to Maryam Gbadamosi-Akindele; maryam.gbadamosi-akindele@va.gov

Academic Editor: Giuseppe Murdaca

A sixty-eight-year-old male with a past medical history of recurrent cocaine use presented to the emergency department with recurrent diarrhea and was found to have a white blood cell (WBC) count of 1.9×10^9/L with agranulocytosis (absolute neutrophil count (ANC) of 95 cell/mm^3). At admission, the patient disclosed that he used cocaine earlier during the day, and a urine drug screen tested positive for this. On hospital day one, the patient was found to have a fever with a maximum temperature of 313.6 K. After ruling out other causes and noting the quick turnaround of his neutropenia after four days of cocaine abstinence, the patient's neutropenia was attributed to levamisole-adulterated cocaine.

1. Introduction

Levamisole is an immunomodulator that is found in almost seventy to eighty percent of cocaine shipments according to the Drug Enforcement Agency (DEA) [1, 2]. There were approximately 1.5 million American cocaine users each month in the year of 2013 making levamisole a relevant public health concern [3]. We present a case of levamisole-cocaine-induced agranulocytosis with the aim to raise awareness regarding the possible complications of this compound.

2. Case Report

A sixty-eight-year-old male presented to the Emergency Department (ED) complaining of recurrent diarrhea and a documented fever of 312 K for one-day duration. The patient had a past medical history of end-stage renal disease on hemodialysis, insulin-dependent type II diabetes mellitus, essential hypertension, and chronic cocaine dependence. On further history, the patient reported the use of cocaine over the past five years with an average use of three times a week but could not specify a certain amount on each time.

The patient disclosed that he had used cocaine earlier that day.

At admission, blood pressure was 106/78, heart rate was 96 beats per minute, respiratory rate was 18, temperature was 312.2 K, and oxygen saturation was 93% on room air. Physical examination showed a thin, malnourished male with right below knee amputation who was in mild distress. No cutaneous manifestations were noticed, and no other abnormalities were appreciated on the rest of the patient's physical examination. Laboratory workup was done and included a complete blood count (CBC) with differential, which showed a WBC count of 1.9×10^9/L (reference range: 4.0–11.0×10^9/L), segmented neutrophils 4% (reference range: 40–70%), bands 1% (reference range: 0–6%), immature granulocytes of 0.0% (reference range: 0.0–0.9%), and lymphocytes 70% (reference range: 16–45%). Basophils, eosinophils, and monocytes were within normal limits. Hemoglobin was 9.8 g/dL (reference range: 12.5–17 g/dL), which was around baseline and was attributed to the patient's end-stage renal disease, and platelet count was 237×10^9/L (reference range: 150–450×10^9/L). A complete metabolic profile was also obtained showing a serum potassium of 3.1 mmol/L (reference range: 3.6–5.0 mmol/L), creatinine of 371.4 μmol/L (reference range: 45–90 μmol/L), blood urea nitrogen of 9.64 mmol/L (reference range: 2.5–7.1 mmol/L), and glomerular filtration rate of 12 with a normal liver function. Urine drug screen was positive for cocaine. Erythrocyte sedimentation rate, C-reactive protein, and urine analysis were within reference range. At that point, isoantibodies including cytoplasmic antineutrophil cytoplasmic antibody (C-ANCA) and perinuclear antineutrophil cytoplasmic antibody (P-ANCA) were not tested because the patient had normal inflammatory markers and no urinary, pulmonary, or cutaneous manifestations.

The patient was admitted to the hospital, and intravenous fluids were initiated along with correction of electrolyte disturbances and symptomatic therapy. The patient's diarrhea resolved during his first admission day, but the patient spiked a fever with a temperature maximum of 313.6 K. A repeat CBC with differential was done and showed a WBC count of 1.0×10^9/L, segmented neutrophils of 3%, bands of 1%, immature granulocytes of 0.0%, and lymphocytes of 44% with normal basophils, eosinophils, and monocytes. The patient's calculated ANC was 40 cells/mm^3, and the decision to start empirical antibiotics and initiate a septic workup was taken. Blood cultures, urine analysis and culture, and stool analysis and culture were all negative. Chest X-ray and chest/abdomen CT scan showed no abnormalities, and ultimately no source of infection was isolated.

Further tests were initiated in an attempt to find a cause for the patient's unexplained neutropenia. Medications were reviewed carefully for possible idiosyncratic drug reactions and bone marrow toxicity, but none of the patient's medications fit such a profile. A viral panel including hepatitis A, B, and C and HIV were all negative. Vitamin B12 level was 681.7 pmol/L (reference range: 216–687 pmol/), folate level was 38.7 nmol/L (reference range: 4.5–45.3 nmol/L), copper level of 11.2 μmol/L (reference range: 9.9–23.1 μmol/L), reticulocyte count of 2.3% (reference range: 0.5–2.3%), lactate dehydrogenase level of 380 IU/L (reference range: 313–680 IU/L), and negative antinuclear antibody test. A peripheral smear showed a decreased number of morphologically unremarkable neutrophils in the background of anemia (Figure 1). The patient refused a bone marrow biopsy.

On the fourth hospital admission day, the patient started to recover on empirical antibiotics and supportive care (see Table 1 and Figure 2, resp.). The thought of an adulterant in cocaine was brought up as the patient's WBC started to improve after abstinence of drug use. Blood and urine testing for levamisole were not performed due to the short half-life of the drug and the fact that it would not have been detected at that point.

Given the patient's clinical picture, laboratory findings, and no alternative cause of his agranulocytosis, the diagnosis of levamisole-cocaine-induced neutropenia was thought to be most appropriate as a diagnosis of exclusion. The patient's white blood cell count and absolute neutrophil count started to recover four to five days after stopping cocaine use which suggested an association.

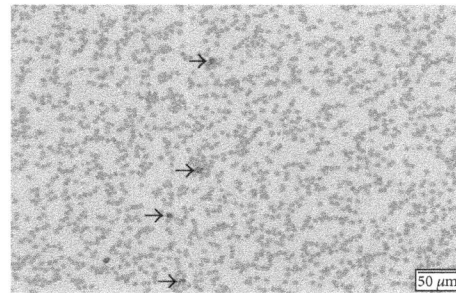

FIGURE 1: Unremarkable neutrophils in the background of anemia. Absolute leukopenia with absolute neutropenia. Black arrows show a decreased number morphologically.

3. Discussion

Levamisole is a broad-spectrum antihelminthic which was first introduced in 1966 and is used currently in veterinary medicine. In humans, the drug was found to have immune-stimulant and anti-inflammatory properties and has been used for the treatment of rheumatoid arthritis, nephrotic syndrome, and other autoimmune diseases. It also showed to be beneficial in the management of lung, colon, and breast cancer. The drug was withdrawn from the US market in 1999 due to safety issues [1, 2]. For the last decade, many cases of levamisole-adulterated cocaine have been reported. These case reports suggested various complications of levamisole including neutropenia, vasculitis with cutaneous involvement, and neurological manifestations [1]. We consider the severe neutropenia in our case to be caused by cocaine adulterated with levamisole after other causes of neutropenia have been excluded.

In assessing similar patients with unexplained neutropenia, it is important to evaluate for idiosyncratic drug reactions. Reviewing new medications which can possibly cause neutropenia such as clozapine, trimethoprim/sulfamethoxazole, sulfasalazine, propylthiouracil, and methimazole can guide diagnosis [4]. When starting a workup in such cases, a differential diagnosis usually includes viral infections such as hepatitis B or C and human immunodeficiency virus (HIV) and atypical presentations of autoimmune diseases such systemic lupus erythematosus (SLE). Myelodysplastic syndrome and aplastic anemia rarely present with isolated neutropenia, but it is still important to keep an open mind for such etiologies. Other causes that need to be evaluated include deficiencies in vitamin B12, folate, and copper. Such causes were all excluded in our case.

The pathogenesis behind neutropenia caused by levamisole is not fully understood [1]. Levamisole is thought to form antigen-antibody complexes that deposit on the surface of neutrophils causing complement fixation, activation, and cytolysis. It increases T-cell activation and proliferation and increases neutrophil mobility, adherence, and chemotaxis [1]. Also, levamisole acts as a hapten increasing the formation of antibodies to granulocyte antigens and triggering an immune response resulting in destruction of leukocytes [1, 4]. Another explanation is that it could serve as a substrate

TABLE 1

Day	1 month prior to admission	0	1	2	3	4	5	6
White blood cell count (4.0–11.0 × 10^9/L)	4.3	1.9	1.0	1.1	1.3	1.8	2.4	3.6
Absolute neutrophil count (ANC), cell/mm^3	—	95	40	88	130	306	528	1008
White blood cell differential (%)								
Segmented neutrophil % (43.0–76.0)	41	4	3	8	9	13	18	23
Bands % (0–6)	0	1	1	0	1	4	4	5
Lymphocyte % (16.0–45.0)	28	70.7	50	52	57.3	63	46	42
Monocyte % (5.0–14)	8	14	12	12	18	16	11	10
Eosinophil % (0.0–5.0)	0	4.0	4.8	4.5	4.2	3.3	3.0	2.5
Basophil % (0.0–1.0)	0	1.0	1.0	0.5	0.7	0.6	0	0

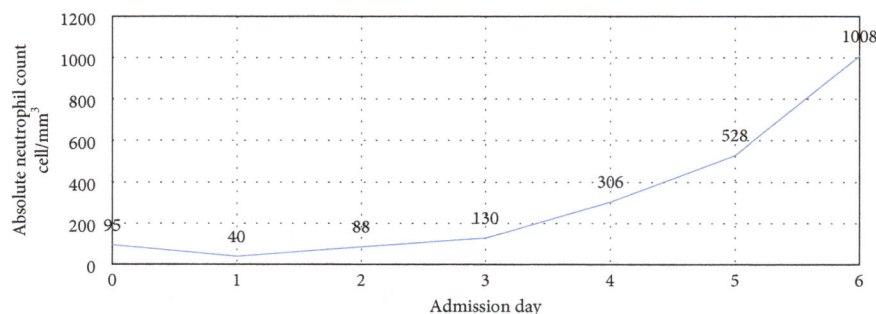

FIGURE 2

for myeloperoxidase to form reactive metabolites that might stimulate autoimmunity [5].

Studies have shown that levamisole use has been associated with multiple isoantibodies including C-ANCA and P-ANCA. Antibodies to double-stranded DNA, cardiolipin, lupus anticoagulant, ribonucleoprotein, antiphospholipids, and antineutrophil cell wall antibodies have also been detected [4, 6]. The presence of such antibodies correlates with the adverse manifestations of levamisole use [1, 4]. Also, research has shown that agranulocytosis recurs with recurrent cocaine use. Genotyping reveals a significant association between HLA-B27 and cocaine-associated agranulocytosis (odds ratio (OR) 9.2; 95% confidence interval (CI)). This does not mean that every patient needs to be tested for genetic predisposition, but clinicians should have a high index of suspicion in these patients and warn them about the possible risks [7].

It is still not known why drug dealers add levamisole to cocaine. Inert adulterants are added to illicit drugs by drug dealers to increase its weight and volume before sale [1]. It has been suggested that levamisole has similar physical properties as cocaine as it can increase norepinephrine transmission through inhibition of norepinephrine reuptake and can be partially metabolized to amphetamine-like compound. Also, it can increase opioid and dopamine concentrations in the cerebral reward pathway making it a favorable adulterant to cocaine potentiating its effect [8, 9].

Levamisole levels can be detected in urine and plasma by gas chromatography mass spectroscopy. The timing is important since the half-life of levamisole is only 5.6 hours and remains detectable for 2-3 days after initial exposure [5, 7].

Bone marrow biopsy in such patients reveals a hypercellular bone marrow with a relative myeloid hypoplasia.

The most common treatment of levamisole-induced neutropenia is the withdrawal of the drug. Granulocyte colony-stimulating factor use results in neutrophil recovery within 2-3 days of administration. However, spontaneous neutrophil recovery after 5–10 days of cessation of levamisole has been previously reported [10]. Supportive care during the period of agranulocytosis and having a low threshold in initiating antimicrobials is of high importance and can prevent life-threatening opportunistic infections.

4. Conclusion

Levamisole should always be on the list of differential diagnoses in patients who are dependent on cocaine and are found to have neutropenic fever. Clinicians should always keep in mind early testing for levamisole in suspected cases. Such patients are at risk of life-threatening opportunistic infections, and an infectious workup together with broad-spectrum antibiotics should be initiated immediately.

Levamisole-cocaine immune-mediated disease is a public health concern in cocaine users. In light of the high number of cocaine users along with the fact that almost 70 to 80% of cocaine has been adulterated with levamisole, physicians should counsel patients about the adverse effects of such compounds. Patients should be aware of the possible signs and symptoms and should be counselled about the increased recurrence risk of these manifestations with continued cocaine use.

Disclosure

The details of this manuscript were presented as a clinical vignette poster in the Society of General Internal Medicine (SGIM) at the Hilton, Washington, DC, on April 20, 2017.

Conflicts of Interest

The authors declare that they have no conflicts of interest regarding the publication of this paper.

Authors' Contributions

Thamer Kassim wrote the manuscript and reviewed it. Lakshmi Chintalacheruvu helped in writing part of the discussion and reviewed the manuscript. Osman Bhatty performed literature review and reviewed the manuscript. Mohammad Selim performed literature review and helped in writing discussion. Osama Diab performed literature review and reviewed the manuscript. Ali Nayfeh performed literature search and review. Jayadev Manikkam Umakanthan performed review of the manuscript. Maryam Gadamosi-Akindele, the mentor of Thamer Kassim, worked with Thamer Kassim on the manuscript and reviewed it.

References

[1] J. A. Buchanan and E. J. Lavonas, "Agranulocytosis and other consequences due to use of illicit cocaine contaminated with levamisole," *Current Opinion in Hematology*, vol. 19, no. 1, pp. 27–31, 2012.

[2] E. Bertol, F. Mari, M. G. Milia, L. Politi, S. Furlanetto, and S. B. Karch, "Determination of aminorex in human urine samples by GC-MS after use of levamisole," *Journal of Pharmaceutical and Biomedical Analysis*, vol. 55, no. 5, pp. 1186–1189, 2011.

[3] Drugabuse.gov, "Nationwide trends," 2017 , https://www.drugabuse.gov/publications/drugfacts/nationwide-trends.

[4] F. Andersohn, C. Konzen, and E. Garbe, "Systematic review: agranulocytosis induced by nonchemotherapy drugs," *Annals of Internal Medicine*, vol. 146, no. 9, pp. 657–65, 2007.

[5] P. A. Dherange, N. Beatty, and A. Al-Khashman, "Levamisole-adulterated cocaine: a case of retiform purpura, cutaneous necrosis and neutropenia," *BMJ Case Reports*, vol. 2015, p. bcr2015211768, 2015.

[6] N. P. Arora, T. Jain, R. Bhanot, and S. K. Natesan, "Levamisole-induced leukocytoclastic vasculitis and neutropenia in a patient with cocaine use: an extensive case with necrosis of skin, soft tissue, and cartilage," *Addiction Science & Clinical Practice*, vol. 7, no. 1, p. 19, 2012.

[7] J. A. Buxton, J. Omura, M. Kuo et al., "Genetic determinants of cocaine-associated agranulocytosis," *BMC Research Notes*, vol. 8, no. 1, p. 240, 2015.

[8] A. Larocque and R. S. Hoffman, "Levamisole in cocaine: unexpected news from an old acquaintance," *Clinical Toxicology*, vol. 50, no. 4, pp. 231–241, 2012.

[9] T. M. Brunt, J. van den Berg, E. Pennings, and B. Venhuis, "Adverse effects of levamisole in cocaine users: a review and risk assessment," *Archives of Toxicology*, vol. 91, no. 6, pp. 2303–2313, 2017.

[10] N. Y. Zhu, D. F. Legatt, and A. R. Turner, "Agranulocytosis after consumption of cocaine adulterated with levamisole," *Annals of Internal Medicine*, vol. 150, no. 4, pp. 287–289, 2009.

25

Biphenotypic Acute Leukemia versus Myeloid Antigen-Positive ALL: Clinical Relevance of WHO Criteria for Mixed Phenotype Acute Leukemia

William A. Hammond,[1,2] **Pooja Advani,**[1] **Rhett P. Ketterling,**[3] **Daniel Van Dyke,**[3]
James M. Foran ⓘ,[1] **and Liuyan Jiang**[4]

[1]*Division of Hematology and Oncology, Mayo Clinic, Jacksonville, FL, USA*
[2]*Baptist MD Anderson Cancer Center, Jacksonville, FL, USA*
[3]*Division of Laboratory Medicine and Pathology, Mayo Clinic, Rochester, MN, USA*
[4]*Division of Laboratory Medicine and Pathology, Mayo Clinic, Jacksonville, FL, USA*

Correspondence should be addressed to James M. Foran; foran.james@mayo.edu

Academic Editor: Stephen Langabeer

Updated WHO criteria define mixed phenotype acute leukemia (MPAL) with more stringent diagnostic criteria than the formerly described entity biphenotypic acute leukemia (BAL). The changes in diagnostic criteria influence management by assigning weight to aberrantly expressed markers and minimizing expression of myeloid markers other than myeloperoxidase (MPO), potentially foregoing consolidative allogeneic transplant for an otherwise "favorable" lymphoid phenotypic leukemia. We present a case of MPO-negative, myeloid antigen-positive acute lymphoblastic leukemia who progressed with refractory phenotypic acute myeloid leukemia while receiving lymphoid-directed therapy and discuss concerns raised by the adoption of the new, more stringent diagnostic criteria for BAL.

1. Introduction

Acute leukemia (AL) refers to a broad category of diseases defined by the clonal, malignant proliferation of hematopoietic progenitor cells with aberrant differentiation and is categorized by the World Health Organization (WHO) as myeloid, lymphoid, or those with ambiguous lineage. Within the category of ambiguous lineage are the mixed phenotype acute leukemias (MPALs) [1]. The term "MPAL" was introduced in the WHO classification 4th edition, 2008, and includes the former clinical entities of bilineal and biphenotypic acute leukemia (BAL). Bilineal refers to two separate, concomitant blast populations with distinctly different lineages, whereas BAL refers to a single blast population with aberrant coexpression of both myeloid- and lymphoid-specific markers. The diagnosis of MPAL is unchanged in the 2017 WHO revised 4th edition [2].

The diagnostic criteria for MPAL are now more stringent and exclude some cases that would formerly have been considered as BAL. Historically, BAL comprises up to 5% of all leukemias [3]; however, when strictly defined by the current WHO criteria, the incidence of MPAL may be as low as 0.5–2.4% [4, 5]. The criteria for MPAL exclude ALs with aberrant expression of antigens of an alternate lineage, which can be observed in as many as one-third of all B-lineage ALL cases when a limited myeloid immunophenotypic panel is applied, including only CD13 and CD33, known as myeloid antigen-positive (My+) ALL [6]. Leukemic blasts may also betray lineage fidelity, often in a consistent or predictable manner, leading to the distinction within the current WHO classification of MPAL with *BCR-ABL1* and with *MLL* (i.e., t[v;11q23]) rearrangements as unique entities. At any point during the course of AL, a new blast population may arise with an antigen-expression profile characteristic of a different lineage, referred to as lineage switch. To illustrate potential pitfalls and challenges of the current revised classification, we report a case of lineage switch from My+ ALL to an AML phenotype during intensive ALL-directed chemotherapy, with persistence of an underlying *CDKN2A* deletion.

2. Case

A 23-year-old man presented in 2014 with a white blood cell count of 34×10^9/L with 87% circulating blasts by manual differential count. Flow cytometric analysis on the peripheral blood (PB) revealed 89.6% blasts by CD45/SSC gating. The blasts expressed CD10, CD19, CD34, HLA-DR, and CD20 (dim); partially expressed CD13, CD15, and CD33; and did not express CD2, CD7, CD56, and CD117. A subsequent bone marrow (BM) biopsy was done the next day but was a dry tap; therefore, flow cytometry and other cytogenetic studies were not performed on the BM sample. Immunohistochemistry (IHC) studies were performed on the BM biopsy showing 95% blasts positive for CD79a, PAX-5, and TdT, and negative for CD20 and myeloperoxidase (MPO). The morphology and immunophenotype of the blasts in the peripheral blood and bone marrow biopsy were consistent with B-lineage lymphoblastic leukemia. We did perform FISH analysis with a B-ALL panel on the peripheral blood specimen which revealed *CDKN2A* (p16 at 9q21) gene deletion on one or both chromosomes 9. Fusion of *BCR* and *ABL1* was not detected. Intensive chemotherapy was initiated according to the CALGB 10403 "Adolescent Young Adult" regimen [7], and the patient achieved complete remission. He then proceeded to consolidation without consideration of allogeneic hematopoietic cell transplantation (allo-HCT) based on standard of care for B-cell ALL with favorable cytogenetic and molecular profile.

However, the patient had prolonged cytopenias during consolidation therapy culminating in treatment delay. In early January of 2015 (approximately 24 weeks after initial diagnosis), the patient's complete blood count revealed 27% blasts. Flow cytometry analysis was performed on the PB; the blasts expressed HLA-DR, CD15, CD33, and CD117; partially expressed CD13 and CD56; and did not express CD2, CD3, CD5, CD7, CD10, CD19, CD20, or CD34. A restaging BM biopsy was performed the same day; unfortunately, it was again a dry tap, so flow cytometric analysis could not be performed. The histology examination of the BM biopsy revealed a hypocellular (30%) marrow with 85% recurrent leukemic blasts. IHC showed the blasts were now positive for MPO, while CD10, PAX-5 CD20, CD79a, and TdT were negative. The overall findings on PB and BM biopsy were consistent with a lineage switch to acute myeloid leukemia (AML) (Figure 1). Although it was a dry tap, a very small amount of aspiration specimen was obtained in the EDTA tube. Despite few marrow spicules on the aspiration smear, cytogenetic analysis and FISH studies were performed. FISH analysis with both B-ALL and AML panels showed persistence of a heterozygous *CDKN2A* deletion, plus the acquisition of a *TP53* deletion, and 7q and 17q duplications. Cytogenetic studies now showed a complex karyotype in

18/20 metaphases, 47,X,-Y,add(1)(p36.1),+18,+add(18)(q23) [12]/47-48,X,-Y,del(1)(p32p36.1),add(11)(p11.2),+18,+18 [cp6]/46,XY [2].

Intensive salvage chemotherapy was initiated with the MEC regimen [8], and nadir BM evaluation was hypocellular without blasts, although FISH demonstrated low-level *CDKN2A* deletion, consistent with minimal residual disease. Ten days later, a rising PB blast percentage prompted another BM biopsy which showed persistence of AL with the same phenotype and FISH with *CDKN2A* deletion. Further intensive chemotherapy was initiated, but the patient ultimately died of respiratory failure and refractory AL.

3. Discussion

AL frequently presents with aberrant expression of antigens despite putative lineage fidelity. My+ ALL describes a heterogeneous group with aberrant expression of a small number of cross-lineage markers (<2 points) by earliest definition from the European Group for the Immunological Characterization of Leukemias (EGIL) [9] and later adopted by the WHO in the 2001 guidelines [10]. The impact of aberrant antigen expression short of BAL has been investigated and does not appear to alter therapy or prognosis but may be useful for monitoring of minimal residual disease [11].

We present a case of AL that formerly would have been considered BAL by the EGIL criteria but was diagnosed as My+ ALL using current WHO criteria, not meeting the criteria for MPAL. The initial blast population expressed sufficient lymphoid (CD79a, CD19, CD10, and TdT) and myeloid (CD13, CD33, and CD15) antigens to qualify as biphenotypic under former terminology; however, in the absence of MPO, the only marker currently considered definitive for myeloid categorization, it could not be considered MPAL. At the time of disease relapse after ALL-directed therapy, a clear lineage switch to an AML phenotype had occurred. This subsequent recurrence suggests that an initial diagnosis of BAL as recognized by the EGIL criteria may have been more clinically applicable for this patient. Figure 2 compares the former and current diagnostic requirements of BAL and MPAL under the EGIL and WHO criteria, respectively, and highlights the stringency of the modern WHO criteria for MPAL.

This case further illustrates an example of lineage switch during active therapy for AL and not secondary AML, which was confirmed by persistence of CDKN2A deletion in both leukemias. The mechanism of phenotypic evolution remains unknown, but the emergence of a second preexisting leukemic population selected by treatment of the primary disease or clonal selection could account for the evolution of this disease. Another theory suggests induced changes within the progenitor cell that may be therapy independent. Lineage switches have been documented in 6–9% of AL cases at relapse, and the time from initial treatment to relapse has been demonstrated to correlate with a lack of response to subsequent treatment, short duration of second remission, and short event-free survival [12].

(a)

(b)

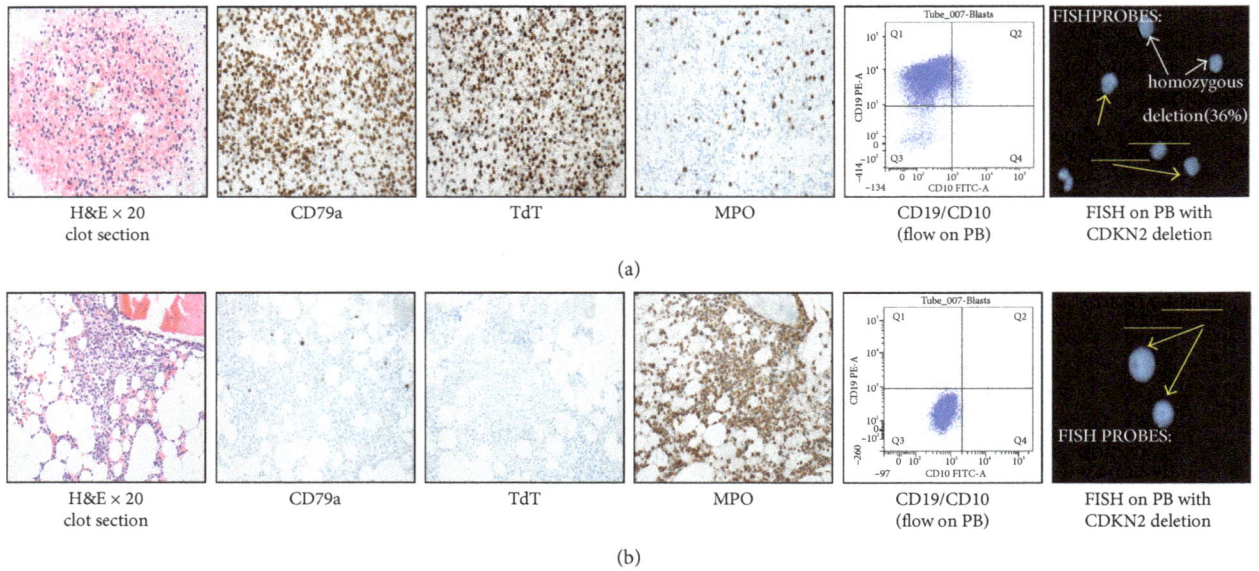

FIGURE 1: Histology and immunohistochemistry (IHC) studies on bone marrow biopsies. Flow cytometry analysis and FISH studies on peripheral blood specimens from (a) diagnosis and (b) relapse at 24 weeks. (a) This series shows the phenotype of B-cell ALL, staining positive for CD79a and TdT but negative for MPO. Flow cytometry shows a blast population that is strongly CD19 positive and weakly CD10 positive. The FISH study shows two blast populations: a heterozygous deletion in 42.5% of nuclei [9p-(CDKN2Ax1,D9Z1x2)] and a homozygous deletion in 36% of nuclei [9p-x2(CDKN2Ax0,D9Z1x2)]. (b) This series demonstrates a myeloid leukemia phenotype with strong MPO staining and lack of CD19 and CD10 expression by flow. The FISH shows persistence of a heterozygous CDKN2A gene deletion [9p-(CDKN2Ax1,D9Z1x2)] present in 75.5% of nuclei tested. ALL, acute lymphoblastic leukemia; CDKN2A, cyclin-dependent kinase inhibitor 2A; FISH, fluorescence in situ hybridization; TdT, terminal deoxynucleotidyl transferase; MPO, myeloperoxidase.

FIGURE 2: Comparison of EGIL criteria for BAL and the 2008 WHO criteria for MPAL. BAL, biphenotypic acute leukemia; EGIL, European Group for the Immunological Characterization of Leukemias; MPAL, mixed phenotype acute leukemia.

Deletion at 9p21 is relatively frequent in adult ALL and is observed in 10–15% of cases. This deletion affects the tumor suppressor gene *CDKN2A*, which encodes for p16^{INK4a} and p14^{ARF} and results in abnormal regulation of the cell cycle by preventing the phosphorylation of the retinoblastoma protein. The prognostic significance of del(9p21) in the large prospective UKALLXII/E2993 trial [13] is associated with superior 5-year overall survival (OS). Conversely, del(9p21) is uncommon in AML, occurs in only 2–5% of cases [14], and portends a poor prognosis with shorter duration of complete response and lower event-free OS [15].

BALs have a worse prognosis and historically have been treated with either myeloid or lymphoid therapy with early consideration of allo-HCT [3, 4]. This patient received lymphoid-directed induction therapy with an intensive AYA regimen, since the *CDKN2A* deletion was not clearly an adverse marker. In retrospect, the emergence of a resistant myeloid clone during ALL-based therapy suggests the designation of BAL may have been appropriate and could have guided therapy, including consideration of early allo-HCT.

This case challenges the current definition of MPAL, which may be too restrictive clinically, and the classification of cases that formerly met the criteria for BAL. The current WHO criteria may not consistently identify all MPAL patients, limiting the clinical utility of this AL designation.

Disclosure

This case was presented as a poster at the 25th Annual Mayo Clinic Hematology/Oncology Reviews, Amelia Island, Florida, July 2015.

Conflicts of Interest

The authors declare that they have no conflicts of interest.

Authors' Contributions

James M. Foran and Liuyan Jiang contributed equally to this work. William A. Hammond was responsible for drafting of the manuscript and study concept and design. Pooja Advani was responsible for drafting of the manuscript. Rhett P. Ketterling and Daniel Van Dyke were responsible for analysis and interpretation of data and critical revision of the manuscript for intellectual content. James M. Foran and Liuyan Jiang were responsible for study concept and design and critical revision of the manuscript for important intellectual content.

Acknowledgments

The authors would like to thank Mayo Clinic Scientific Publications, Florida, for their assistance in manuscript preparation.

References

[1] S. Swerdlow, E. Campo, N. Harris et al., *WHO Classification of Tumours of Haematopoietic and Lymphoid Tissues*, International Agency for Research on Cancer, Lyon, France, 4th edition, 2008.

[2] S. Swerdlow, E. Campo, N. Harris et al., "WHO classification of tumours of haematopoietic and lymphoid tissues," in *WHO Classification of Tumours*, vol. 2, International Agency for Research on Cancer, Lyon, France, 4th edition, 2017.

[3] A. Aribi, C. Bueso-Ramos, E. Estey et al., "Biphenotypic acute leukaemia: a case series," *British Journal of Haematology*, vol. 138, no. 2, pp. 213–216, 2007.

[4] E. Matutes, W. F. Pickl, M. Van't Veer et al., "Mixed-phenotype acute leukemia: clinical and laboratory features and outcome in 100 patients defined according to the WHO 2008 classification," *Blood*, vol. 117, no. 11, pp. 3163–3171, 2011.

[5] L. Yan, N. Ping, M. Zhu et al., "Clinical, immunophenotypic, cytogenetic, and molecular genetic features in 117 adult patients with mixed-phenotype acute leukemia defined by WHO-2008 classification," *Haematologica*, vol. 97, no. 11, pp. 1708–1712, 2012.

[6] M. S. Czuczman, R. K. Dodge, C. C. Stewart et al., "Value of immunophenotype in intensively treated adult acute lymphoblastic leukemia: cancer and leukemia Group B study 8364," *Blood*, vol. 93, no. 11, pp. 3931–3939, 1999.

[7] W. Stock, S. M. Luger, A. S. Advani et al., "Favorable outcomes for older adolescents and young adults (AYA) with acute lymphoblastic leukemia (ALL): early results of US intergroup trial C10403," *Blood*, vol. 124, no. 21, p. 796, 2014.

[8] S. Amadori, W. Arcese, G. Isacchi et al., "Mitoxantrone, etoposide, and intermediate-dose cytarabine: an effective and tolerable regimen for the treatment of refractory acute myeloid leukemia," *Journal of Clinical Oncology*, vol. 9, no. 7, pp. 1210–1214, 1991.

[9] M. C. Bene, G. Castoldi, W. Knapp et al., "Proposals for the immunological classification of acute leukemias: European Group for the Immunological Characterization of Leukemias (EGIL)," *Leukemia*, vol. 9, no. 10, pp. 1783–1786, 1995.

[10] E. S. Jaffe, N. Harris, H. Stein, and J. Vardiman, *World Health Organization Classification of Tumours: Pathology and Genetics of Tumours of Haematopoietic and Lymphoid Tissues*, IARC, Lyon, France, 2001.

[11] S. Faderl, S. O'Brien, C. H. Pui et al., "Adult acute lymphoblastic leukemia: concepts and strategies," *Cancer*, vol. 116, no. 5, pp. 1165–1176, 2010.

[12] E. Dorantes-Acosta and R. Pelayo, "Lineage switching in acute leukemias: a consequence of stem cell plasticity?," *Bone Marrow Research*, vol. 2012, Article ID 406796, 18 pages, 2012.

[13] A. V. Moorman, C. J. Harrison, G. A. Buck et al., "Karyotype is an independent prognostic factor in adult acute lymphoblastic leukemia (ALL): analysis of cytogenetic data from patients treated on the Medical Research Council (MRC) UKALLXII/ Eastern Cooperative Oncology Group (ECOG) 2993 trial," *Blood*, vol. 109, no. 8, pp. 3189–3197, 2007.

[14] H. G. Drexler, "Review of alterations of the cyclin-dependent kinase inhibitor INK4 family genes p15, p16, p18 and p19 in human leukemia-lymphoma cells," *Leukemia*, vol. 12, no. 6, pp. 845–859, 1998.

[15] S. Faderl, H. M. Kantarjian, E. Estey et al., "The prognostic significance of p16(INK4a)/p14(ARF) locus deletion and MDM-2 protein expression in adult acute myelogenous leukemia," *Cancer*, vol. 89, no. 9, pp. 1976–1982, 2000.

26

Concurrent Diagnosis of Chronic Myeloid Leukemia and Follicular Lymphoma

Amy G. Starr [ID],[1] **Sushma R. Jonna,**[2] **Joeffrey J. Chahine,**[1] **Bhaskar V. Kallakury,**[1] **and Chaitra S. Ujjani**[2]

[1]*MedStar Georgetown University Hospital, Department of Pathology, 3800 Reservoir Rd NW, Medical Dental Building, SE 200, Washington, DC 20007, USA*
[2]*Lombardi Comprehensive Cancer Center, Department of Hematology and Oncology, MedStar Georgetown University Hospital, 3800 Reservoir Rd. NW, Washington, DC 20007, USA*

Correspondence should be addressed to Amy G. Starr; amygstarr@gmail.com

Academic Editor: Kazunori Nakase

Lymphadenopathy in chronic myeloid leukemia (CML) is usually due to extramedullary involvement with accelerated or blast phases of the disease. The occurrence of non-Hodgkin lymphoma (NHL) as a synchronous malignancy with CML is rare. We report a case of a 73-year-old male who presented with dyspnea and right-sided lower extremity edema in the setting of leukocytosis. Bone marrow evaluation indicated a chronic phase chronic myeloid leukemia (CML), confirmed by molecular testing. Imaging of the chest for persistent dyspnea revealed supraclavicular and mediastinal lymphadenopathy. Biopsy of the cervical node showed expanded lymphoid follicles with atypical germinal centers that were positive for CD10, BCL-2, and BCL-6, consistent with follicular lymphoma (FL). Nodal PCR demonstrated clonal IGH and IGK gene rearrangements, and FISH analysis was positive for IGH-BCL-2 fusion. Together, these tests supported the diagnosis of FL. Additionally, the lymph node showed paracortical expansion by maturing pan-hematopoietic elements, no blastic groups, and positive RT-PCR analysis for BCR-ABL1, indicating concomitant involvement by chronic phase-CML. To our knowledge, this is the first reported case of a patient with a concurrent diagnosis of CML and FL.

1. Introduction

The diagnosis of synchronous myeloid and lymphoid malignancies is a rare occurrence. The most commonly reported combination is of Philadelphia chromosome-negative myeloproliferative neoplasms (MPNs) and chronic lymphocytic leukemia (CLL) [1]. Laurenti et al. published the largest case series ($n = 46$), finding that patients typically initially present with CLL and then subsequently develop an MPN [2]. The occurrence of chronic myeloid leukemia (CML) with a lymphoid malignancy is uncommon but has been noted with various non-Hodgkin lymphoma (NHL) histologies [3–6]. To our knowledge, this is the first reported case of a patient with a concomitant diagnosis of CML and follicular lymphoma (FL).

2. Case

A 73-year-old Caucasian male presented with three weeks of dyspnea, headache, and lower extremity edema. Initial labs were significant for marked leukocytosis with increase in myeloid precursors and rare blasts: white blood cell (WBC) 156 k/μL, neutrophils 103 k/μL, monocytes 7.1 k/μL, eosinophils 1.6 k/μL, basophils 0, and blasts 12 k/μL. Other cell lines were normal with hemoglobin of 12.6 gm/dL and platelets of 242 k/μL. Uric acid was elevated at 9.0 ml/dL, and lactate dehydrogenase was 860 units/L.

A bone marrow biopsy was performed and revealed a chronic myeloproliferative neoplasm. H&E stained slides of the core showed marked hypercellularity (99%) with profound myeloid hyperplasia and complete maturation to segmented neutrophils. Immature myeloid cells of all stages were appropriately present, without dysplasia or increased blasts. A moderate amount of reticulin fibrosis was seen. Giemsa stain of the aspirate confirmed the biopsy findings with blast count of less than 5%. By flow cytometric analysis, myeloid cells in the blast gate expressing CD34 accounted for less than 1% of total cells. Molecular diagnostic testing of the aspirate indicated the presence of the BCL-ABL1 p210-type transcript by RT-PCR with an international scale-normalized (ISN) copy number of 35.27%. Fluorescence in situ hybridization (FISH) testing for BCR-ABL1 fusion was present in 89% of cells. Together, these findings were consistent with a diagnosis of chronic phase-CML.

Given the symptoms of intermittent dyspnea in the absence of anemia, the patient underwent further evaluation. Stress echocardiogram indicated a normal left ventricular ejection fraction. Computed tomography (CT) chest with contrast enhancement revealed mediastinal, cervical, and supraclavicular adenopathy, without evidence of pulmonary embolism.

The patient subsequently underwent an excisional biopsy of the cervical lymph node, which revealed involvement with CML and FL (Figure 1). Atypical follicles with abnormal germinal centers and paracortical expansion by maturing pan-hematopoietic elements without blastic groups were noted. Immunohistochemistry (IHC) analysis showed that the atypical germinal centers expressed the pan-B cell marker CD20 and the germinal center marker CD10. There was coexpression of BCL2 and BCL6. The findings were consistent with low-grade follicular lymphoma, with fewer than 15 centroblasts per high-power field. PCR analysis for immunoglobulin heavy chain and kappa light chain gene rearrangements indicated monoclonality. Fluorescence in situ hybridization detected the IGH-BCL-2 translocation confirming follicular lymphoma.

IHC and flow cytometric analysis of the paracortical pan-myeloid hyperplasia showed no evidence of increased myeloblasts. Qualitative RT-PCR of the node detected the presence of the CML-type Mbcr (p210) fusion protein, and quantitative RT-PCR showed an ISN copy number of BCR-ABL transcripts of 0.642%, confirming nodal involvement by chronic phase-CML. Given the unusual presentation of concomitant CML and FL, further testing was done to evaluate for other abnormalities. PD-L1 expression was low (10%) using the 22C3 clone (Dako), and EBV was negative both by IHC for the viral latent membrane protein 1 (LMP1) and by Epstein–Barr encoding region in situ hybridization (EBER).

3. Clinical Course

The patient was initiated on imatinib for treatment of CML. It was chosen over the other available tyrosine kinase inhibitors due to drug interactions with his other medications. As he had no indications for treatment of the FL, he was clinically monitored with the watch-and-wait approach. Imatinib was well tolerated and only briefly held for thrombocytopenia. By three months of treatment, the WBC normalized to 5.1 k/μL, and BCR-ABL1 by RT-PCR of peripheral blood decreased to an ISN value of 30%. His

symptoms of dyspnea resolved. At 6 months, bone marrow biopsy was normocellular, consistent with complete morphologic remission. Flow cytometric analysis confirmed the absence of increased myeloblasts or involvement by FL. He achieved a partial cytogenetic remission, as karyotyping indicated persistence of Philadelphia chromosome in 15% of cells. BCR-ABL1 by RT-PCR of peripheral blood showed an ISN value of 1.15%. Repeat PET scan to reassess lymphadenopathy showed stable disease. He is currently continuing on imatinib for CML and is being followed clinically for FL.

4. Discussion

The diagnosis of both myeloid and lymphoid neoplasms in a single patient, whether simultaneous or sequential, is extremely rare, with an overall incidence of less than 1% [1]. The majority of cases (66%) have sequential presentations while only 34% present concurrently [2]. Here, we present the third known case of a patient with nodal involvement by both FL and chronic phase-CML. Both previously documented cases occurred in patients with CML who developed follicular lymphoma after initial diagnosis [6, 7].

Extramedullary disease (EMD) in CML, including nodal involvement, typically occurs in the accelerated phase (AP) or blast phase (BP), which accounts for 15% of new CML diagnoses [8, 9]. The most common sites of extramedullary involvement are bone, lymph nodes, skin, soft tissues, and the central nervous system [10]. In a study by Inverardi et al., half of the patients were in chronic phase (CP) CML at the time EMD was diagnosed, and the other half were in AP or BP. Those patients that were in CP-CML progressed to BP CML within 4 months, implying that extramedullary disease may herald impending blast crisis even if blast transformation was not present initially [10]. These early studies evaluated patients before the benefit of tyrosine kinase inhibitors (TKIs) was well understood. The clinical course of patients with CML has evolved since the advent of TKIs, which have significantly impacted the prognosis of the disease. In spite of this, physicians should closely monitor patients with evidence of EMD, as they may be at higher risk for blast formation. In the present case, the patient's lymphadenopathy was concerning for EMD leading to a lymph node biopsy. Evaluation for AP and BP was confounded by the unexpected finding of FL. Further analysis by molecular testing confirmed lymph node involvement by CP-CML without any increase in blast cells.

Postulations regarding pathogenesis for the dual presentations of myeloid and lymphoid malignancies include genetic instability, specific chemotherapy drugs, radiotherapy, and environmental exposures as predisposing factors. Genetic mutations of oncogenes, such as those of the RAS family, or tumor suppressor genes, such as p53, are noted in patients with CML and NHL [11–14] and theoretically predispose to multiple malignancies. In a recent study, data from the randomized control trial, CML study IV, were analyzed to evaluate the impact of long-term use of TKIs in the development of secondary malignancies. Patients with CML on TKIs had a significantly higher standard incidence

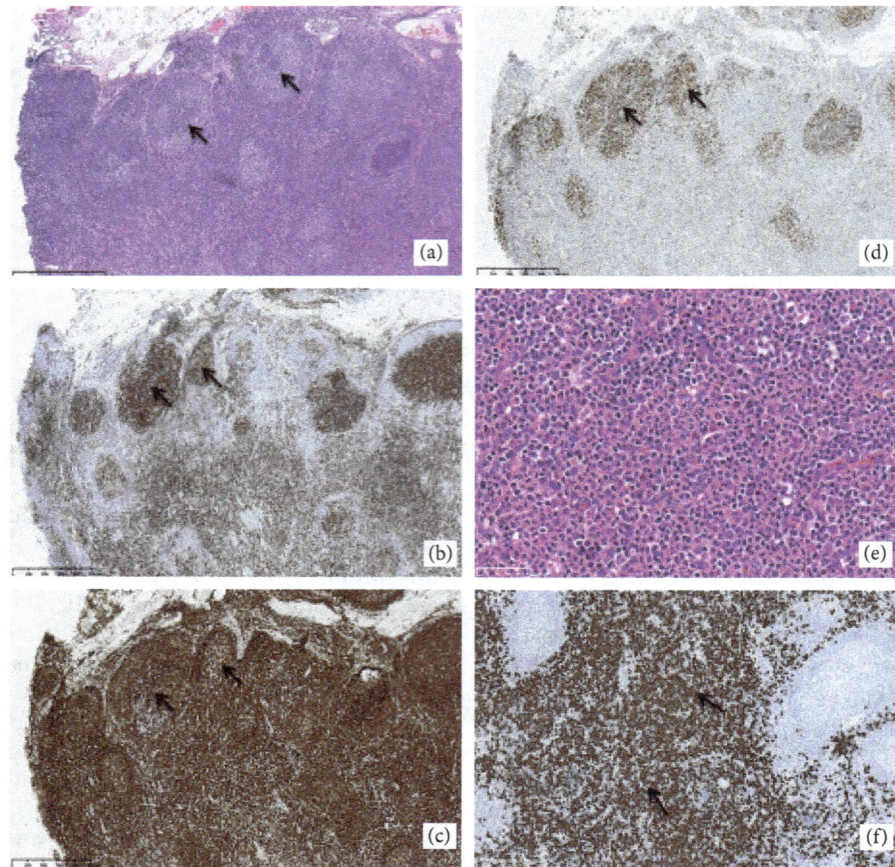

FIGURE 1: Lymph node histology and immunohistochemistry. (a) H&E section of lymph node showing atypical follicles (arrow). (b) CD10 immunostain highlighting FL cells within atypical germinal centers (arrow). (c) BCL-2 immunostain highlighting FL cells (arrow). (d) BCL-6 immunostain highligting FL cells (arrow). (e) Higher magnification of the area of paracortical expansion by neoplastic CML cells. (f) CD15 highlighting neoplastic CML cells (arrow). (a–d) 10x objective magnification, (e) 40x objective magnification, and (f) 20x objective magnification.

ratio of 3.33 in males and 4.29 in females for development of NHL compared with a matched German population. The median time from diagnosis of CML to the diagnosis of another malignancy was 2.4 years [15]. The effect of TKIs on DNA repair mechanisms is thought to be a potential mechanism for this finding based on preclinical studies [16]. In a recently published case report, a patient experiencing a complete cytogenetic response with imatinib for CML developed FL three years after initiation of the first generation TKI. He received rituximab monotherapy for the FL, resulting in a partial remission. Although he continued to receive imatinib, eventually achieving a major molecular remission, he subsequently lost this deeper response after another three years, followed by a progression of FL. Treatment with a second-generation TKI resulted not only in a major molecular remission of the CML, but also a complete remission for the FL [7]. As our patient had concurrent nodal involvement by CP-CML and FL at initial presentation, the presence of these two malignancies may represent independent events.

Pathologists and oncologists must be aware of the possibility of concurrent hematologic malignancies.

Lymphadenopathy in a patient with CML may represent blast crisis, but a distinct lymphoid malignancy is also possible. When this is suspected on morphologic examination, further evaluation using ancillary techniques including immunohistochemistry, flow cytometry, and PCR-based assays offer conclusive and accurate diagnosis. As the management of each of the synchronous malignancies often differs, this distinction is important for clinicians to make treatment decisions. Future investigations to evaluate the pathogenesis of the dual occurrence of myeloid and lymphoid malignancies are warranted to better understand and manage patients.

Disclosure

The abstract of this case report was presented as a poster at the College of American Pathologists' 2017 Annual Meeting.

Conflicts of Interest

The authors declare that they have no conflicts of interest.

References

[1] G. Hauck, D. Jonigk, H. Kreipe, and K. Hussein, "Simultaneous and sequential concurrent myeloproliferative and lymphoproliferative neoplasms," *Acta Haematologica*, vol. 129, no. 3, pp. 187–196, 2013.

[2] L. Laurenti, M. Tarnani, I. Nichele et al., "The coexistence of chronic lymphocytic leukemia and myeloproliperative neoplasms: a retrospective multicentric GIMEMA experience," *American Journal of Hematology*, vol. 86, no. 12, pp. 1007–1012, 2011.

[3] P. Pathak, Y. Li, B. A. Gray, W. S. May Jr., and M. J. Markham, "Synchronous occurrence of chronic myeloid leukemia and mantle cell lymphoma," *Case Reports in Hematology*, vol. 2017, Article ID 7815095, 4 pages, 2017.

[4] S. Alsop, W. G. Sanger, K. S. Elenitoba-Johnson, and M. S. Lim, "Chronic myeloid leukemia as a secondary malignancy after ALK-positive anaplastic large cell lymphoma," *Human Pathology*, vol. 38, no. 10, pp. 1576–1580, 2007.

[5] R. Ichinohasama, I. Miura, N. Takahashi et al., "Ph-negative non-Hodgkin's lymphoma occurring in chronic phase of Ph-positive chronic myelogenous leukemia is defined as a genetically different neoplasm from extramedullary localized blast crisis: report of two cases and review of the literature," *Leukemia*, vol. 14, no. 1, pp. 169–182, 2000.

[6] R. Martoia, T. Lamy, P. Delmaire, J. P. Algayres, Y. Rougier, and A. Laurens, "Occurrence of non-Hodgkin's lymphoma in chronic myeloid leukemia," *La Revue de Médecine Interne*, vol. 8, no. 5, pp. 471–474, 1987.

[7] S. I. Fujiwara, Y. Shirato, T. Ikeda et al., "Successful treatment of follicular lymphoma with second-generation tyrosine kinase inhibitors administered for coexisting chronic myeloid leukemia," *International Journal of Hematology*, vol. 107, no. 6, pp. 712–715, 2018.

[8] S. Faderl, M. Talpaz, Z. Estrov, S. O'Brien, R. Kurzrock, and H. M. Kantarjian, "The biology of chronic myeloid leukemia," *New England Journal of Medicine*, vol. 341, no. 3, pp. 164–172, 1999.

[9] G. Specchia, G. Palumbo, D. Pastore, D. Mininni, A. Mestice, and V. Liso, "Extramedullary blast crisis in chronic myeloid leukemia," *Leukemia Research*, vol. 20, no. 11-12, pp. 905–908, 1996.

[10] D. Inverardi, M. Lazzarino, E. Morra et al., "Extramedullary disease in Ph'-positive chronic myelogenous leukemia: frequency, clinical features and prognostic significance," *Haematologica*, vol. 75, pp. 146–148, 1990.

[11] T. Nedergaard, P. Guldberg, E. Ralfkiaer, and J. Zeuthen, "A one-step DGGE scanning method for detection of mutations in the K-, N-, and H-ras oncogenes: mutations at codons 12, 13 and 61 are rare in B-cell non-Hodgkin's lymphoma," *International Journal of Cancer*, vol. 71, no. 3, pp. 364–369, 1997.

[12] C. Hirsch-Ginsberg, A. C. LeMaistre, H. Kantarjian et al., "RAS mutations are rare events in Philadelphia chromosome-negative/bcr gene rearrangement-negative chronic myelogenous leukemia, but are prevalent in chronic myelomonocytic leukemia," *Blood*, vol. 76, pp. 1214–1219, 1990.

[13] S. Nakatsuka, T. Hongyo, M. Syaifudin, T. Nomura, N. Shingu, and K. Aozasa, "Mutations of p53, c-kit, K-ras, and beta-catenin gene in non-Hodgkin's lymphoma of adrenal gland," *Japanese Journal of Cancer Research*, vol. 93, no. 3, pp. 267–274, 2002.

[14] K. Tanaka, K. Takauchi, M. Takechi, T. Kyo, H. Dohy, and N. Kamada, "High frequency of RAS oncogene mutation in chronic myeloid leukemia patients with myeloblastoma," *Leukemia & Lymphoma*, vol. 13, no. 3-4, pp. 317–322, 1994.

[15] M. B. Miranda, M. Lauseker, M. P. Kraus et al., "Secondary malignancies in chronic myeloid leukemia patients after imatinib-based treatment: long-term observation in CML Study IV," *Leukemia*, vol. 30, no. 6, pp. 1255–1262, 2016.

[16] L. Brown and N. McCarthy, "DNA repair: a sense-abl response?," *Nature*, vol. 387, no. 6632, pp. 450-451, 1997.

27

PAX5-Negative Classical Hodgkin Lymphoma: A Case Report of a Rare Entity

Elham Vali Betts,[1] **Denis M. Dwyre,**[1] **Huan-You Wang,**[2] **and Hooman H. Rashidi**[1]

[1]*Department of Pathology and Laboratory Medicine, University of California, Davis, Davis, CA, USA*
[2]*Department of Pathology, University of California, San Diego, La Jolla, CA, USA*

Correspondence should be addressed to Elham Vali Betts; evali@ucdavis.edu and Hooman H. Rashidi; hrashidi@ucdavis.edu

Academic Editor: Sudhir Tauro

Classical Hodgkin lymphoma (CHL) is recognized as a B-cell neoplasm arising from germinal center or postgerminal center B-cells. The hallmark of CHL is the presence of CD30 (+) Hodgkin and Reed-Sternberg (HRS) cells with dim expression of PAX5. Nearly all of the HRS cells are positive for PAX5. However, a small minority of HRS cells may lack PAX5 expression, which can cause a diagnostic dilemma. Herein we describe two cases of PAX5-negative CHL and review of the English literature on this very rare entity. It is crucial to be aware of this phenomenon, which in some cases may lead to misdiagnosis and may ultimately adversely affect patient's management.

1. Introduction

Classical Hodgkin lymphoma (CHL) per WHO 2008 is a clonal lymphoid neoplasm. CHL contains Reed-Sternberg (RS) cells in a background of a nonneoplastic inflammatory infiltrate including lymphocytes, eosinophils, neutrophils, histiocytes, and plasma cells [1]. Kanzler et al. microdisected and analyzed the RS cells from frozen tissue and showed nearly all RS cells carry immunoglobulin (Ig) heavy and light chain rearrangement, which supported the B-cell origin of these neoplasms [2]. Moreover, identical IgHV gene rearrangement was detected between RS cells of a given case, which showed the monoclonality of these cells [2]. RS cells show somatic hypermutation in the IgHV gene and since these mutations occur in the proliferating B-cells in germinal centers (GC), they are recognized to arise from GC or post-GC B-cells. The RS cells therefore are expected to express B-cell specific markers. According to WHO, the most specific B-cell marker is CD19 and since PAX5 is closely tied to this molecule, nearly all of the RS cells are reported to express PAX5 by immunohistochemistry. RS cells, however, are typically negative for CD19 [3]. The PAX5 acts as a transcriptional factor that is expressed by B-cells and its binding sites serve as promotors for certain B-cell-specific genes such as those that promote CD19 expression [4]. The expression of PAX5 is reduced and in rare cases of CHL, PAX5 expression is absent in RSC. This has been postulated to be caused by compromised B-cell specific transcription machinery and inactivity of immunoglobulin promoters, which results in low levels to absent expression of several B-cell-restricted transcription factors such as PAX5 and OCT2 [5]. Hence, the PAX5 negative cases of CHL are extremely rare and pose a major diagnostic challenge for hematopathologists. In review of the English literature, no known large case series of PAX5 negative CHL cases are noted and it is extremely important to have a review of the literature on this extremely rare entity.

2. Case Presentation

2.1. Case 1. A 22-year-old male presented with a neck mass, night sweats, and weight loss. The excisional biopsy showed an effaced node involved by a nodular lymphohistiocytic infiltrate separated by fibrocollagenous bands. Among the background inflammatory cells were large atypical lymphoid cells with one to more nuclei, prominent nucleoli, and abundant pale cytoplasm, resembling Hodgkin Reed-Sternberg (HRS) cells (Figure 1(a)). These large atypical cells were positive for CD30 and focally positive for CD15.

(a)

(b)

(c)

(d)

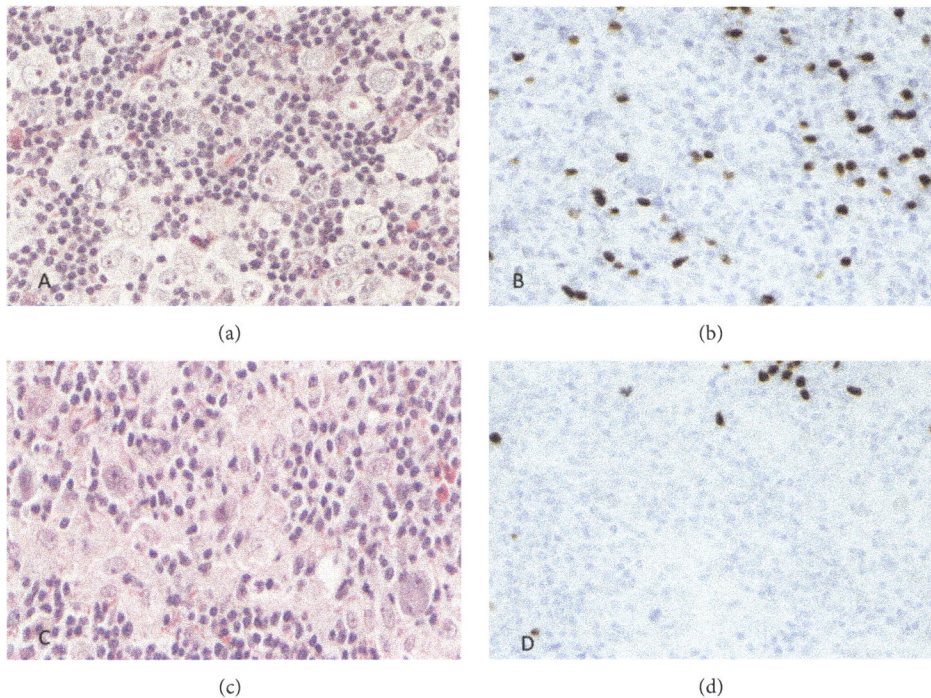

FIGURE 1: (a and c) Large atypical lymphoid cells with one to more nuclei, prominent nucleoli, and abundant cytoplasm consistent with RS cells and Hodgkin cells on the hematoxylin and eosin stain. (b and d) The large atypical cells are negative for PAX5 expression.

They were negative for PAX5 (Figure 1(b)), OCT2, BOB1, CD20, BCL6, CD2, CD3, CD4, CD5, CD7, CD8, and ALK1. T-cell gene rearrangement was negative which along with negative expression of pan-T-cell markers and ALK excludes anaplastic large cell lymphoma (ALCL). The H&E histology along with the immunohistochemical profile confirmed the suspected morphologic diagnosis of a CHL, nodular sclerosis subtype. Patient has been receiving treatment and has undergone allogeneic bone marrow transplant.

2.2. Case 2. A 53-year-old HIV-negative male presented with discomfort at the base of the neck, which was unresponsive to antibiotic therapy. A mass was noted, and a fine needle aspiration (FNA) was performed of the mass. The FNA showed scattered large atypical lymphoid cells. On a follow-up excisional biopsy, H&E sections of a lymph node showed an effaced nodal architecture with prominent nonnecrotizing granulomas and a mixed infiltrate of small lymphoid cells, histiocytes, and eosinophils with intermingled large atypical cells. The majority of the large cells were mononucleated cells with prominent large cherry red nucleoli and moderate to abundant eosinophilic cytoplasm, consistent with Hodgkin cells (Figure 1(c)). Occasional classical binucleated RS cells were also noted. These large cells were positive for CD30, CD15 (subset), CD79a (small subset), and MUM1 but were negative for CD20, CD45, OCT2, PAX5 (Figure 1(d)), CD2, CD3, CD4, CD5, CD7 CD8, granzyme-B, perforin, and ALK1. In this case expression of CD79a in a subset of RSC indicates the B-cell origin of the CD30 positive malignant cells. The T-cell gene rearrangement was negative which along with

negative expression of the T-cell markers, ALK, and cytotoxic markers excludes ALCL. No acid fast organisms were noted by AFB stain. Subsequently, a diagnosis of a CHL, mixed cellularity subtype was rendered. Patient has undergone six cycles of chemotherapy and has been responding well to the treatment.

3. Discussion

PAX5 negative CHLs are extremely rare since CHL is believed to be a B-cell neoplasm. PAX5 is a nuclear transcription factor and, among the hematopoietic malignancies, the expression of this marker is mostly restricted to B-cells [6, 7]. The gene expression of PAX5 is increased during B-cell maturation and PAX5 expression has been shown to regulate B-cell proliferation and immunoglobulin secretion [6]. Hence, the absence of PAX5 in CHL is a very unusual finding and warrants further investigation. A study by Desouki et al. showed five of 39 cases of CHL were negative for PAX5 by immunohistochemical staining; of the five CHL cases noted in this study, two were mixed cellularity, two were nodular sclerosis, and one CHL was not otherwise specified [6]. Hertel et al. showed 4 cases of PAX5-negative classical Hodgkin lymphoma nodular sclerosis and one case of CHL, mixed cellularity type from 18 cases evaluated in the study [5]. In another study performed by Johri et al. one case out of 24 cases of CHL lacked expression of PAX5 [8]. A study by Foss et al. showed 3 cases of CHL without expression of PAX5 by immunohistochemistry out of 31 cases that were evaluated [9]. In a study performed by Nguyen et al., they showed two

TABLE 1: PAX5-negative HRS cells in different variants of CHL.

Reported cases of PAX5-negative CHL	
	PAX5-negative CHL
Desouki et al.	
MCHL[1]	2
NSHL[2]	2
LRHL[3]	0
CHL, NOS[4]	1
Total	5
Hertel et al.	
NSHL	4
MCHL	1
Johri et al.	
CHL	1
Nguyen et al.	
CHL	2
Vali Betts et al.	
CHL, NS type[5]	1
CHL, MC type[6]	1

[1]Mixed cellularity CHL, [2]nodular sclerosis CHL, [3]lymphocyte rich CHL, [4]CHL, not otherwise specified, [5]CHL, nodular sclerosis type, and [6]CHL, mixed cellularity type.

cases of PAX5 negative from 74 cases of CHL evaluated in their study [10] (Table 1).

In the differential diagnoses of PAX5 negative CHL, ALCL (a T-cell lymphoma) has to be considered and ruled out, typically by immunohistochemical staining and gene rearrangement studies. Unlike HRS cells in CHL, large cells in ALCL are commonly positive for CD45 and may express EMA [11]. In ALK positive ALCL, the tumor cells may have loss of many of the pan T-cell markers in addition to being positive for ALK1 staining. In the ALK negative ALCL cases, the tumor cells nearly always express CD2 and most are CD4 positive [11]. Cytotoxic markers, such as perforin and granzyme-B, are expressed in ALCL. Additionally, T-cell receptor gene rearrangement studies are helpful in such cases as molecular findings indicative of a clonally restricted T-cell population would strongly favor a form of T-non-Hodgkin lymphoma (T-NHL)/ALCL over CHL. ALCL should be negative for PAX5. However, rare cases of ALCL with expression of PAX5 have been reported [12, 13]. PAX5 expression in these cases has been reported to be due to extra copies of PAX5 and not PAX5 rearrangement [13]. It is important to be aware of both of these entities, PAX5-negative CHL and PAX5-positive ALCL, and use extensive immunohistochemical stains along with gene rearrangement studies to define the origin of the neoplastic cells.

The clinical significance of the lack of PAX5 staining in CHL is unknown. A very small study of PAX5-negative CHL cases suggested that patients with PAX5-negative CHL may have worse clinical outcomes, when compared to typical PAX5-positive CHL. These patients are more prone to relapse or short-ended progression free survival [11]. The study was very small and a larger evaluation of patients with this rare entity would need to be studied before making a definitive

assessment of such potential prognostic significance. Additionally, the diagnosis of a PAX5-negative CHL should be done with extreme caution and only when other mimickers have been definitively ruled out.

Conflicts of Interest

The authors declare that they have no conflicts of interest.

Acknowledgments

The authors would like to thank DR. Elaine S. Jaffe of NCI for her expert opinions on these two cases.

References

[1] H. Stein, G. Delsol, SA. Pileri, LM. Weiss, S. Poppema, and ES. Jaffe, "WHO classification of hematopoietic and lymphoid tissue, International Agency for Research on Cancer," Lyon, France, 2008.

[2] H. Kanzler, R. Küppers, M.-L. Hansmann, and K. Rajewsky, "Hodgkin and Reed-Sternberg cells in Hodgkin's disease represent the outgrowth of a dominant tumor clone derived from (crippled) germinal center B cells," Journal of Experimental Medicine, vol. 184, no. 4, pp. 1495–1505, 1996.

[3] F. G. Haluska, A. M. Brufsky, and G. P. Canellos, "The cellular biology of the Reed-Sternberg cell," Blood, vol. 84, no. 4, pp. 1005–1019, 1994.

[4] H. Kaneko, T. Ariyasu, R. Inoue et al., "Expression of Pax5 gene in human haematopoietic cells and tissues: Comparison with immunodeficient donors," Clinical and Experimental Immunology, vol. 111, no. 2, pp. 339–344, 1998.

[5] C. B. Hertel, X.-G. Zhou, S. J. Hamilton-Dutoit, and S. Junker, "Loss of B cell identity correlates with loss of B cell-specific transcription factors in Hodgkin/Reed-Sternberg cells of classical Hodgkin lymphoma," Oncogene, vol. 21, no. 32, pp. 4908–4920, 2002.

[6] M. M. Desouki, G. R. Post, D. Cherry, and J. Lazarchick, "PAX-5: a valuable immunohistochemical marker in the differential diagnosis of lymphoid neoplasms," Clinical Medicine and Research, vol. 8, no. 2, pp. 84–88, 2010.

[7] L. Krenacs, A. W. Himmelmann, L. Quintanilla-Martinez et al., "Transcription factor B-cell-specific activator protein (BSAP) is differentially expressed in B cells and in subsets of B-cell lymphomas," Blood, vol. 92, no. 4, pp. 1308–1316, 1998.

[8] N. Johri, S. C. U. Patne, M. Tewari, and M. Kumar, "Diagnostic utility of PAX5 in Hodgkin and non-Hodgkin lymphoma: A study from Northern India," Journal of Clinical and Diagnostic Research, vol. 10, no. 8, pp. XCO4–XCO7, 2016.

[9] H.-D. Foss, R. Reusch, G. Demel et al., "Frequent expression of the B-cell-specific activator protein in Reed- Sternberg cells of classical Hodgkin's disease provides further evidence for its B-cell origin," Blood, vol. 94, no. 9, pp. 3108–3113, 1999.

[10] T. D. T. Nguyen, J. L. Frater, J. Klein et al., "Expression of TIA1 and PAX5 in Classical Hodgkin Lymphoma at Initial Diagnosis May Predict Clinical Outcome," Applied Immunohistochemistry and Molecular Morphology, vol. 24, no. 6, pp. 383–391, 2016.

[11] E. S. Jaffe, "Anaplastic large cell lymphoma: The shifting sands of diagnostic hematopathology," Modern Pathology, vol. 14, no. 3, pp. 219–228, 2001.

[12] D. M. Ong, K. D. Cummins, A. Pham, and G. Grigori-adis, "PAX5-expressing ALK-negative anaplastic large cell lymphoma with extensive extranodal and nodal involvement," *BMJ Case Reports*, vol. 2015, Article ID 211159, 2015.

[13] A. L. Feldman, M. E. Law, D. J. Inwards, A. Dogan, R. F. McClure, and W. R. MacOn, "PAX5-positive T-cell anaplastic large cell lymphomas associated with extra copies of the PAX5 gene locus," *Modern Pathology*, vol. 23, no. 4, pp. 593–602, 2010.

28

Molecular Profiling: A Case of *ZBTB16-RARA* Acute Promyelocytic Leukemia

Stephen E. Langabeer,[1] **Lisa Preston,**[1] **Johanna Kelly,**[2] **Matt Goodyer,**[3] **Ezzat Elhassadi,**[3] **and Amjad Hayat**[3]

[1]*Cancer Molecular Diagnostics, St. James's Hospital, Dublin 8, Ireland*
[2]*Department of Clinical Genetics, Our Lady's Children Hospital, Dublin 12, Ireland*
[3]*Department of Haematology, Galway University Hospital, Galway, Ireland*

Correspondence should be addressed to Stephen E. Langabeer; slangabeer@stjames.ie

Academic Editor: Massimo Gentile

Several variant *RARA* translocations have been reported in acute promyelocytic leukemia (APL) of which the t(11;17)(q23;q21), which results in a *ZBTB16-RARA* fusion, is the most widely identified and is largely resistant to therapy with all-trans retinoic acid (ATRA). The clinical course together with the cytogenetic and molecular characterization of a case of ATRA-unresponsive *ZBTB16-RARA* APL is described. Additional mutations potentially cooperating with the translocation fusion product in leukemogenesis have been hitherto unreported in *ZBTB16-RARA* APL and were sought by application of a next-generation sequencing approach to detect those recurrently found in myeloid malignancies. This technique identified a solitary, low level mutation in the *CEBPA* gene. Molecular profiling of additional mutations may provide a platform to individualise therapeutic management in patients with this rare form of APL.

1. Introduction

Acute promyelocytic leukemia (APL) is a distinct form of acute myeloid leukemia (AML) characterized by the balanced translocation t(15;17)(q24;q21) that results in production of the *PML-RARA* oncogene. Retinoid-based therapy in combination with either anthracyclines or arsenic trioxide results in favorable rates of complete remission and overall survival, provided that the patient can be supportively managed through the initial coagulopathy [1]. However, a small proportion of patients harbor variant translocations that result in fusion of *RARA* to one of a number of alternative partner genes [2, 3]. The most often reported of these variant translocations is the t(11;17)(q23;q21) which results in the fusion of the zinc finger gene *ZBTB16* (formerly *PLZF*) to the *RARA* locus [4, 5]. The bone marrow morphology of patients with *ZBTB16-RARA* APL tends to be distinct from those patients with either classical or the hypogranular variant of APL [6]. Identification of the *ZBTB16-RARA* fusion is critical for therapeutic purposes as these patients are generally resistant to differentiating retinoid therapy, specifically all-trans retinoic acid (ATRA) [7], and treatment should be with standard AML regimens according to current recommendations [8].

In murine models of APL, induction of *PML-RARA* expression in myeloid stem cells results in a myeloproliferative disease that subsequently develops into leukemia with promyelocytic features after a relatively long latency implicating the requirement for further cooperating mutations to fully recapitulate the APL phenotype [9, 10]. The development and application of whole exome sequencing and targeted exome sequencing have led to the identification of several cooperating mutations in APL and demonstrates the clonal and subclonal acquisition of mutational events in conjunction with the driver *PML-RARA* oncogene [11, 12]. A similar pattern of these cooperative mutations appears to exist within patients with APL and those with other types of AML [13]. Whether these additional mutations have a prognostic impact is unclear [14]. However, identification of these mutations may allow targeted intervention [15]. To date, the pattern

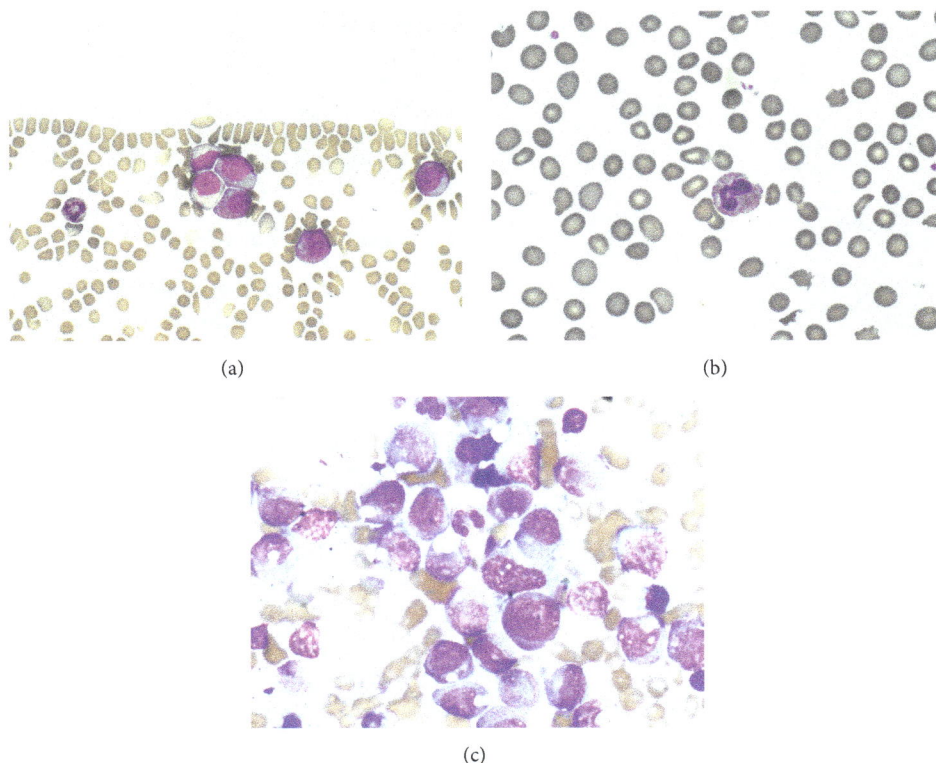

FIGURE 1: (a) Peripheral blood promyelocytes; (b) peripheral blood pseudo-Pelger-Huet neutrophils; (c) bone marrow effacement by promyelocytes at diagnosis.

of cooperating mutations in patients with *ZBTB16-RARA* APL has not been investigated. Characterization of a patient with this uncommon cytogenetic variant of APL is described with subsequent application of a targeted next-generation sequencing (NGS) approach to identify allied mutational events.

2. Case Report

An 81-year-old female presented with a short history of back pain with a physical examination proving unremarkable. Full blood count revealed pancytopenia (hemoglobin 8.8 g/dl, neutrophils 1.8×10^9/L, and platelets 140×10^9/L) and abnormal circulating promyelocytes that constituted 40% of nucleated cells. A coagulation screen was only mildly deranged with a prothrombin time of 15.1 seconds, an activated partial thromboplastin time of 29.4 seconds, and fibrinogen of 3.2 g/L. Peripheral blood promyelocytes, which accounted for 40% of nucleated cells, had regular nuclei, were hypergranular and lacked Auer rods (Figure 1(a)) with increased numbers of pseudo-Pelger-Huet neutrophils noted (Figure 1(b)). Immunophenotyping detected autofluorescent blasts that expressed MPO, CD13, CD14, and CD33 but lacked CD34 and HLA-DR expression. The bone marrow was effaced by promyelocytes (Figure 1(c)) which stained strongly positive for Sudan Black. The patient commenced ATRA with a progressive concurrent increase noted in both peripheral blood myeloblasts and promyelocytes (white cell count

40.5×10^9/L), thrombocytopenia (platelets 92×10^9/L), and coagulopathy (fibrinogen 0.7 g/L) despite intensive blood product support. The chest findings were more consistent with aspiration and therefore no response to ATRA with differentiation syndrome excluded. Hydroxyurea and idarubicin were initiated in an attempt to achieve cytoreduction; however, progressive respiratory compromise and worsening coagulopathy led to the patients' death due to pulmonary hemorrhage ten days after presentation.

Cytogenetic G-band analysis identified an aberration involving 17q in 4/13 metaphases analysed. Metaphase fluorescent in situ hybridisation studies revealed a rearrangement involving *RARA* at 17q12 and confirmed the partner chromosome to be 11q, thus identifying the t(11;17) translocation with a full karyotype of 46,XX,add(17)(q21)[4]/46,XX[9].ish der(11)t(11;17)(q23;q21)(RARA+).nuc ish(PMLx2, RARAx3)[142/200]. A standardised reverse transcription-PCR approach [16] did not detect *PML-RARA* transcripts, but, using primers previously described [7], a *ZBTB16-RARA* fusion transcript, consistent with fusion of *ZBTB16* exon 3 fused to *RARA* exon 2, was detected and confirmed by Sanger sequencing (Figure 2). The reciprocal *RARA-ZBTB16* fusion was not detected.

An NGS approach utilising a gene panel to detect additional mutations cooperating with the *ZBTB16-RARA* fusion in propagating APL was retrospectively employed. Amplicon libraries covering thirty commonly mutated genes implicated in myeloid malignancies were generated using genomic

ZBTB16 exon 3 ——→✕←—— RARA exon 2

ACACAGGCAGACCCATACTGCCATTGAGACCCAGAGCAGCA

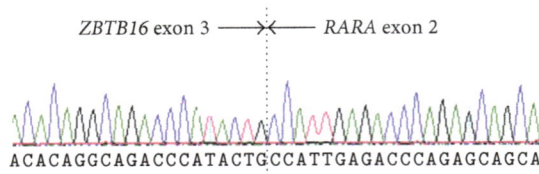

FIGURE 2: Sanger sequencing demonstrating fusion of *ZBTB16* exon 3 to *RARA* exon 2.

DNA from the diagnostic bone marrow aspirate using an Ion AmpliSeq™ approach (Thermo Fisher Scientific, Paisley, UK). A single in-frame *CEBPA* p.P189delP mutation was detected (c.564–566 delGCC; reference sequence GRCh37: 19:33792755-7) with an allele frequency of 6.2%.

3. Discussion

Several rare variant *RARA* translocations have been described in APL among which the *ZBTB16-RARA* is the most frequent. Identification of the t(11;17) at the cytogenetic and/or the *ZBTB16-RARA* fusion at the cytogenetic and molecular levels, respectively, is paramount as, in the case described herein, *ZBTB16-RARA* APL is generally unresponsive to ATRA therapy, although it must be noted that some response to initial ATRA therapy has been documented in very rare cases and always in combination with other agents [17–19]. Although distinctive morphological features have been ascribed to *ZBTB16-RARA* APL [6], the peripheral blood and bone marrow morphology in this case more closely resembled that of typical APL, an aspect infrequently reported [20].

The NGS approach adopted herein detected only one additional mutation in *CEBPA* which encodes a transcription factor involved in cell fate decisions for myeloid cell differentiation [21]. This gene is recurrently mutated in types of AML other than APL, but mutations at this codon have been rarely documented [22]. Although no constitutional material was available and therefore not analysed in tandem, the low allele frequency implies that this is an acquired, somatic mutation of *CEBPA* and not a single nucleotide polymorphism. How *CEBPA* mutations might cooperate with the *ZBTB16-RARA* fusion in leukemogenesis is unclear; however, one study has demonstrated that CEBPA protein activity is severely impaired in leukemic promyelocytes with the t(11;17) translocation and that the reciprocal RARA-ZBTB16 protein inhibits myeloid cell differentiation through its interaction with CEBPA [23]. It is acknowledged that this NGS approach is limited to those commonly mutated genes in myeloid malignancies and that a greater coverage of both other genes and additional exons of those genes within this panel may prove more informative.

In conclusion, rapid identification and comprehensive molecular profiling are vital for future appropriate tailoring of therapy in patients with this rare form of APL.

Disclosure

Current address of Matt Goodyer is Service d'Hématologie, Hôpital du Valais, 1950 Sion, Switzerland, and current address of Ezzat Elhassadi is Department of Haematology, University Hospital Waterford, Waterford, Ireland.

Conflicts of Interest

The authors declare that there are no conflicts of interest regarding the publication of this paper.

Acknowledgments

The authors are grateful to Kathleen Brosnan, Cancer Molecular Diagnostics, St. James's Hospital, Dublin, Ireland, for technical assistance with next-generation sequencing.

References

[1] L. Cicconi and F. Lo-Coco, "Current management of newly diagnosed acute promyelocytic leukemia," *Annals of Oncology*, vol. 27, no. 8, pp. 1474–1481, 2016.

[2] J. Adams and M. Nassiri, "Acute promyelocytic leukemia a review and discussion of variant translocations," *Archives of Pathology and Laboratory Medicine*, vol. 139, no. 10, pp. 1308–1313, 2015.

[3] W. Yan and G. Zhang, "Molecular characteristics and clinical significance of 12 fusion genes in acute promyelocytic leukemia: a systematic review," *Acta Haematologica*, vol. 136, no. 1, pp. 1–15, 2016.

[4] S.-J. Chen, A. Zelent, J.-H. Tong et al., "Rearrangements of the retinoic acid receptor alpha and promyelocytic leukemia zinc finger genes resulting from t(11;17)(q23;q21) in a patient with acute promyelocytic leukemia," *Journal of Clinical Investigation*, vol. 91, no. 5, pp. 2260–2267, 1993.

[5] J. D. Licht, C. Chomienne, A. Goy et al., "Clinical and molecular characterization of a rare syndrome of acute promyelocytic leukemia associated with translocation (11;17)," *Blood*, vol. 85, no. 4, pp. 1083–1094, 1995.

[6] D. Sainty, V. Liso, A. Cantù-Rajnoldi, and et al., "A new morphological classification system for acute promyelocytic leukemia distinguishes cases with underlying PLZF/RARA gene rearrangements," *Blood*, vol. 96, no. 4, pp. 1287–1296, 2000.

[7] F. Guidez, W. Huang, J. H. Tong et al., "Poor response to all-trans retinoic acid therapy in a t(11;17) PLZF/RAR alpha patient," *Leukemia*, vol. 8, no. 2, pp. 312–317, 1994.

[8] M. A. Sanz, D. Grimwade, M. S. Tallman et al., "Management of acute promyelocytic leukemia: recommendations from an expert panel on behalf of the European LeukemiaNet," *Blood*, vol. 113, no. 9, pp. 1875–1891, 2009.

[9] L. M. Kelly, J. L. Kutok, I. R. Williams et al., "PML/RARα and FLT3-ITD induce an APL-like disease in a mouse model," *Proceedings of the National Academy of Sciences of the United States of America*, vol. 99, no. 12, pp. 8283–8288, 2002.

[10] L. D. Wartman, D. E. Larson, Z. Xiang et al., "Sequencing a mouse acute promyelocytic leukemia genome reveals genetic events relevant for disease progression," *Journal of Clinical Investigation*, vol. 121, no. 4, pp. 1445–1455, 2011.

[11] J. S. Welch, T. J. Ley, D. C. Link et al., "The origin and evolution of mutations in acute myeloid leukemia," *Cell*, vol. 150, no. 2, pp. 264–278, 2012.

[12] V. Madan, P. Shyamsunder, and L. Han, "Comprehensive mutational analysis of primary and relapse acute promyelocytic leukemia," *Leukemia*, vol. 30, no. 8, pp. 1672–1681, 2016.

[13] L. Riva, C. Ronchini, M. Bodini et al., "Acute promyelocytic leukemias share cooperative mutations with other myeloid-leukemia subgroups," *Blood Cancer Journal*, vol. 3, no. 9, p. e147, 2013.

[14] R. Dillon and D. Grimwade, "Prognostic significance of additional cytogenetic abnormalities and FLT3 mutations in acute promyelocytic leukemia," *Leukemia & Lymphoma*, vol. 55, no. 7, pp. 1444–1446, 2014.

[15] C. Lai, J. E. Karp, and C. S. Hourigan, "Precision medicine for acute myeloid leukemia," *Expert Review of Hematology*, vol. 9, no. 1, pp. 1–3, 2016.

[16] J. J. M. Van Dongen, E. A. Macintyre, J. A. Gabert et al., "Standardized RT-PCR analysis of fusion gene transcripts from chromosome aberrations in acute leukemia for detection of minimal residual disease. Report of the BIOMED-1 concerted action: investigation of minimal residual disease in acute leukemia," *Leukemia*, vol. 13, no. 12, pp. 1901–1928, 1999.

[17] D. J. Culligan, D. Stevenson, Y.-L. Chee, and D. Grimwade, "Acute promyelocytic leukaemia with t(11;17)(q23;q12-21) and a good initial response to prolonged ATRA and combination chemotherapy," *British Journal of Haematology*, vol. 100, no. 2, pp. 328–330, 1998.

[18] J. H. Jansen, M. C. de Ridder, W. M. C. Geertsma et al., "Complete remission of t(11;17) positive acute promyelocytic leukemia induced by all-trans retinoic acid and granulocyte colony-stimulating factor," *Blood*, vol. 94, no. 1, pp. 39–45, 1999.

[19] M. C. Petti, F. Fazi, M. Gentile et al., "Complete remission through blast cell differentiation in PLZF/RARα-positive acute promyelocytic leukemia: In vitro and in vivo studies," *Blood*, vol. 100, no. 3, pp. 1065–1067, 2002.

[20] S. B. Han, J. Lim, Y. Kim, H. Kim, and K. Han, "A variant acute promyelocytic leukemia with t(11;17)(q23;q12); ZBTB16-RARA showing typical morphology of classical acute promyelocytic leukemia," *The Korean Journal of Hematology*, vol. 45, no. 2, pp. 133–135, 2010.

[21] E. Ohlsson, M. B. Schuster, M. Hasemann, and B. T. Porse, "The multifaceted functions of C/EBPα in normal and malignant haematopoiesis," *Leukemia*, vol. 30, no. 4, pp. 767–775, 2016.

[22] L.-I. Lin, C.-Y. Chen, D.-T. Lin et al., "Characterization of CEBPA mutations in acute myeloid leukemia: Most patients with CEBPA mutations have biallelic mutations and show a distinct immunophenotype of the leukemic cells," *Clinical Cancer Research*, vol. 11, no. 4, pp. 1372–1379, 2005.

[23] N. Girard, M. Tremblay, M. Humbert et al., "RARα-PLZF oncogene inhibits C/EBPα function in myeloid cells," *Proceedings of the National Academy of Sciences of the United States of America*, vol. 110, no. 33, pp. 13522–13527, 2013.

29

The Relationship between Multiple Myeloma with Renal Failure and Metastatic Calcification

Takanori Fukuta ⓘ, Takayuki Tanaka, Yoshinori Hashimoto, and Hiromi Omura

Department of Hematology, Tottori Prefectural Central Hospital, Tottori, Japan

Correspondence should be addressed to Takanori Fukuta; takanori.fukuta@jfcr.or.jp

Academic Editor: Alessandro Gozzetti

While cases of multiple myeloma (MM) with metastatic calcification have been reported, the mechanisms for this calcification have yet to be explained. We observed a case of MM in a patient with end-stage renal failure who developed vascular and pulmonary calcification. A 51-year-old male was diagnosed with Bence-Jones type MM and required maintenance hemodialysis. He was treated with bortezomib-dexamethasone, vincristine-doxorubicin-dexamethasone, the M2 protocol, and lenalidomide-dexamethasone (Rd) therapy. During the sixth cycle of Rd therapy, he complained of pain in both lower legs. Well-demarcated ulcers with severe pain had developed on the right lower leg, both exterior thighs, and penis. We found that the patient's serum intact parathyroid hormone level was elevated, while it had previously been permissively controlled. Computed tomography scan showed widespread centrilobular opacities of the bilateral lungs and high-density lesions along small blood vessels in the trunk and all four extremities. Histological calcifications were identified in small blood vessels and the alveolar walls. The risk of metastatic calcification in MM appears to be associated with renal failure, but not with MM itself.

1. Introduction

Multiple myeloma (MM) is a clonal plasma cell proliferative disorder with symptoms related to bone marrow infiltration, impaired hematopoiesis, or end-organ damage, which ultimately leads to renal failure, bone lesions, and hypercalcemia.

Metastatic calcification is the deposition of calcium salts in systemic organs. Calcific uremic arteriolopathy (CUA), a type of metastatic calcification, is a rare condition characterized by cutaneous artery calcinosis, leading to skin ischemia and ulceration. The term "calciphylaxis" is also used to describe such lesions, but it was originally used to describe hypersensitivity [1].

Cases of MM with metastatic calcification have been previously reported, but the mechanism for this calcification is unclear. Here we describe a patient with MM and end-stage renal failure who developed vascular and pulmonary calcification, and we examine the relationship between MM and calcification.

2. Case Presentation

A 51-year-old male was referred to our hospital because of a three-month history of gradually progressing renal failure.

During his first hospitalization, he complained of lumbar pain. On physical examination, he had conjunctival pallor and severe percussion tenderness of his back. No skin lesions or neurological deficits were seen. Laboratory test results were as follows: hemoglobin, 8.7 g/dL; creatinine, 7.01 mg/dL; total protein, 7.4 g/dL; albumin, 3.2 g/dL; calcium, 14.8 mg/dL; phosphate, 6.2 mg/dL; beta-2-microglobulin, 27.9 mg/L; IgG, 341 mg/dL; IgA, 21 mg/dL; IgM, 18 mg/dL; free kappa light chain, 99,900 mg/L; and free lambda light chain, 9.7 mg/L. Chest X-ray results were normal. Computed tomography (CT) showed vertebral compression fractures of Th8 and L1 and bilateral pleural effusions without calcified lesions. Urine immunoelectrophoresis showed a positive result for the Bence-Jones protein. Bone marrow aspiration revealed plasma cell proliferation (65% of total nucleated cells, Figure 1) with expression of CD38 and CD56, absence of CD19 and CD20, and an MIB-1 labeling index of 25%. Chromosomal analysis of the bone marrow by G-banding showed a normal 46,XY karyotype, but fluorescence in situ hybridization revealed the abnormalities del(13q) and t(4;14). He was diagnosed with Bence-Jones protein type MM (stage III according to the International Staging System, and stage IIIB according to the Durie–Salmon classification system).

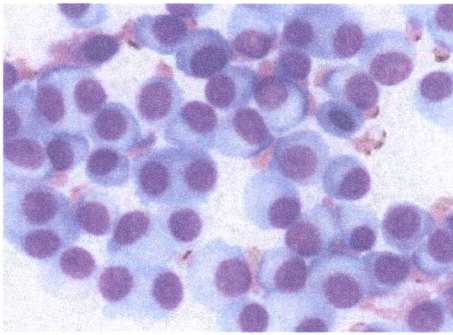

FIGURE 1: Morphology of the plasma cells in a bone marrow smear (May–Giemsa staining).

We began treatment with intravenous fluids and intramuscular injections of calcitonin to treat the severe hypercalcemia. Simultaneously, he received bortezomib-dexamethasone (Bd) therapy (subcutaneous injection of 1.3 mg/(m^2·day) bortezomib plus 20 mg/day dexamethasone orally on days 1, 4, 8, and 11). Unexpectedly, he experienced severe acute heart failure on day 8, and temporarily required the support of a mechanical ventilator. Bd therapy was discontinued during the first treatment cycle. Because renal function had not improved, maintenance hemodialysis was initiated. Subsequently, we continued MM treatment with two cycles of vincristine-doxorubicin-dexamethasone (0.4 mg/body of vincristine and 9 mg/m^2 of doxorubicin on days 1 to 4; and 40 mg/body of dexamethasone on days 1 to 4, 9 to 12, and 17 to 20 of a 28-day cycle) and the M2 protocol (multiple chemotherapeutic agents, not including proteasome inhibitors), followed by lenalidomide-dexamethasone (Rd) therapy (5 mg/day lenalidomide on days 1 to 21 plus 20 mg/body dexamethasone on days 1, 8, 15, 22 of a 28-day cycle).

About four months after starting Rd therapy, the patient suffered from myoclonus-like movement of the lower extremities. During the sixth cycle of Rd therapy, he complained of pain in both lower legs, but did not have skin lesions or tenderness. He had been taking loxoprofen, fentanyl (patch and buccal tablet), mecobalamin, ferrous fumarate, lansoprazole, amlodipine, furosemide, alfacalcidol, and darbepoetin alfa. It was unlikely that his pain was drug-induced.

The patient's serum creatinine kinase level was elevated to 1,268 U/L. Diffusion-weighted and short tau inversion recovery magnetic resonance imaging revealed diffuse high signal intensity in the crural muscles (Figure 2(a)). A muscle biopsy was performed on the right tibial anterior muscles (Figure 3) and 40 mg/day prednisolone was prescribed by a neurologist because of suspected polymyositis/dermatomyositis. However, typical pathologic findings of polymyositis/dermatomyositis, like lymphocyte infiltration around muscle fibers, were absent and vessel calcification was noted. Prednisolone was ineffective against his symptoms. During steroid administration, well-demarcated ulcers developed on the right lower leg, both exterior thighs, and the penis. These ulcers gradually worsened (Figure 4) and the patient experienced severe pain, especially during dialysis or exercise. He could not continue dialysis because of this exacerbation of pain. Moreover, muscle atrophy of his lower limbs impaired his daily activities. The administration of 40 mg/day prednisolone was continued

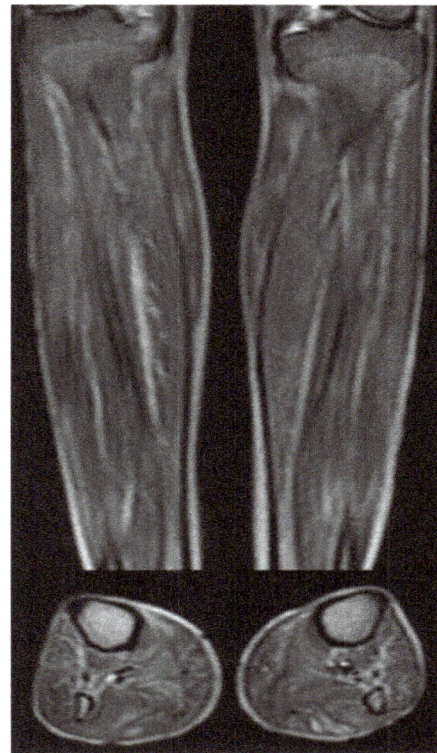

(a)

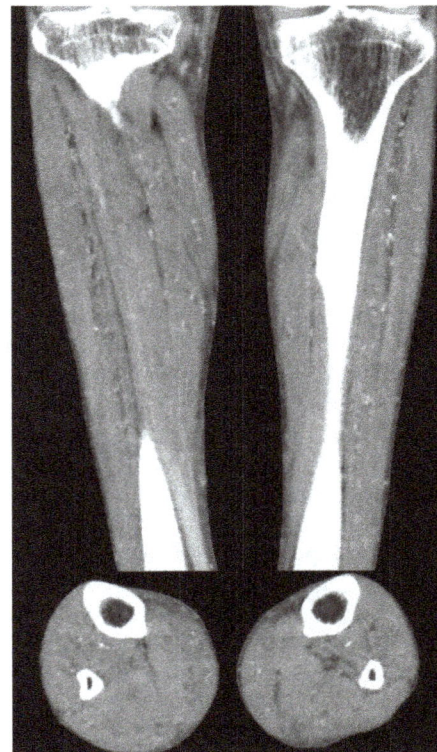

(b)

FIGURE 2: MRI/CT image of lower legs. (a) STIR (short tau inversion recovery) magnetic resonance image showing high-signal intensity areas in the lower leg muscles. These lesions had high DWI signals and normal ADC values. The muscle structure was intact. (b) Noncontrast enhanced computed tomography showing high density areas along the vessels.

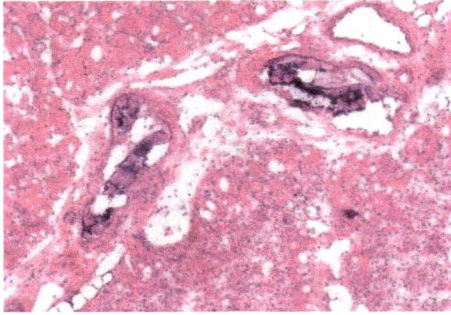

FIGURE 3: Muscle biopsy of the right anterior tibial muscle (hematoxylin-eosin staining). Calcifications are observed in the vascular walls among the muscular bundles. Muscle fibers are slightly basophilic, and myophagia is also observed.

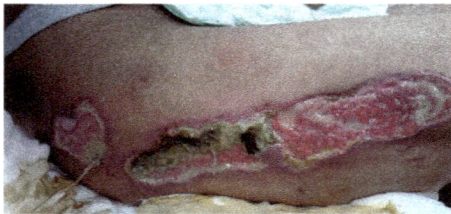

FIGURE 4: Refractory ischemic skin ulcers of the right exterior thigh due to vascular calcification. This wound later reached the fascia.

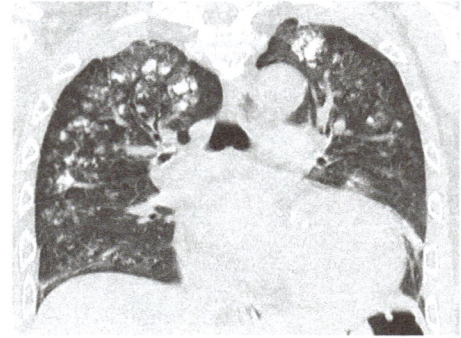

(a)

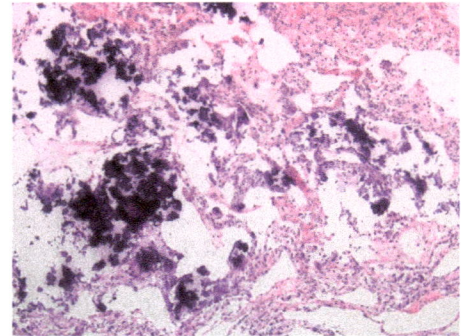

(b)

FIGURE 5: (a) Computed tomography of the lungs. Calcifications were observed in both the lungs, especially in the upper fields. (b) Transbronchial lung biopsy specimen (hematoxylin-eosin staining). Basophilic fine calcific substances were observed along the alveolar wall.

for 42 days and was then stopped on the 84th day after tapering. The patient's serum intact parathyroid hormone (PTH) level was 429 pg/mL, while previously it was permissively controlled within the range of 140–250 pg/mL. Before dialysis, his levels of serum albumin, calcium, and phosphate were 4.0 g/dL, 7.4 mg/dL, and 7.9 mg/dL, respectively. He was diagnosed with secondary hyperparathyroidism (HPT). We could not exclude a relationship between MM and HPT, although his free light chain ratio was decreasing.

CT showed widespread centrilobular opacities of both lungs (Figure 5(a)) and high-density lesions along small blood vessels in the trunk and extremities (Figure 2(b)), but the mediastinum, abdominal organs, and large vessels like the thoracic and abdominal aorta were intact. A pulmonary function test demonstrated restrictive impairment with reduced diffusion capacity: the predicted forced vital capacity was 48.6%, the forced expiratory volume of the first breath was 87.9%, and the predicted diffusing capacity of lung for carbon monoxide was 67.1%. ^{99m}Tc-hydroxymethylene diphosphonate scintigraphy revealed abnormal diffuse accumulation in both upper lung fields (Figure 6). Echography revealed no enlargement of the parathyroid glands.

Next, a transbronchial lung biopsy was performed, and microscopy confirmed the presence of calcifications of the alveolar walls (Figure 5(b)) and of a small vessel in the right anterior tibial muscle (Figure 3). However, pathological calcification was absent from the right exterior thigh ulcer. Healing of the skin biopsy wound was delayed.

The patient was ultimately diagnosed with muscle and skin ischemia from CUA. He was treated with cinacalcet, and his intact PTH levels fell to a normal range. He underwent four

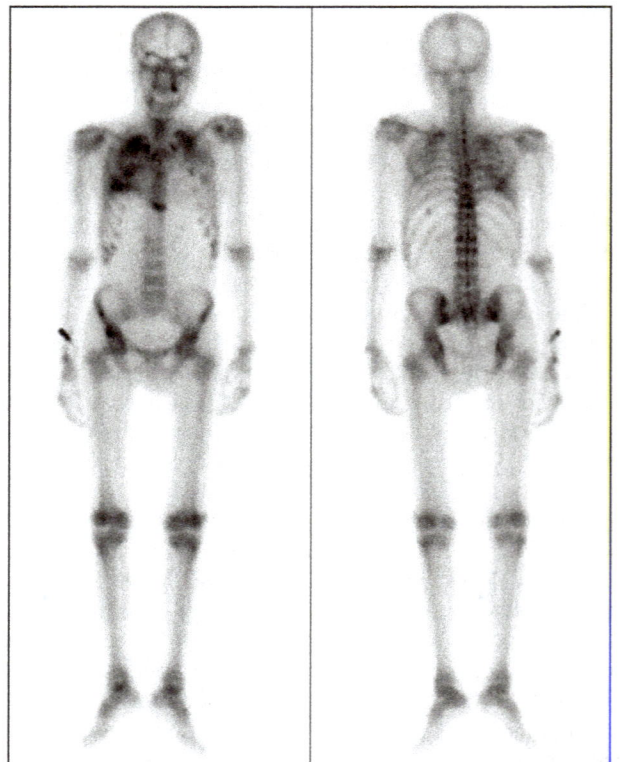

FIGURE 6: ^{99m}Tc-hydroxymethylene diphosphonate scintigraphy. Accumulation in both of the upper lung fields was detected.

TABLE 1: Data for patients with multiple myeloma plus lung or vessel calcifications.

Age	Sex	Immunoglobulin chain	Cr (mg/dL)	Corrected Ca (mg/dL)	P (mg/dL)	Intact PTH (pg/mL)	Lung lesions**	Pathological vessel calcifications	Reference
45	M	Lambda	2.6	12.3	NA	NA	+		[9]
57	F	IgA lambda	7.44	7.5	11.9	149	+	+	[10]
52	F	IgG kappa	Normal	18.4*	Normal	Normal	+		[11]
35	F	IgG kappa	1.66	13.8*	NA	NA	+	+	[12]
44	M	Nonsecretory	Elevated	Elevated	NA	NA	+		[13]
42	M	IgG lambda	Normal	Normal	Normal	NA		+	[14]
60	F	Kappa	5	18*	11.4	NA	+	+	[15]
52	M	Kappa	2.56	20*	5.82	NA		+	[16]
54	F	Nonsecretory	4.9	16.4	7.7	Normal	+		[17]
49	M	NA	7	12.8	NA	NA	+		[18]
51	F	IgG kappa	15.3	12.5	6.6	NA	+	+	[19]
66	F	IgA lambda	2.75	12.8*	NA	NA	+		[20]
66	F	IgA lambda	1.92	18.0*	NA	NA	+		[20]
47	M	NA	Elevated	Elevated	NA	NA	+		[21]
70	M	IgG	4	17.5*	5.2	NA	+		[22]
62	M	IgG	8.6	12*	NA	NA	+		[22]
57	M	IgA kappa	7.3	16.7	5.7	NA	+	+	[23]
51	F	IgG	2.01	14.1*	NA	NA	+	+	[24]
55	M	IgA lambda	3.1	14.6*	3.4	NA	+	+	[25]
53	M	Lambda	3	14.4*	4.9	<100	+		[26]
56	M	IgA lambda	3.3	17.5	NA	NA	+		[27]
63	M	NA	NA	16.4*	NA	NA	+		[28]
74	F	IgG lambda	NA	Normal	Normal	Normal			[29]
55	M	NA	NA	Elevated	NA	NA	+		[30]
37	M	NA	4.9	13.1*	7.2	NA	+		[31]
73	F	IgG kappa	3.5	15.3	5.8		+		[32]
65	M	IgG kappa	1.8	14.7	4.4	NA		+	[33]
67	M	IgA lambda	4.9	12.5	Normal	NA			[34]
51	M	Kappa	7.01	15.6	6.2	429	+	+	Our case

The blank spaces for "lung lesions on CXR/CT/scintigram or histology finding" and "pathological vessel calcifications" mean that these findings were not described. M: male; F: female; NA: not available. *Not corrected; **findings on CXR/CT/scintigram or histology.

additional cycles of Rd therapy, but ulcer infections occurred repeatedly in both thighs, occasionally progressing to sepsis. He has since been monitored closely for MM, without treatment, for four months. Meanwhile, the ulcers have achieved epithelialization after topical treatment, but his serum free light chain ratio level increased from 290 to 1532. He is currently undergoing Pd therapy (2 mg/day pomalidomide on days 1 to 21, plus 4 mg/day dexamethasone on days 1, 8, 15, and 22 of a 28-day cycle) without any adverse events. Since severe heart failure occurred during the combined regimen with bortezomib, we have avoided administering proteasome inhibitors. His disease is stable according to the International Myeloma Working Group criteria.

3. Discussion

In this case, metastatic calcification occurred in an MM patient with end-stage renal failure and secondary HPT. Melosalgia triggered the diagnosis of CUA. Histological calcifications were observed in small blood vessels and the alveolar walls. Cutaneous ulcers were found symmetrically in our patient, on both lower limbs and the penis, which were accompanied by strong pain exacerbated by dialysis and exertion. This symptom is consistent with ischemia: dialysis reduces the circulating plasma volume, while exertion increases oxygen demand. Clinicians should avoid biopsy for the definite diagnosis of suspected CUA based on clinical presentations, because such lesions may exhibit delayed wound healing. CUA causes a high mortality rate due to sepsis from wound infection [2]. The myoclonus-like movement of the lower extremities of our patient might have been another consequence of ischemia.

The mineral and bone metabolism of patients with renal failure should be controlled to improve prognosis. Recently, the term "chronic kidney disease-mineral and bone disorder" has been used for the condition traditionally called renal osteodystrophy. Complex abnormalities of calcium, phosphate, and PTH are all part of chronic kidney disease-mineral and bone disorder.

The relationship between MM and HPT is unclear. Hussain et al. described 30 cases of MM with primary HPT and reported that this condition is more common in females, its effects are observed in various types of MM immunoglobulin chains, and it does not coincide with the appearance of HPT. Unfortunately, the frequency of renal failure in these patients is not currently available [3]. Our hypothesis is that the main risk factor for HPT is not MM, but renal failure. Secondary HPT is common within dialysis populations. For example, Hedgeman et al. reported that the prevalence of secondary HPT within dialysis populations ranges from about 30 to 50% [4].

Interestingly, our patient developed metastatic pulmonary calcification, depositions of calcium in the pulmonary parenchyma, and pathologically identified calcifications of the alveolar walls, but not of lung small vessels. CT images showed a relatively strong deposition of calcium in the upper lung zone, which is typical of metastatic pulmonary calcification. It has been reported that the ventilation-perfusion ratio of the lung apex is higher than that of the base; therefore, the partial pressure of carbon dioxide in the artery is low and its pH is high. This environment appears to facilitate tissue calcification [5]. These lung lesions often do not cause respiratory failure and they are difficult to detect by chest radiography [5]. Kaltreider et al. found just 13 cases of interstitial pulmonary calcification in a series of 7,221 autopsies [6]. In contrast, metastatic pulmonary calcification was observed in 60% (9/15) [7] to 75% (42/56) [8] of chronic dialysis patients in an autopsy series. Chronic dialysis thus appears to carry a high risk of lung calcification.

To clarify the relationship between MM and metastatic calcification, PubMed was searched using the terms "multiple myeloma," and "metastatic calcification," and we then added other appropriate articles published between 1980 and 2015. Table 1 shows data from 29 MM patients with metastatic calcification or CUA. Twenty-four of the patients (92%, excluding three with unclear renal function) presented renal insufficiency, and 26 (90%) developed hypercalcemia. Calcification of both the lungs and vessels were confirmed in eight patients (28%). PTH values were available in few cases. The type of immunoglobulin light and heavy chains observed were not uniform. These previous reports indicate that myeloma does not seem to have a primary role in metastatic calcification. We hypothesize that renal failure, not only in patients requiring dialysis, is a fundamental cause of calcinosis in MM patients.

The risk of metastatic calcification in MM appears to have a strong relationship with renal failure, but not with MM itself. Metastatic calcification, such as CUA and metastatic pulmonary calcification, is rare complication in MM patients, even in those with renal failure. However, clinicians should be aware of this condition, because it can induce organ injury or lethal outcomes.

Conflicts of Interest

The authors declare that there are no conflicts of interest regarding the publication of this article.

References

[1] H. Selye, G. Gabbiani, and R. Strebel, "Sensitization to calciphylaxis by endogenous parathyroid hormone," *Endocrinology*, vol. 71, no. 4, pp. 554–558, 1962.

[2] S. M. Roe, L. D. Graham, W. B. Brock, and D. E. Barker, "Calciphylaxis: early recognition and management," *American Surgeon*, vol. 60, no. 2, pp. 81–86, 1994.

[3] N. Hussain, M. Khan, A. Natarajan et al., "A case of multiple myeloma coexisting with primary hyperparathyroidism and review of the literature," *Case Reports in Oncological Medicine*, vol. 2013, Article ID 420565, 8 pages, 2013.

[4] E. Hedgeman, L. Lipworth, K. Lowe et al., "International burden of chronic kidney disease and secondary hyperparathyroidism: a systematic review of the literature and available data," *International Journal of Nephrology and Renovascular Disease*, vol. 2015, Article ID 184321, 15 pages, 2015.

[5] E. D. Chan, D. V. Morales, C. H. Welsh, M. T. McDermott, and M. I. Schwarz, "Calcium deposition with or without bone formation in the lung," *American Journal of Respiratory and Critical Care Medicine*, vol. 165, no. 12, pp. 1654–1669, 2002.

[6] H. B. Kaltreider, G. L. Baum, G. Bogaty, M. D. McCoy, and M. Tucker, "So-called "metastatic" calcification of the lung," *American Journal of Medicine*, vol. 46, no. 2, pp. 188–196, 1969.

[7] J. D. Conger, W. S. Hammond, A. C. Alfrey et al., "Pulmonary calcification in chronic dialysis patients. Clinical and pathologic studies," *Annals of Internal Medicine*, vol. 83, no. 3, pp. 330–336, 1975.

[8] D. C. Kuzela, W. E. Huffer, J. D. Conger, S. D. Winter, and W. S. Hammond, "Soft tissue calcification in chronic dialysis patients," *American Journal of Pathology*, vol. 86, no. 2, pp. 403–424, 1977.

[9] S. R. Surani, S. Surani, A. Khimani, and J. Varon, "Metastatic pulmonary calcification in multiple myeloma in a 45-year-old man," *Case Reports in Pulmonology*, vol. 2013, Article ID 341872, 3 pages, 2013.

[10] K. Ueki, S. Yamada, A. Tsuchimoto et al., "Rapid progression of vascular and soft tissue calcification while being managed for severe and persistent hypocalcemia induced by denosumab treatment in a patient with multiple myeloma and chronic kidney disease," *Internal Medicine*, vol. 54, no. 20, pp. 2637–2642, 2015.

[11] C. K. Weber, J. M. Friedrich, E. Merkle et al., "Reversible metastatic pulmonary calcification in a patient with multiple myeloma," *Annals of Hematology*, vol. 72, no. 5, pp. 329–332, 1996.

[12] S. Cagirgan, N. Soyer, F. Vural et al., "Metastatic pulmonary calcinosis and leukocytoclastic vasculitis in a patient with multiple myeloma," *Turkish Journal of Haematology*, vol. 29, no. 4, pp. 397–400, 2012.

[13] H. Kempter, G. Hagner, A. N. Savaser, H. Huben, and C. Minguillon, "Metastatic pulmonary calcification in a patient with nonsecretory multiple myeloma," *Respiration*, vol. 49, no. 1, pp. 77–80, 1986.

[14] R. F. Raper and L. S. Ibels, "Osteosclerotic myeloma complicated by diffuse arteritis, vascular calcification and extensive cutaneous necrosis," *Nephron*, vol. 39, no. 4, pp. 389–392, 1985.

[15] C. Crippa, S. Ferrari, M. Drera et al., "Pulmonary calciphylaxis and metastatic calcification with acute respiratory failure in multiple myeloma," *Journal of Clinical Oncology*, vol. 28, no. 9, pp. e133–e135, 2010.

[16] E. Sullivan and C. Hoyle, "Calciphylaxis, occurring 10 weeks after hypercalcaemia, in a patient with multiple myeloma," *British Journal of Haematology*, vol. 155, no. 2, p. 136, 2011.

[17] A. J. Chaves Alvarez, A. Herrera Saval, J. Marquez Enriquez, and F. Camacho Martinez, "Metastatic calcinosis cutis in multiple myeloma," *British Journal of Dermatology*, vol. 142, no. 4, pp. 820–822, 2000.

[18] E. Marchiori, N. L. Muller, A. S. Souza et al., "Unusual manifestations of metastatic pulmonary calcification: high-resolution CT and pathological findings," *Journal of Thoracic Imaging*, vol. 20, no. 2, pp. 66–70, 2005.

[19] R. H. Poe, C. Kamath, M. A. Bauer et al., "Acute respiratory distress syndrome with pulmonary calcification in two patients

with B cell malignancies," *Respiration*, vol. 56, no. 1-2, pp. 127–133, 1989.

[20] H. Nilsson-Ehle, C. Holmdahl, M. Suurkula, and J. Westin, "Bone scintigraphy in the diagnosis of skeletal involvement and metastatic calcification in multiple myeloma," *Acta Medica Scandinavica*, vol. 211, no. 6, pp. 427–432, 1982.

[21] G. L. Arbona, S. Antonmattei, M. R. Tetalman, and J. D. Scheu, "Tc-99m-diphosphonate distribution in a patient with hypercalcemia and metastatic calcifications," *Clinical Nuclear Medicine*, vol. 5, no. 9, p. 422, 1980.

[22] M. Salvatori, V. Valenza, A. Ursitti, and G. Menichella, "Bone scan demonstration of metastatic calcification in multiple myeloma," *Rays*, vol. 12, no. 1, pp. 63–66, 1987.

[23] P. Morassi, G. Paladini, G. Mazzanti et al., "Bone scintigraphy in the diagnosis of pulmonary calcification in multiple myeloma," *European Journal of Nuclear Medicine and Molecular Imaging*, vol. 11, no. 8, pp. 327–329, 1985.

[24] J. L. Coolens, P. Devos, and M. De Roo, "Diffuse pulmonary uptake of ^{99m}Tc bone-imaging agents: case report and survey," *European Journal of Nuclear Medicine and Molecular Imaging*, vol. 11, no. 1, pp. 36–42, 1985.

[25] F. Cardellach, J. Rabasseda, A. Pujol et al., "Detection of metastatic calcification in lungs and stomach with radionuclide in multiple myeloma," *Thorax*, vol. 37, no. 7, pp. 552-553, 1982.

[26] Y. Hirose, J. Tachibana, S. Sugai et al., "Metastatic calcification in the stomach demonstrated by a bone scan in Bence Jones lambda myeloma," *Japanese Journal of Medicine*, vol. 26, no. 1, pp. 72–75, 1987.

[27] M. Ito, C.-T. Hsu, S. Shikuwa et al., "Multiple myeloma in alcoholic liver cirrhosis," *Tohoku Journal of Experimental Medicine*, vol. 157, no. 1, pp. 39–44, 1989.

[28] J. H. Liou, L. C. Cho, and Y. H. Hsu, "Paraneoplastic hypercalcemia with metastatic calcification–clinicopathologic studies," *Kaohsiung Journal of Medical Sciences*, vol. 22, no. 2, pp. 85–88, 2006.

[29] N. Kerk, V. Meyer, and T. Goerge, "Calciphylaxis induced by acquired protein S deficiency in a patient with multiple myeloma - effective treatment with low-molecular-weight heparin," *Journal der Deutschen Dermatologischen Gesellschaft*, vol. 10, no. 7, pp. 518-519, 2012.

[30] T. Kanoh, H. Uchino, I. Yamamoto, and K. Torizuka, "Soft-tissue uptake of technetium-99m MDP in multiple myeloma," *Clinical Nuclear Medicine*, vol. 11, no. 12, pp. 878-879, 1986.

[31] M. Livingood and S. A. Newman, "An unusual presentation of perforating metastatic calcinosis cutis," *SkinMed*, vol. 11, no. 5, pp. 314-315, 2013.

[32] B. A. Eagel, S. A. Stier, and C. Wakem, "Non-osseous bone scan abnormalities in multiple myeloma associated with hypercalcemia," *Clinical Nuclear Medicine*, vol. 13, no. 12, pp. 869-873, 1988.

[33] M. M. Cooper, "Metastatic calcification: an unusual cause of lower intestinal hemorrhage," *New York State Journal of Medicine*, vol. 88, no. 7, pp. 389-390, 1988.

[34] S. Wynchank, A. J. Brendel, F. Leccia et al., "Transient intense gastric fixation of 99mTc-MDP," *European Journal of Nuclear Medicine and Molecular Imaging*, vol. 8, no. 10, pp. 458–460, 1983.

30

Simultaneous Occurrence of Rosai–Dorfman Disease and Nodal Marginal Zone Lymphoma in a Patient with Sjögren's Syndrome

Vadim R. Gorodetskiy [ID],[1] Wolfram Klapper,[2] Natalya A. Probatova,[3] Vladimir I. Vasilyev,[1] and Elena V. Rozhnova[4]

[1]*Department of Intensive Methods of Therapy, V.A. Nasonova Research Institute of Rheumatology, Kashirskoye Shosse 34A, Moscow 115522, Russia*
[2]*Department of Pathology, Hematopathology Section and Lymph Node Registry, Christian-Albrecht University Kiel and University Hospital Schleswig-Holstein, 24105 Kiel, Germany*
[3]*Department of Pathology, N.N. Blokhin Russian Cancer Research Center, Kashirskoye Shosse 24, Moscow 115478, Russia*
[4]*Department of Therapeutic Dentistry, I.M. Sechenov First Moscow State Medical University, Trubetskaya, 8, Building 2, Moscow 119991, Russia*

Correspondence should be addressed to Vadim R. Gorodetskiy; gorodetskiyblood@mail.ru

Academic Editor: Kiyotaka Kawauchi

We present an exceptionally rare case of co-occurrence of Rosai–Dorfman disease (RDD) and nodal marginal zone lymphoma (NMZL) in a 60-year-old Caucasian female with a 20-year course of Sjögren's syndrome (SS). In response to treatment for lymphoma, the patient presented a short positive response, followed by a rapid progression of the disease accompanied by the development of the peripheral facial nerve palsy. We failed to detect Epstein–Barr virus (EBV) in the NMZL/RDD sample by EBV-encoded RNA (EBER) in situ hybridization but identified genomic DNA of EBV by polymerase chain reaction. A second biopsy revealed EBV-positive diffuse large B-cell lymphoma (DLBCL), not otherwise specified. The identical clonal immunoglobulin heavy chain gene rearrangements in the NMZL and DLBCL pointed to their clonal relationship. Though the role of EBV in the pathogenesis of some lymphomas is well-known, there have been only few cases of EBV-induced transformation of low-grade B-cell lymphoma into high-grade lymphoma and no cases of a patient with an NMZL background. To our knowledge, this is the first report of a concomitant occurrence of RDD and NMZL in a SS patient.

1. Introduction

Sjögren's syndrome (SS) is a systemic autoimmune disease characterized by chronic inflammation of the exocrine glands, mainly the salivary and lacrimal glands [1]. Among autoimmune diseases, SS is known to have the highest incidence of lymphomas [2]. The latest World Health Organization (WHO) classification distinguishes three subtypes of B-cell marginal zone lymphoma (MZL) according to the sites involved: extranodal marginal zone of mucosa-associated lymphoid tissue (MALT) lymphoma, splenic MZL (SMZL), and nodal MZL (NMZL) [3]. MZL, particularly MALT lymphoma of the salivary glands, is the most common histological type of lymphoma encountered in the setting of SS [4–6].

Rosai–Dorfman disease (RDD, sinus histiocytosis with massive lymphadenopathy) is a rare idiopathic histiocytic disorder [7]. While the pathogenesis of RDD remains elusive, the new histiocytic society has classified this disease into the following categories: familial, classical (nodal), extranodal, neoplasia-associated, and immune disease-associated [8]. Although a few hundred publications related to RDD can be found in the literature, only 28 cases of RDD associated with non-Hodgkin and Hodgkin lymphomas have been reported to date. Furthermore, the simultaneous occurrence of RDD and NMZL is extremely rare, and to the best of our knowledge, only two cases of this kind have been documented [9, 10]. The association of RDD with autoimmune diseases has also been reported; however, we were able to find only two documented cases describing the co-occurrence of SS and RDD [11, 12]. This report presents an exceptionally rare case of simultaneous occurrence of RDD and NMZL in a female with SS.

2. Case Presentation

In February 2013, a 60-year-old Caucasian woman was admitted to the V. A. Nasonova Research Institute of Rheumatology with complaints of weakness, weight loss of 25 kg over 2 years, dryness of the eyes and mouth, and enlargement of the cervical and axillary lymph nodes. Her medical history was consistent with a 20-year course of SS. Since May 2011, she had experienced numbness in her feet followed by the development of Raynaud's syndrome and recurrent purpura on the shins. Increasing and decreasing lymphadenopathy involving the neck and axillae was observed over 2 years. Within 3 months before admission, she was taking 4 mg of methylprednisolone every other day.

At the time of admission, peripheral blood counts were as follows: hemoglobin 13.6 g/dl, platelets 224×10^9/L, and white blood cells 6.7×10^9/L, with 85% neutrophils, 8% lymphocytes, and 7% of monocytes. Laboratory data showed that electrolytes and renal and liver function were within the normal range. The serum lactate dehydrogenase level was elevated to 593 IU/L (normal <378). Ophthalmic examination revealed that the patient had keratoconjunctivitis sicca (with filamentous keratitis), with a Schirmer's test score of <1 mm/5 min and tear break-up time of 3-4 sec (OD) and 8 sec (OS). Dental examination of the submandibular and parotid salivary glands showed no salivation (sialometry: 0 mL). A labial salivary gland biopsy showed marked focal lymphocytic sialadenitis with focus score of 4 foci per 4 mm^2. Anti-SSA/Ro antibody level exceeded 200 U/ml (normal < 25), antinuclear antibody level was 1: 640 (normal < 1:160) with homogeneous and speckled patterns, and rheumatoid factor level was 885 IU/mL (normal < 20). Based on the clinical, serological, and pathological features, the diagnosis of SS was confirmed.

Protein electrophoresis and immunofixation of the patient's serum showed monoclonal immunoglobulin (Ig) M kappa (1.5 g/L) and a decrease in polyclonal IgG and IgA levels. The monoclonal Ig had the property of cryoglobulin. Urine protein electrophoresis and immunofixation assays detected the presence of monoclonal free kappa type light chains (0.06 g/24 h). Increased β2-microglobulin and C-reactive protein levels were noted to be as high as 5.99 mg/L (normal < 2.4) and 47.7 mg/L (normal < 6.0), respectively. In addition, the C4 complement level was reduced to 0.02 g/L (normal range 0.1–0.4). A full staging computerized tomography (CT) scan showed multiple enlarged lymph nodes in the neck, axillary, mediastinal, lung hilar, abdominal, and retroperitoneal spaces, with a fusion of the conglomerates (maximum size of 4.1×2.4 cm) and mild splenomegaly (measuring $8.2 \times 13.3 \times 15.2$ cm). Additionally, bilateral lymphangitis was found in the lung parenchyma, and the patient had developed moderate bilateral hydrothorax with compression of basal segments of the lower lobes.

Histologic examination of the right axillary lymph node revealed a completely effaced architecture (Figure 1(a)). The sinus system was open and filled with pleomorphic histiocytic cells, some of which showed emperipolesis of peripheral blood cells (Figure 1(b)). Immunohistochemical staining showed the expression of CD68 (Figure 1(c)) and CD163 in these histiocytic cells accompanied by coexpression of S100 (Figure 1(d)), while the staining result was negative for CD1a and Langerin. The lymph node tissue showed an infiltrate consisting of partly nodular and partly diffused pattern of CD20-positive and CD10-negative B-lymphocytes and extensive plasma cell infiltration (Figure 1(e)). The plasma cells showed positive staining for light kappa chain (Figure 1(f)), IgM heavy chain (Figure 1(g)), and MUM1 (Figure 1(h)). However, they did not stain positive for the expression of CD138, VS38c, CD56, and Cyclin-D1. Ki-67, a marker of cell proliferation, was expressed in 5–7% of the cells of the sinuses and up to 50% of the cells within the intervening cords of the lymph node (Figure 1(i)). We failed to detect Human herpesvirus-8 by immunohistochemistry and EBV-encoded RNA (EBER) in situ hybridization (EBER-ISH), but the DNA of the EBV was detected in the sample by the polymerase chain reaction (PCR). Further, sequence analysis of lymph node tissue showed no mutations within the codon 265 of the MYD88 gene and somatic mutations in KRAS and MAP2K1. Histological and cytological analysis revealed no infiltration of bone marrow by lymphocytes and plasma cells. Thus, the patient was diagnosed with concomitant RDD and plasmacytic marginal zone lymphoma. After six cycles of MDB (melphalan [Alkeran] + dexamethasone + bortezomib), a partial response was achieved according to the data of the CT scan. As follow-up analyses, electrophoresis and immunofixation of serum proteins were performed that failed to detect any presence of monoclonal IgM kappa. Electrophoresis followed by immunofixation of concentrated urine proteins showed secretion of the monoclonal free kappa type light chains in trace amounts. In November 2013, a month after the end of chemotherapy, a fast-growing firm mass developed in the left mandibular fossa spreading anteriorly to the parotid area. Soon, peripheral paralysis of the facial nerve occurred (Figure 2). Histological examination of this mass revealed a necrotic tissue interspersed with foci of small lymphoid cells with scarce large tumor cells, mainly with round and oval nuclei containing nucleoli and pyroninophilic cytoplasm. Large tumor cells were also present as perivascular and perineural clusters (Figure 3(a)). Small lymphoid cells were predominantly T lymphocytes (CD3+) and expressed either CD4 or CD8, approximately in equal proportions. Large lymphoid cells expressed CD20 (Figure 3(b)), CD79α, CD30 (Figure 3(c)), light kappa chain (Figure 3(d)), IgM heavy chain (Figure 3(e)), PAX5, and MUM1 (Figure 3(f)). Expression of Ki-67 was observed in nearly 60% of tumor cells. The EBER-ISH demonstrated the presence of EBV-positive large lymphocytes (Figure 3(g)). EBV-positive diffuse large B-cell lymphoma, not otherwise specified (DLBCL, NOS) was diagnosed.

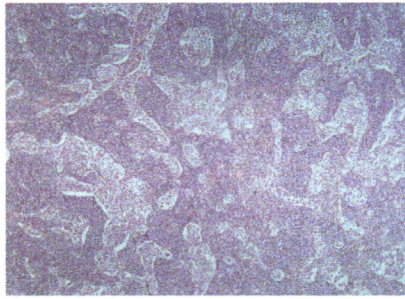
(a)

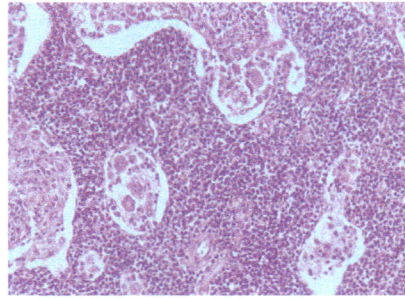
(b)

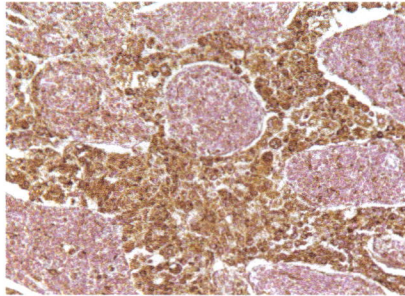
(c)

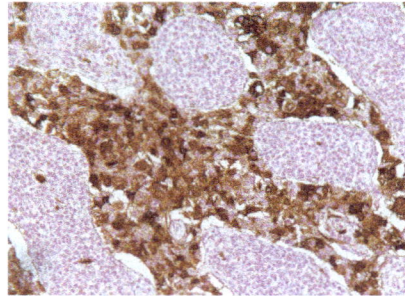
(d)

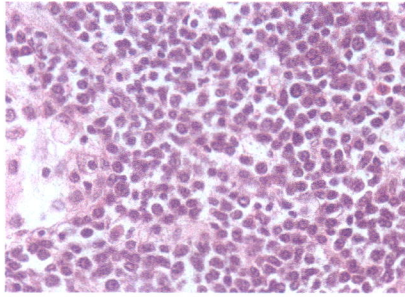
(e)

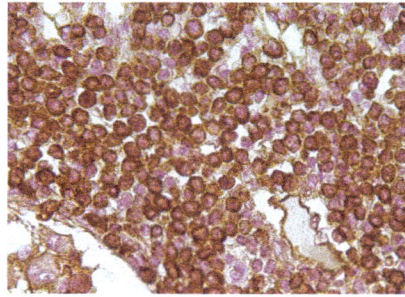
(f)

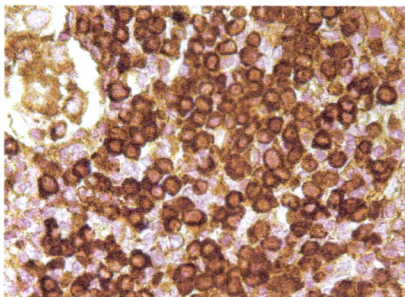
(g)

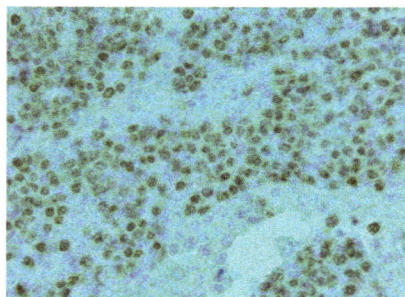
(h)

FIGURE 1: Continued.

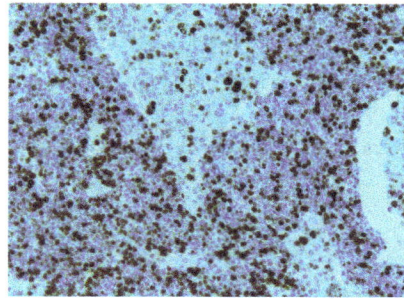

(i)

FIGURE 1: (a) The lymph node shows a completely effaced architecture. The sinus system is open and filled with partly pleomorphic histiocytic cells (×50, hematoxylin and eosin stain (H&E)). (b) The partly pleomorphic histiocytic cells are present in the sinuses, while the intervening cords exhibit a marked plasmacytosis (×200, H&E). (c) The histiocytic cells express CD68 (×200). (d) The histiocytic cells show nuclear and cytoplasmic positivity for S100 (×200). (e) The mature plasma cells (Marschalko type) present in the intervening cords (×630, H&E). (f) Monomorphic expression of light kappa chain in plasma cells (×630). (g) Monomorphic expression of IgM in plasma cells (×630). (h) Expression of MUM1 in plasma cells (×630). (i) Ki-67 is expressed in 5–7% of the cells of the sinuses and up to 50% of cells within the intervening cords of the lymph node (×200).

Multiplex BIOMED-2 PCR fragment assays were used to study rearrangements of the Ig heavy chain (IGH) gene in NMZL and DLBCL samples. IGH framework 1, 2, and 3 assays (Tube A, Tube B, and Tube C) were used to detect Vh-Jh rearrangements. Identical clonal patterns between the NMZL and DLBCL were demonstrated (Figure 4). The resulting condition was considered a transformation of NMZL into an EBV-positive DLBCL, NOS. R-CHOP (rituximab, cyclophosphamide, doxorubicin, vincristine, and prednisone) immunochemotherapy was prescribed to the patient. Unfortunately, a few days following the completion of the first cycle, the patient suddenly lost consciousness and died. No postmortem study was performed.

3. Discussion

In the current study, the patient experienced SS for a long time and had SS-associated lymphoma risk factors, such as purpura, low levels of complement component C4, and cryoglobulinemia. Clinical data suggested the development of lymphoma, while RDD was an accidental finding. In our patient, the prominent sinuses were occupied with large histiocytes exhibiting emperipolesis and expressing CD68 and CD163 with coexpression of S100, remaining negative for CD1a and Langerin; these characteristics allowed for the diagnosis of RDD. We believe that the lymphoplasmacytic infiltrate that was composed of sheets of plasma cells within the intervening cords could be erroneously attributed to RDD. However, monotypic expression of IgM kappa by plasma cells indicated their neoplastic nature, and this finding was consistent with the presence of monoclonal IgM kappa in the serum. The admixed B-lymphocytes, which do not form physiological B-cell follicles, allowed us to classify this lymphoma as MZL with extensive plasmacytic differentiation. The lack of MYD88 mutation and any signs of bone marrow involvement argued against a diagnosis of lymphoplasmacytic lymphoma. Further, our patient showed

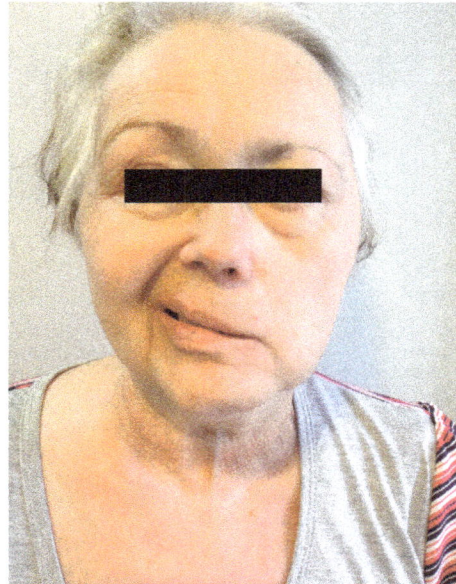

FIGURE 2: Left-sided peripheral facial nerve palsy with an inability to wrinkle the forehead and nose, unequal lid fissures, and inability to lift the corner of the mouth.

an absence of the enlarged salivary glands, minimal enlargement of the spleen, generalized lymphadenopathy, and the lack of bone marrow involvement, confirming the diagnosis of NMZL. A less favorable diagnosis was the MALT lymphoma of the salivary gland with a secondary lymph node involvement or SMZL.

The phenomenon of the lack of CD138 expression in malignant plasma cells of MZL with plasmacytic differentiation has been described previously [13, 14]. In our case, morphologically mature malignant plasma cells (Marschalko type) in the intervening cords also exhibited an

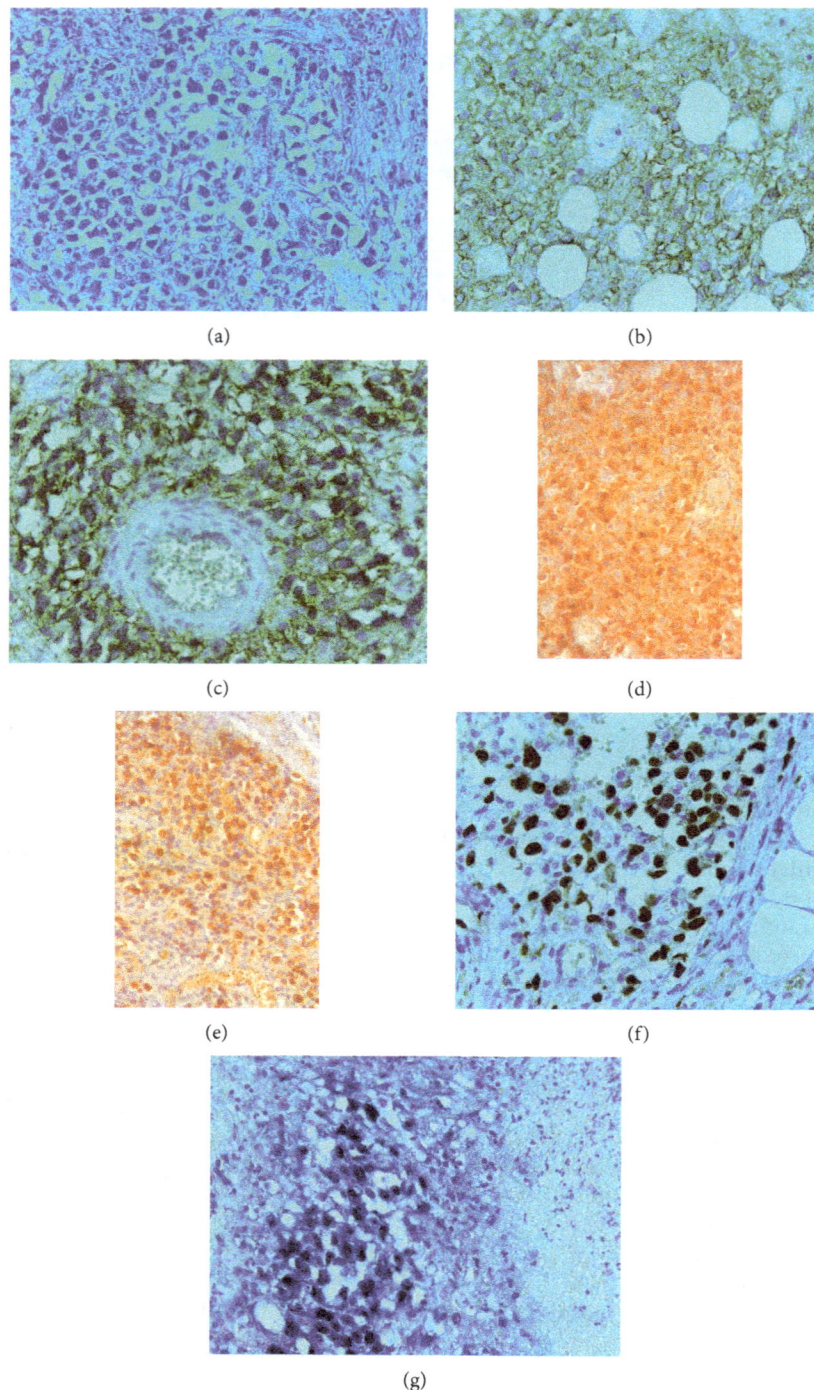

(a)

(b)

(c)

(d)

(e)

(f)

(g)

FIGURE 3: (a) The focus of large lymphoid cells, surrounded by necrotic tissue (×400, H&E). B–F. Immunostaining of the large tumor cells expressing CD20. (b) (×400), CD30 (c) (×400), light kappa chain. (d) (×200), IgM. (e) (×200), MUM1. (f) (×400). (g) Detection of EBV-positive large lymphocytes using EBER in situ hybridization.

aberrant plasma cell-related antigen profile. They did not express CD138 and VS38c, recognized markers for plasma cells. Some studies have shown that the CD138-negative plasma cells form a distinct subpopulation of malignant plasma cells, possibly representing more primitive and highly proliferative cells than CD138-positive cells [15–18].

These data can explain the high index of proliferative activity that was observed in MZL cells of our patient.

In 10% of patients with RDD, an immunological disease is diagnosed [9]. However, to our best knowledge, the co-occurrence of SS and RDD has been described only in two cases. Drosos et al. described a 55-year-old man with

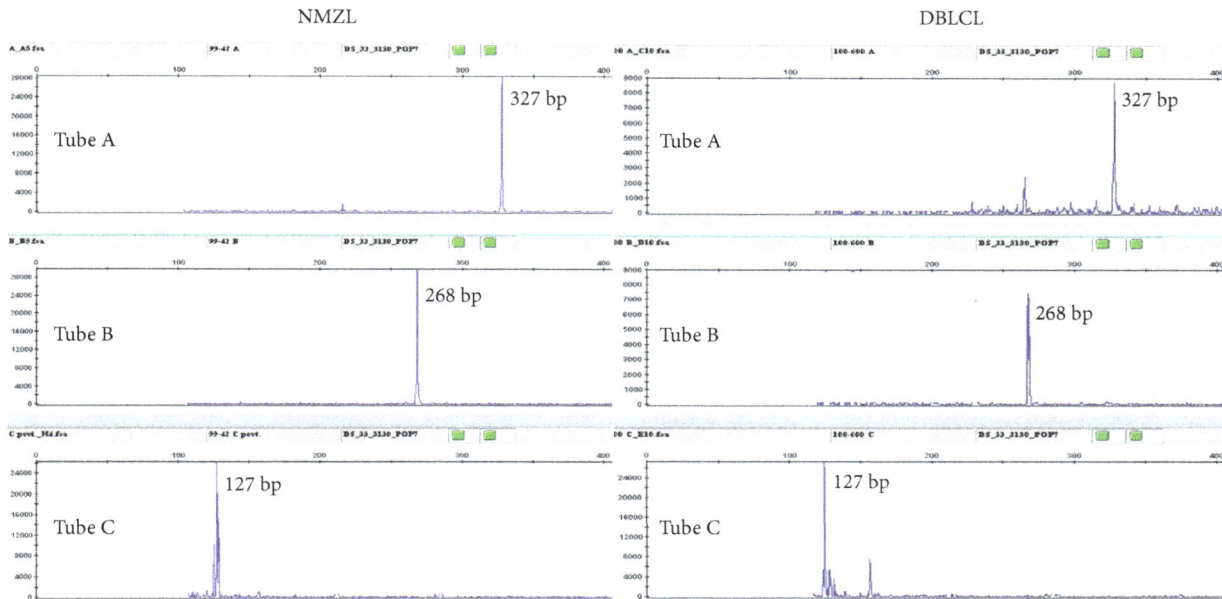

FIGURE 4: B-cell clonality analysis with IGHV FR1-IGHJ (Tube A), IGHV FR2-IGHJ (Tube B), and IGHV FR3-IGHJ (Tube C). PCR products demonstrate an identical clonal pattern between the NMZL and DLBCL.

primary SS who developed RDD after 6 years of being diagnosed with SS [11]. Another report by Maia et al. presented the case of a 40-year-old female with SS diagnosed 8 months following RDD diagnosis [12]. In both these cases, the diagnosis of RDD was established by lymph node biopsy. In our case, RDD was diagnosed in a 60-year-old woman 20 years after the SS diagnosis. The possibility of whether the association between SS and RDD is a coincidence or has a pathogenetic relationship remains to be determined.

After reviewing all the relevant literature, we found 28 case reports of RDD in association with both non-Hodgkin and Hodgkin lymphoma, but none of them had concomitant SS. Only two cases of simultaneous occurrence of RDD and NMZL have been documented. Pang et al. described a case of an 80-year-old woman with subcutaneous lymph node of the arm, and Akria at al. studied a 50-year-old man with abdominal lymphadenopathy who was also diagnosed with autoimmune hemolytic anemia [9, 10]. In both cases, as observed with our patient, RDD and NMZL were localized in the same lymph node. Given the rarity of association between RDD and lymphoma as well as the lack of evidence for clonality in RDD, it may be suggested that the RDD represents an unusual histiocytic response to lymphoma or RDD, and lymphoma arises independently in response to a common, unknown till now, etiological agent.

Multiplex PCR fragment assays showed identical clonal patterns between the NMZL and DLBCL, indicating clonal identity between the two lymphomas. However, such identical clonal relationship does not necessarily indicate a linear disease progression [19, 20]. It is possible to hypothesize that DLBCL was not a consequence of the transformation of NMZL and that both lymphomas in our case originated from a common precursor cell population. However, the expression of the same IgM kappa by tumor cells of both lymphomas suggests that DLBCL was a consequence of the clonal evolution of NMZL.

Evidence has shown that samples identified as EBV negative by immunohistochemistry and EBER-ISH demonstrated the presence of EBV-microRNAs and EBV genome [21]. In our case, we also failed to detect EBER-ISH in the lymph node affected by MZL and RDD, and only the PCR showed the presence of DNA EBV in this sample. However, tumor lymphocytes of DLBCL were EBV-positive. It can be assumed that after chemotherapy, the reactivation of EBV occurred, which became the trigger responsible for the transformation of NMZL into DLBCL. Although an association between EBV infection and lymphoma development is well-established, very few cases of EBV-induced transformation of the low-grade B-cell lymphoma into high-grade lymphoma have been described [22–29]. To our knowledge, this is the first documented case of EBV-induced transformation of the NMZL into DLBCL.

In conclusion, the current study describes an exceptionally rare case of simultaneous occurrence of RDD and NMZL in a patient with SS. We further believe that in the presented case, reactivation of a latent EBV infection by immunosuppressive therapy within a preexisting NMZL led to the development of the secondary EBV-positive DLBCL, NOS.

Conflicts of Interest

The authors declare that there is no conflict of interest regarding the publication of this article.

Acknowledgments

We would like to thank Dr. V. Dengin, Ph.D., for the English translation.

References

[1] R. I. Fox, F. V. Howell, R. C. Bone, and P. E. Michelson, "Primary Sjogren syndrome: clinical and immunopathologic features," *Seminars in Arthritis and Rheumatism*, vol. 14, no. 2, pp. 77–105, 1984.

[2] E. Zintzaras, M. Voulgarelis, and H. M. Moutsopoulos, "The risk of lymphoma development in autoimmune diseases: a meta-analysis," *Archives of Internal Medicine*, vol. 165, no. 20, pp. 2337–2344, 2005.

[3] S. H. Swerdlow, E. Campo, N. L. Harris et al., *WHO Classification of Tumours of Haematopoietic and Lymphoid Tissues*, IARC Press, Lyon, France, 2017.

[4] M. Voulgarelis, U. G. Dafni, D. A. Isenberg et al., "Malignant lymphoma in primary Sjogren's syndrome: a multicenter, retrospective, clinical study by the European concerted action on sjogren's syndrome," *Arthritis & Rheumatism*, vol. 42, no. 8, pp. 1765–1772, 1999.

[5] A. G. Tzioufas, "B-cell lymphoproliferation in primary sjogren's syndrome," *Clinical and Experimental Rheumatology*, vol. 14, no. 14, pp. S65–S70, 1996.

[6] B. Royer, D. Cazals-Hatem, J. Sibilia et al., "Lymphomas in patients with Sjogren's syndrome are marginal zone B-cell neoplasms, arise in diverse extranodal and nodal sites, and are not associated with viruses," *Blood*, vol. 90, no. 2, pp. 766–775, 1997.

[7] E. Foucar, J. Rosai, and R. F. Dorfman, "Sinus histiocytosis with massive lymphadenopathy (Rosai-Dorfman disease): review of the entity," *Seminars in Diagnostic Pathology*, vol. 7, no. 1, pp. 19–73, 1990.

[8] J. F. Emile, O. Alba, S. Fraitag et al., "Revised classification of histiocytoses and neoplasms of the macrophage-dendritic cell lineages," *Blood*, vol. 127, no. 22, pp. 2672–2681, 2016.

[9] C. S. Pang, D. D. Grier, and M. W. Beaty, "Concomitant occurrence of sinus histiocytosis with massive lymphadenopathy and nodal marginal zone lymphoma," *Archives of Pathology & Laboratory Medicine*, vol. 135, no. 3, pp. 390–393, 2011.

[10] L. Akria, V. Sonkin, A. Braester, H. I. Cohen, C. Suriu, and A. Polliack, "Rare coexistence of Rosai-Dorfman disease and nodal marginal zone lymphoma complicated by severe life-threatening autoimmune hemolytic anemia," *Leukemia & Lymphoma*, vol. 54, no. 7, pp. 1553–1556, 2013.

[11] A. A. Drosos, A. N. Georgiadis, Z. M. Metafratzi, P. V. Voulgari, S. C. Efremidis, and M. Bai, "Sinus histiocytosis with massive lymphadenopathy (Rosai-Dorfman disease) in a patient with primary sjogren's syndrome," *Scandinavian Journal of Rheumatology*, vol. 33, no. 2, pp. 119–122, 2004.

[12] R. C. Maia, E. de Meis, S. Romano, J. A. Dobbin, and C. E. Klumb, "Rosai-Dorfman disease: a report of eight cases in a tertiary care center and a review of the literature," *Brazilian Journal of Medical and Biological Research*, vol. 48, no. 1, pp. 6–12, 2015.

[13] S. E. Coupland, M. Hellmich, C. Auw-Haedrich, W. R. Lee, I. Anagnostopoulos, and H. Stein, "Plasmacellular differentiation in extranodal marginal zone B cell lymphomas of the ocular adnexa: an analysis of the neoplastic plasma cell phenotype and its prognostic significance in 136 cases," *British Journal of Ophthalmology*, vol. 89, no. 3, pp. 352–359, 2005.

[14] H. J. Meyerson, J. Bailey, J. Miedler, and F. Olobatuyi, "Marginal zone B cell lymphomas with extensive plasmacytic differentiation are neoplasms of precursor plasma cells," *Cytometry Part B: Clinical Cytometry*, vol. 80, no. 2, pp. 71–82, 2011.

[15] D. Joshua, A. Peterson, R. Brown, B. Pope, L. Snowdon, and J. Gibson, "The labelling index of primitive plasma cells determines the clinical behaviour of patients with myelomatosis," *British Journal of Haematology*, vol. 94, no. 1, pp. 76–81, 1996.

[16] B. Pope, R. Brown, J. Gibson, E. Yuen, and D. Joshua, "B7-2-positive myeloma:incidence, clinical characteristics, prognostic significance and implications for tumour therapy," *Blood*, vol. 96, no. 4, pp. 1274–1279, 2000.

[17] W. Matsui, C. Huff, Q. Wang et al., "Characterisation of clonogenic multiple myeloma cells," *Blood*, vol. 103, no. 6, pp. 2332–2336, 2004.

[18] S. Reid, S. Yang, R. Brown et al., "Characterisation and relevance of CD138-negative plasma cells in plasma cell myeloma," *International Journal of Laboratory Hematology*, vol. 32, no. 6p1, pp. e190–e196, 2010.

[19] J. Fitzgibbon, S. Iqbal, A. Davies et al., "Genome-wide detection of recurring sites of uniparental disomy in follicular and transformed follicular lymphoma," *Leukemia*, vol. 21, no. 7, pp. 1514–1520, 2007.

[20] H. Liu, Q. Yan, B. Nuako-Bandoh et al., "Richter transformation: clonal identity does not indicate a linear disease progression," *British Journal of Haematology*, vol. 157, no. 1, pp. 136–139, 2012.

[21] L. Mundo, M. R. Ambrosio, M. Picciolini et al., "Unveiling another missing piece in EBV-driven lymphomagenesis: EBV-encoded microRNAs expression in EBER-negative Burkitt lymphoma cases," *Frontiers in Microbiology*, vol. 8, p. 229, 2017.

[22] J. E. Strunk, C Schuttler, J Ziebuhr et al., "Epstein-barr virus–induced secondary high-grade transformation of sjogren's syndrome–related mucosa-associated lymphoid tissue lymphoma," *Journal of Clinical Oncology*, vol. 31, no. 17, pp. e265–e268, 2013.

[23] T. Terasawa, H. Ohashi, M. Utsumi et al., "Case of epstein-barr virus-associated transformation of mantle cell lymphoma," *American Journal of Hematology*, vol. 73, no. 3, pp. 194–199, 2003.

[24] J. Tao and L. Kahn, "Epstein-Barr virus–associated high-grade B-cell lymphoma of mucosal-associated lymphoid tissue in a 9-year-old boy," *Archives of Pathology & Laboratory Medicine*, vol. 124, no. 10, pp. 1520–1524, 2000.

[25] D. Rubin, S. D. Hudnall, A. Aisenberg, J. O. Jacobson, and N. L. Harris, "Richter's transformation of chronic lymphocytic leukemia with Hodgkin's-like cells is associated with Epstein-Barr virus infection," *Modern Pathology*, vol. 7, no. 1, pp. 91–98, 1994.

[26] T. Petrella, N. Yaziji, F. Collin et al., "Implication of the epstein-barr virus in the progression of chronic lymphocytic leukaemia/small lymphocytic lymphoma to hodgkin-like lymphomas," *Anticancer Research*, vol. 17, no. 5B, pp. 3907–3913, 1997.

[27] M. P. Menon, L. Hutchinson, J. Garver, E. S. Jaffe, and B. A. Woda, "Transformation of follicular lymphoma to epstein-barr virus–related hodgkin-like lymphoma," *Journal of Clinical Oncology*, vol. 31, no. 5, pp. e53–e56, 2013.

[28] S. M. Ansell, C. Y. Li, R. V. Lloyd, and R. L. Phyliky, "Epstein-Barr virus infection in Richter's transformation," *American Journal of Hematology*, vol. 60, no. 2, pp. 99–104, 1999.

[29] M. R. Ambrosio, G. D. Falco, A. Gozzetti et al., "Plasmablastic transformation of a pre-existing plasmacytoma: a possible role for reactivation of epstein barr virus infection," *Haematologica*, vol. 99, no. 11, pp. e235–237, 2014.

31

Multiple Liver Nodules Mimicking Metastatic Disease as Initial Presentation of Multiple Myeloma

Andrew C. Tiu (iD),[1] Rashmika Potdar,[2] Vivian Arguello-Gerra,[3] and Mark Morginstin[2]

[1]Department of Medicine, Einstein Medical Center, Philadelphia, PA, USA
[2]Division of Hematology and Medical Oncology, Einstein Medical Center, Philadelphia, PA, USA
[3]Department of Pathology and Laboratory Medicine, Einstein Medical Center, Philadelphia, PA, USA

Correspondence should be addressed to Andrew C. Tiu; tiuandre@einstein.edu

Academic Editor: Masayuki Nagasawa

Multiple myeloma is a malignant clonal proliferation of plasma cells in the bone marrow preceded by monoclonal gammopathy of undetermined significance. Initial presentation of multiple myeloma as extramedullary spread in soft tissues particularly in the liver is uncommon. We report a case of a 74-year-old African American female who presented with epigastric pain, hematemesis, elevated alkaline phosphatase, and gamma-glutamyl transferase. Initial impression was peptic ulcer disease; however, ultrasound and CT scan of the abdomen showed multiple liver nodules and perihepatic lymphadenopathy suggestive of metastatic disease. Biopsy of the liver nodules showed CD138 and kappa light chain-restricted positive cells consistent with extramedullary spread of multiple myeloma to the liver. The patient achieved partial response after 6 months of treatment with Velcade, cyclophosphamide, and dexamethasone (VCD). Due to severe neutropenia from cyclophosphamide, regimen was switched to Velcade, Revlimid, and dexamethasone (VRD) which resulted to very good partial response in 1 year which eventually persisted after 4 years. No controlled prospective studies have defined the standard treatment for multiple myeloma with extramedullary spread particularly to the liver. Treatment of multiple myeloma with extramedullary disease follows guidelines for multiple myeloma.

1. Introduction

Multiple myeloma (MM) is a malignant clonal proliferation of plasma cells in the bone marrow preceded by monoclonal gammopathy of undetermined significance (MGUS) [1]. MM is commonly diagnosed with CRAB criteria (hypercalcemia, renal insufficiency, anemia, and bone lesions) from end-organ damage by light chain deposition, plasma cell proliferation, and interaction of the plasma cells with the microenvironment. Soft tissue involvement of MM is referred to as extramedullary myeloma (EM).

EM has been described since the 19th century with a spectrum of presentations depending on the location of the tumor most commonly in organs containing reticuloendothelial cells such as liver, kidney, skin, and lymph nodes. There were no clear clinical implications or prognostic significance at that time [2]. With advanced imaging techniques such as PET/CT scan, EMs are diagnosed promptly. In 1,003 consecutive MM patients, incidence of EM was 13%, 7% at diagnosis and 6% during follow-up [3]. In another case series, in

936 patients treated for MM, only 66 presented initially as EM with liver involvement in 21% [4]. Overall, the incidence of EM is higher at relapse than at diagnosis [3, 5].

The mechanism of extramedullary involvement by multiple myeloma has been extensively reviewed by Bladé et al. [5] *vide infra*. Multiple reports have described how EMs are associated with multiple cytogenetic abnormalities in younger patients which lead to poor survival rate and progression-free survival despite the novel agents [3, 4]. Our case report focused on an elderly patient with kappa light chain MM presenting as multiple nodules in the liver. She was diagnosed in January 2013. This report emphasized the rarity of liver involvement in MM, the presentation of MM as extramedullary involvement at diagnosis, and partial response to novel agents bortezomib and lenalidomide for five years.

2. Case Description

A 74-year-old African American female with past medical history of atrial flutter s/p ablation, osteoarthritis, and peptic

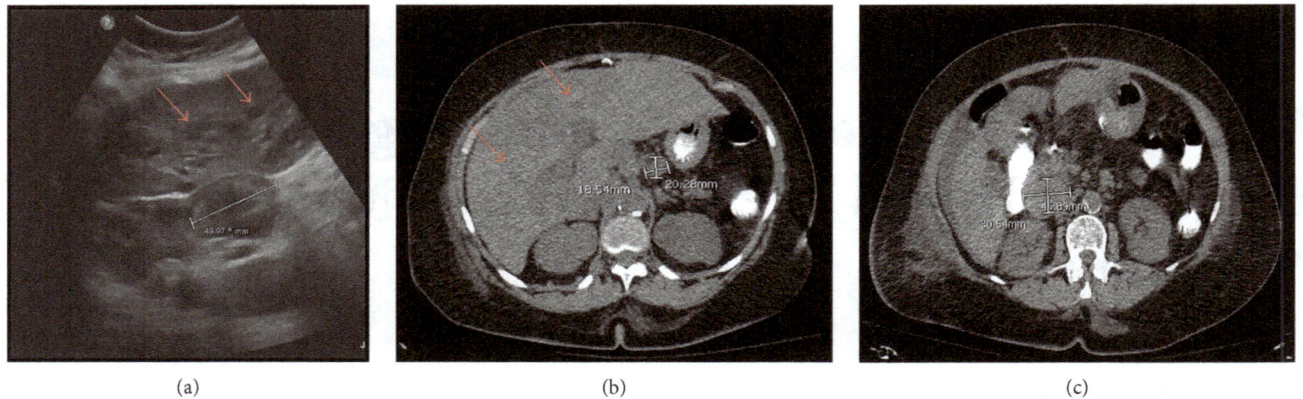

FIGURE 1: (a) Ultrasound of the liver showing 5 cm enlarged perihepatic lymph node with multiple hypoechoic nodules in the liver (red arrows); (b, c) CT scan showing multiple hypodense nodules in the liver parenchyma (red arrows) with marked enlarged perihepatic lymph nodes.

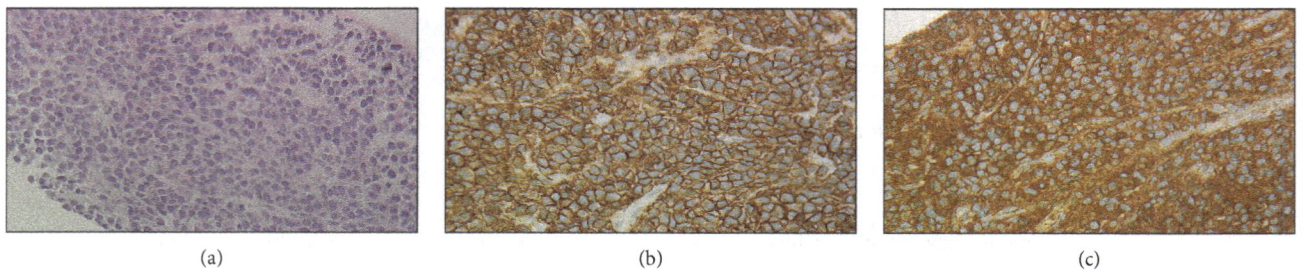

FIGURE 2: (a) Liver fine-needle aspirate (FNA) and core biopsy (400x objective) showing a monomorphic population of plasma cells with eccentric nuclei and clock-faced chromatin. Hepatocytes are not present. (b) Liver FNA immunohistochemical staining (400x objective) revealed CD138, highlighting plasma cells. (c) Kappa light surface antigen showing all plasma cells positive for stain and proving clonality.

ulcer disease s/p Roux-en-Y gastrojejunostomy initially presented with epigastric pain and hematemesis with elevated alkaline phosphatase and gamma-glutamyl transferase. Review of systems was unremarkable. Family history was pertinent for breast cancer and lung cancer of her aunt and mother, respectively. She is a 15-pack-year smoker. Physical examination was unremarkable for hepatosplenomegaly and jaundice.

Admission labs included hemoglobin 8.3 g/dL, calcium 9.0 mg/dL, BUN 35 mg/dL, creatinine 2.0 mg/dL, total bilirubin 0.7 mg/dL, ALT 16 IU/L, and AST 21 IU/L. The elevated creatinine levels were initially attributed to hypovolemia. Esophagogastroduodenoscopy revealed gastric and jejunal ulcer while ultrasound of the hepatobiliary tract showed multiple hypoechoic liver nodules occupying at least 50% of the parenchyma and perihepatic lymphadenopathy (Figure 1(a)). CT abdomen and pelvis confirmed the innumerable liver lesions without any colonic mass and perihepatic lymphadenopathy (Figures 1(b) and 1(c)). Colonoscopy was attempted to rule out colon cancer which has metastasized to the liver but was unsuccessful. CT colonography subsequently failed to show any colonic masses or polyps.

Percutaneous biopsy of the liver nodule and perihepatic lymph node both confirmed the CD138 and kappa light chain-restricted positive cells consistent with plasmacytoma (Figure 2). There was no morphological suspicion for amyloidosis; thus, Congo red stain was not done. Labs revealed kappa light chain of 8280 mg/L, lambda light chain of 2.48 mg/L, and kappa/lambda ratio of 3338. Serum and urine immunofixation both confirmed the presence of a monoclonal kappa light chain clone and absence of a heavy chain component. The quantitative immunoglobulin levels were as follows: IgA 57 mg/dL, IgM 25 mg/dL, and IgG 366 mg/dL. There were no osteolytic lesions on skeletal survey. MRI of the brain and CT thorax with contrast were negative.

Bone marrow biopsy showed at least 30–40% kappa clonal plasma cells with positive CRAB criteria (hemoglobin and creatinine) confirming the diagnosis of light chain multiple myeloma (Figure 3). Fluorescence in situ hybridization (FISH) from the bone marrow showed normal (46,XX) karyotype and positive for hyperdiploidy of chromosomes 7, 9, 11, 14, and 17 with partial deletion of IgH gene. Bone marrow flow cytometry interpretation was limited due to hemodilution, processing of the sample, and clotting. There were no circulating plasma cells detected at diagnosis. According to Revised International Staging System (R-ISS) for multiple myeloma, the patient had stage III (β2-microglobulin level was 9.1 mg/L and LDH was 423 IU/L, without high-risk chromosomal abnormalities). This prognosticated a median progression-free survival of 29 months and overall

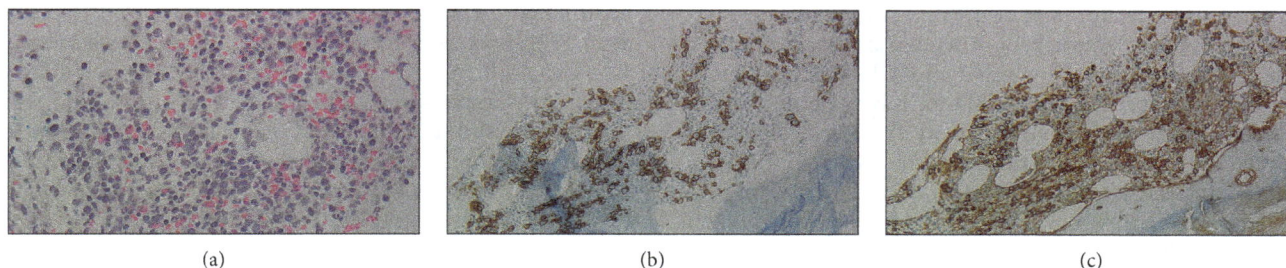

FIGURE 3: (a) Bone marrow (objective 400x) showing increased cellularity with increased scattered plasma cells intermixed with hematopoietic elements. (b, c) Bone marrow immunohistochemical staining showing CD138 and kappa light surface antigen (200x objective), highlighting scattered clonal plasma cells occupying 30–40% of total cellularity.

survival of 43 months. It should be noted that R-ISS does not take EM localizations into account.

Treatment was started with CyBorD: weekly dexamethasone 40 mg, bortezomib 1.5 mg/m^2, and cyclophosphamide 500 mg. This regimen was adopted from the multiple myeloma prognosis scoring from the R-ISS, given that the patient had R-ISS stage III with high LDH placing her at higher risk. Despite her older age, CyBorD was offered given that the patient had good baseline functional capabilities (independent and ambulatory). She also had no poorly controlled comorbid conditions.

After 6 months of treatment with CyBorD regimen, serum free light chains decreased: kappa 1690 mg/L, lambda 1.7 mg/L, and kappa/lambda ratio 994. Repeat bone marrow biopsy showed a decrease to 10% kappa clonal plasma cells, while repeat FISH showed negativity for myeloma markers such as aneusomy for chromosomes 7, 9, 11, and 17, deletion of RB1 and TP53 genes, and IgH gene rearrangement. Repeat flow cytometry showed small plasma cell clone with similar immunophenotype as the prior study. Repeat CT abdomen showed interval decrease in size of the hepatic nodules and perihepatic lymph nodes approximately 70%. In retrospect (in year 2013), this constituted a partial response according to the International Myeloma Working Group (IMWG). It should be noted that recommendations from IMWG were published on March 14, 2016 (3 years later).

Now, the patient was offered autologous stem cell transplantation; however, the patient refused, so CyBorD was continued. After 1 year, cyclophosphamide was stopped due to severe neutropenia. VRD regimen with low-dose lenalidomide 10 mg daily (21 days/28 days cycle) was started. The patient was continued on weekly bortezomib and dexamethasone. Lower dose of lenalidomide was used considering the patient's age and comorbidities. Because of severe diarrhea and rash, lenalidomide dose was further reduced to 2.5 mg daily in a stepwise manner. The patient's dexamethasone dose was reduced to 20 mg weekly due to gastric ulcer.

The patient was able to achieve very good partial response by IMWG criteria after one year of shifting regimens from CyBorD to VRD. Serum free light chains were as follows: kappa 37 mg/L, lambda 15.1 mg/L, and kappa/lambda ratio 2.45. Repeat bone marrow examination was not done; however, repeat CT abdomen showed complete disappearance of the hepatic nodules and perihepatic lymphadenopathy. Skeletal survey did not show any bone lesions.

The patient has achieved very good partial response by IMWG criteria after 4 years on the VRD regimen: kappa 65.7 mg/L, lambda 24.5 mg/L, and kappa/lambda ratio 2.68. The quantitative immunoglobulin levels were as follows: IgA 228/dL, IgM 27 mg/dL, and IgG 1067 mg/dL. The patient is presently continued on the same regimen. Unfortunately, PET/CT scan was not done at diagnosis or during the course of the disease. Currently, PET scan is the preferred imaging technique for EM.

3. Discussion

Soft tissue involvement of multiple myeloma particularly on the liver is rare as emphasized by the incidence described by Talamo et al. in 2,584 patients, wherein only 11 patients had liver involvement [6]. The pattern of plasma cell infiltration was described as either diffuse sinusoidal, nodular, portal, or mixed [7–11], while the mechanisms of extramedullary spread included decreased expression of adhesion molecules, downregulation of chemokine receptors, downregulation of tetraspanins, increased heparanase-1 expression, angiogenesis, and mutations in alternative or classical nuclear factor-κB pathways [12]. The morphology of EMs is usually immature or plasmablastic with a shift from secreting intact immunoglobulins to free light chains (*light chain escape phenomenon*) like the case of our patient [13, 14].

Liver involvement in extramedullary myeloma is found as hypoechoic nodules on CT scan and ultrasound similar to our patient [15–17]. Rarely, it may present as hyperechoic nodules on ultrasound and hypervascular lesions on CT [18, 19]. These lesions are seen on MRI as high signal intensity on T1-weighted images and out-of-phase spoiled gradient echo [20].

The treatment of this archaic disease is still a moving target considering newer diagnostic criteria, new staging system, and more effective therapeutics [21]. Extramedullary myeloma is one of the special circumstances where treatment is not well defined due to its rarity, molecular, and proliferative heterogeneity. Initial treatment depends on risk stratification and prognostication [22]. Currently, there are two scoring systems, namely, the Revised International Staging System (R-ISS) [23] and the Mayo Stratification for Myeloma and Risk-adapted Therapy (mSMART 2.0) [24]. R-ISS comprised 3 common cytogenetic markers [del(17p) and/or t(4;14) and/or t(14;16)] while mSMART included additional molecular markers. It should be noted that both these prognostic scoring systems do not take EM localizations into account. Furthermore, mSMART has not been formally validated. For instance, in our patient, there is a discrepancy between the results of the scoring systems, wherein R-ISS is at high risk because of elevated LDH levels, while mSMART is at standard risk because of the absence of high-risk cytogenetic markers. High-risk cytogenetics is not always necessary for EM as patients without extramedullary involvement may also have high-risk cytogenetics [25]. The authors aired on the side of caution by utilizing R-ISS (high risk) in the initial management of the patient. The decision was supported by the natural history of extramedullary myeloma conferring poor prognosis as described by Varettoni et al. [3].

The current initial treatment for multiple myeloma relies on whether the patient is a transplant candidate. Velcade, Revlimid, and dexamethasone (VRD) is the standard frontline regimen, while carfilzomib replaces Velcade (KRD) if the patient has high-risk features [26, 27]. Four cycles is the duration for both induction regimens for transplant-eligible patients while 12–18 cycles is the typical duration for transplant-ineligible patients [21, 22]. For high-risk patients, carfilzomib- or bortezomib-based maintenance is utilized for 2 years after the initial treatment. Multidrug combinations such as VDT-PACE for 2 cycles (Velcade, dexamethasone, thalidomide-cisplatin, doxorubicin, cyclophosphamide, and etoposide) can also be utilized for multiple extramedullary myelomas prior to autologous stem cell transplantation (ASCT) or after aggressive relapse [28, 29]. This is usually followed by bortezomib maintenance.

Ideally, carfilzomib should be utilized in the initial treatment in our patient due to high-risk features; however, this was not yet available in 2013. Instead, CyBorD also known as VCD regimen was used [30, 31]. Currently, VCD is utilized for patients who are frail, ≥75 years old, and at intermediate risk [21]. Due to toxicity from cyclophosphamide, the authors chose to shift to VRD regimen [31, 32], which unexpectedly deepened the response from partial response to very good partial response after 1 year [33]. To date, the role of the continuous therapy with 2 different regimens is unclear. The choice of the continued VRD regimen was balanced between the wishes of the patient refusing transplant, elderly age, multiple controlled comorbidities, the toxicity of the previous regimen, the improved response with the current regimen, and the toxicity of the current regimen.

The addition of lenalidomide (Revlimid) may have been responsible for the improvement in response as documented by a few case reports. Xie et al. successfully treated secondary multiple myeloma with extramedullary liver plasmacytoma in a renal transplant patient with RCD regimen (Revlimid, cyclophosphamide, dexamethasone) [34]. Similarly, Felici et al. utilized the RCD regimen on a patient with bilateral retro-orbital localization [35]. In two patients with bortezomib-resistant extramedullary myeloma, Revlimid and dexamethasone (RD) regimen was an effective treatment according to Ito et al. [36]. CRVD (cyclophosphamide, Revlimid, Velcade, dexamethasone) was able to attain radiologic partial response in a patient

with hepatic extramedullary disease as reported by Saboo et al. [37]. Bortezomib (Velcade) was originally observed to be efficacious against EM; however, these reports suffered from few sample sizes without adequate controlled trials [38, 39]. Velcade and Revlimid may have synergistic effects which potentially explain their efficacy [40]. The VDT-PACE regimen may not be an option for the patient due to potential toxicities and decreased quality of life.

Defining the best therapeutic regimen to manage the development and progression of extramedullary myeloma remains a challenge. What is certain is that newer agents can improve outcome [41–47]. For every regimen that is started, continued monitoring of response to treatment is warranted. [18F]-FDG PET/CT is the recommended imaging modality especially for hepatic lesions of extramedullary myeloma [37].

4. Conclusion

The approach to a patient with multiple liver nodules is a diagnostic challenge. Once imaging and diagnostic tests ruled out common causes of multiple liver nodules such as primary hepatobiliary cancer, metastatic disease from colorectal cancer, and infection, we can then pursue investigating other infiltrative diseases to the liver such as hematologic malignancies. The presence of anemia, kidney dysfunction, and altered albumin-globulin ratio made the authors suspect multiple myeloma. Our patient had no specific physical examination findings that would suggest a hematologic malignancy such as hepatosplenomegaly, lymphadenopathy, and skeletal pain. Furthermore, there were no specific imaging features for extramedullary myeloma involvement of the liver. Ultimately, biopsy was done to confirm the diagnosis.

EMs are not always associated with high-risk cytogenetic abnormality. Because of the patient's older age, multiple comorbidities, higher $\beta 2$-microglobulin levels, kappa light chain monoclonal gammopathy, extramedullary involvement of the liver, and no high-risk cytogenetics, the risk stratification and treatment options become more complex and must be individualized. There are no clear prognostication factors as to which patients with multiple myeloma have higher risk of presenting as extramedullary disease due to infrequent incidence of EM on diagnosis and the molecular and cytogenetic heterogeneity of MM. The challenge is that most patients who are newly diagnosed have no known risk factors and risk stratification must be continued throughout therapy as these dictate changes in the management. Close follow-up is therefore warranted in this patient to monitor relapse and end-organ damage from MM.

Consent

Written informed consent was obtained from the patient for the anonymized information to be published in this article.

Conflicts of Interest

The authors declare no potential conflicts of interest with respect to the research, authorship, and/or publication of this article.

References

[1] O. Landgren, R. A. Kyle, R. M. Pfeiffer et al., "Monoclonal gammopathy of undetermined significance (MGUS) consistently precedes multiple myeloma: a prospective study," *Blood*, vol. 113, no. 22, pp. 5412–5417, 2009.

[2] R. Perez-Soler, R. Esteban, E. Allende, C. Tornos Salomo, A. Julia, and J. Guardia, "Liver involvement in multiple myeloma," *American Journal of Hematology*, vol. 20, no. 1, pp. 25–29, 1985.

[3] M. Varettoni, A. Corso, G. Pica, S. Mangiacavalli, C. Pascutto, and M. Lazzarino, "Incidence, presenting features and outcome of extramedullary disease in multiple myeloma: a longitudinal study on 1003 consecutive patients," *Annals of Oncology*, vol. 21, no. 2, pp. 325–330, 2010.

[4] S. Z. Usmani, C. Heuck, A. Mitchell et al., "Extramedullary disease portends poor prognosis in multiple myeloma and is over-represented in high-risk disease even in the era of novel agents," *Haematologica*, vol. 97, no. 11, pp. 1761–1767, 2012.

[5] J. Bladé, C. F. de Larrea, and L. Rosiñol, "Extramedullary involvement in multiple myeloma," *Haematologica*, vol. 97, no. 11, pp. 1618-1619, 2012.

[6] G. Talamo, F. Cavallo, M. Zangari et al., "Clinical and biological features of multiple myeloma involving the gastrointestinal system," *Haematologica*, vol. 91, no. 7, pp. 964–967, 2006.

[7] A. J. Gordon and J. Churg, "Visceral involvement in multiple myeloma," *New York State Journal of Medicine*, vol. 49, no. 3, p. 282, 1949.

[8] F. B. Thomas, K. P. Clausen, and N. J. Greenberger, "Liver disease in multiple myeloma," *Archives of Internal Medicine*, vol. 132, no. 2, pp. 195–202, 1973.

[9] M. W. Pasmantier and H. A. Azar, "Extraskeletal spread in multiple plasma cell myeloma. A review of 57 autopsied cases," *Cancer*, vol. 23, no. 1, pp. 167–174, 1969.

[10] S. B. Kapadia, "Multiple myeloma: a clinicopathologic study of 62 consecutively autopsied cases," *Medicine*, vol. 59, no. 5, pp. 380–392, 1980.

[11] K. Oshima, Y. Kanda, Y. Nannya et al., "Clinical and pathologic findings in 52 consecutively autopsied cases with multiple myeloma," *American Journal of Hematology*, vol. 67, no. 1, pp. 1–5, 2001.

[12] J. Bladé, C. Fernández de Larrea, L. Rosiñol, M. T. Cibeira, R. Jiménez, and R. Powles, "Soft-tissue plasmacytomas in multiple myeloma: incidence, mechanisms of extramedullary spread, and treatment approach," *Journal of Clinical Oncology*, vol. 29, no. 28, pp. 3805–3812, 2011.

[13] M. A. Dawson, S. Patil, and A. Spencer, "Extramedullary relapse of multiple myeloma associated with a shift in secretion from intact immunoglobulin to light chains," *Haematologica*, vol. 92, no. 1, pp. 143-144, 2007.

[14] A. Kühnemund, P. Liebisch, K. Bauchmüller et al., "'Light-chain escape-multiple myeloma'-an escape phenomenon from plateau phase: report of the largest patient series using LC-monitoring," *Journal of Cancer Research and Clinical Oncology*, vol. 135, no. 3, pp. 477–484, 2009.

[15] H. Huang, F. Bazerbachi, H. Mesa, and P. Gupta, "Asymptomatic multiple myeloma presenting as a nodular hepatic lesion: a case report and review of the literature," *Ochsner Journal*, vol. 15, no. 4, pp. 457–467, 2015.

[16] K. Chemlal, A. Couvelard, M. J. Grange et al., "Nodular lesions of the liver revealing multiple myeloma," *Leukemia and Lymphoma*, vol. 33, no. 3-4, pp. 389–392, 1999.

[17] R. Thiruvengadam, R. B. Penetrante, H. J. Goolsby, Y. N. Silk, and Z. P. Bernstein, "Multiple myeloma presenting as space-occupying lesions of the liver," *Cancer*, vol. 65, no. 12, pp. 2784–2786, 1990.

[18] M. Z. Simmons, J. A. Miller, C. D. Levine, W. J. Glucksman, and R. H. Wachsberg, "Myelomatous involvement of the liver: unusual ultrasound appearance," *Journal of Clinical Ultrasound*, vol. 25, no. 3, pp. 145–148, 1997.

[19] C. H. Tan, M. Wang, W. J. Fu, and R. Vikram, "Nodular extramedullary multiple myeloma: hepatic involvement presenting as hypervascular lesions on CT," *Annals of the Academy of Medicine*, vol. 40, no. 7, pp. 329–331, 2011.

[20] N. L. Kelekis, R. C. Semelka, D. M. Warshauer, and S. Sallah, "Nodular liver involvement in light chain multiple myeloma: appearance on US and MRI," *Clinical Imaging*, vol. 21, no. 3, pp. 207–209, 1997.

[21] S. V. Rajkumar, "Multiple myeloma: 2016 update on diagnosis, risk-stratification and management," *American Journal of Hematology*, vol. 91, no. 7, pp. 719–734, 2016.

[22] S. V. Rajkumar and S. Kumar, "Multiple myeloma: diagnosis and treatment," *Mayo Clinic Proceedings*, vol. 91, no. 1, pp. 101–119, 2016.

[23] A. Palumbo, H. Avet-Loiseau, S. Oliva et al., "Revised international staging system for multiple myeloma: a report from International Myeloma Working Group," *Journal of Clinical Oncology*, vol. 33, no. 26, pp. 2863–2869, 2015.

[24] J. R. Mikhael, D. Dingli, V. Roy et al., "Management of newly diagnosed symptomatic multiple myeloma: updated mayo stratification of myeloma and risk-adapted therapy (mSMART) consensus guidelines 2013," *Mayo Clinic Proceedings*, vol. 88, no. 4, pp. 360–376, 2013.

[25] L. Rosiñol, A. Oriol, A. I. Teruel et al., "Programa para el Estudio y la Terapéutica de las Hemopatías Malignas/Grupo Español de Mieloma (PETHEMA/GEM) group. Superiority of bortezomib, thalidomide, and dexamethasone (VTD) as induction pretransplantation therapy in multiple myeloma: a randomized phase 3 PETHEMA/GEM study," *Blood*, vol. 120, no. 8, pp. 1589–1596, 2012.

[26] A. J. Jakubowiak, "Evolution of carfilzomib dose and schedule in patients with multiple myeloma: a historical overview," *Cancer Treatment Reviews*, vol. 40, no. 6, pp. 781–790, 2014.

[27] A. J. Jakubowiak, D. Dytfeld, K. A. Griffith et al., "A phase 1/2 study of carfilzomib in combination with lenalidomide and low-dose dexamethasone as a frontline treatment for multiple myeloma," *Blood*, vol. 120, no. 9, pp. 1801–1809, 2012.

[28] B. Barlogie, E. Anaissie, F. van Rhee et al., "Incorporating bortezomib into upfront treatment for multiple myeloma: early results of total therapy 3," *British Journal of Haematology*, vol. 138, no. 2, pp. 176–185, 2007.

[29] F. van Rhee, J. Szymonifka, E. Anaissie et al., "Total therapy 3 for multiple myeloma: prognostic implications of cumulative dosing and premature discontinuation of VTD maintenance components, bortezomib, thalidomide, and dexamethasone, relevant to all phases of therapy," *Blood*, vol. 116, no. 8, pp. 1220–1227, 2010.

[30] C. B. Reeder, D. E. Reece, V. Kukreti et al., "Cyclophosphamide, bortezomib and dexamethasone induction for newly diagnosed multiple myeloma: high response rates in a phase II clinical trial," *Leukemia*, vol. 23, no. 7, pp. 1337–1341, 2009.

[31] S. Kumar, I. Flinn, P. G. Richardson et al., "Randomized, multicenter, phase 2 study (EVOLUTION) of combinations of bortezomib, dexamethasone, cyclophosphamide, and lenalidomide in previously untreated multiple myeloma," *Blood*, vol. 119, no. 19, pp. 4375–4382, 2012.

[32] P. G. Richardson, E. Weller, S. Lonial et al., "Lenalidomide, bortezomib, and dexamethasone combination therapy in patients

with newly diagnosed multiple myeloma," *Blood*, vol. 116, no. 5, pp. 679–686, 2010.

[33] S. Kumar, B. Paiva, K. C. Anderson et al., "International Myeloma Working Group consensus criteria for response and minimal residual disease assessment in multiple myeloma," *The Lancet Oncology*, vol. 17, no. 8, pp. e328–e346, 2016.

[34] X. Xie, W. Wu, Y. Zhu et al., "Successful treatment with lenalidomide of secondary multiple myeloma with extramedullary liver plasmacytoma in a renal transplant recipient: a case report and review of the literature," *Oncology Letters*, vol. 10, no. 5, pp. 2931–2936, 2015.

[35] S. Felici, N. Villivà, G. Balsamo, and A. Andriani, "Efficacy of lenalidomide in association with cyclophosphamide and dexamethasone in multiple myeloma patient with bilateral retro-orbital localisation," *Ecancermedicalscience*, vol. 7, p. 331, 2013.

[36] C. Ito, Y. Aisa, A. Mihara, and T. Nakazato, "Lenalidomide is effective for the treatment of bortezomib-resistant extramedullary disease in patients with multiple myeloma: report of 2 cases," *Clinical Lymphoma Myeloma and Leukemia*, vol. 13, no. 1, pp. 83–85, 2013.

[37] S. S. Saboo, F. Fennessy, L. Benajiba, J. Laubach, K. C. Anderson, and P. G. Richardson, "Imaging features of extramedullary, relapsed, and refractory multiple myeloma involving the liver across treatment with cyclophosphamide, lenalidomide, bortezomib, and dexamethasone," *Journal of Clinical Oncology*, vol. 30, no. 20, pp. e175–e179, 2012.

[38] F. Patriarca, S. Prosdocimo, V. Tomadini, A. Vasciaveo, B. Bruno, and R. Fanin, "Efficacy of bortezomib therapy for extramedullary relapse of myeloma after autologous and non-myeloablative allogeneic transplantation," *Haematologica*, vol. 90, no. 2, pp. 278-279, 2005.

[39] E. Paubelle, P. Coppo, L. Garderet et al., "Complete remission with bortezomib on plasmocytomas in an end-stage patient with refractory multiple myeloma who failed all other therapies including hematopoietic stem cell transplantation: possible enhancement of graft-vs-tumor effect," *Leukemia*, vol. 19, no. 9, pp. 1702–1704, 2005.

[40] P. G. Richardson, E. Weller, S. Jagannath et al., "Multicenter, phase I, dose-escalation trial of lenalidomide plus bortezomib for relapsed and relapsed/refractory multiple myeloma," *Journal of Clinical Oncology*, vol. 27, no. 34, pp. 5713–5719, 2009.

[41] S. K. Kumar, S. V. Rajkumar, A. Dispenzieri et al., "Improved survival in multiple myeloma and the impact of novel therapies," *Blood*, vol. 111, no. 5, pp. 2516–2520, 2008.

[42] A. K. Stewart, S. V. Rajkumar, M. A. Dimopoulos et al., "Carfilzomib, lenalidomide, and dexamethasone for relapsed multiple myeloma," *New England Journal of Medicine*, vol. 372, no. 2, pp. 142–152, 2015.

[43] J. San Miguel, K. Weisel, P. Moreau et al., "Pomalidomide plus low-dose dexamethasone versus high-dose dexamethasone alone for patients with relapsed and refractory multiple myeloma (MM-003): a randomised, open-label, phase 3 trial," *The Lancet Oncology*, vol. 14, no. 11, pp. 1055–1066, 2013.

[44] J. F. San-Miguel, V. T. Hungria, S. S. Yoon et al., "Panobinostat plus bortezomib and dexamethasone versus placebo plus bortezomib and dexamethasone in patients with relapsed or relapsed and refractory multiple myeloma: a multicentre, randomised, double-blind phase 3 trial," *The Lancet Oncology*, vol. 15, no. 11, pp. 1195–1206, 2014.

[45] S. Lonial, M. Dimopoulos, A. Palumbo et al., "Elotuzumab therapy for relapsed or refractory multiple myeloma," *New England Journal of Medicine*, vol. 373, no. 7, pp. 621–631, 2015.

[46] A. Palumbo, A. Chanan-Khan, K. Weisel et al., "Daratumumab, bortezomib, and dexamethasone for multiple myeloma," *New England Journal of Medicine*, vol. 375, no. 8, pp. 754–766, 2016.

[47] P. Moreau, T. Masszi, N. Grzasko et al., "Oral ixazomib, lenalidomide, and dexamethasone for multiple myeloma," *New England Journal of Medicine*, vol. 374, no. 17, pp. 1621–1634, 2016.

32

Improvement of Cardiac Vegetations in Antiphospholipid Syndrome with Enoxaparin and Corticosteroids after Rivaroxaban Failure

Eric Granowicz [ID][1] and Kiyon Chung [ID][2]

[1]Scripps Mercy Hospital, Department of Internal Medicine, San Diego, CA, USA
[2]Scripps Mercy Hospital, Department of Cardiology, San Diego, CA, USA

Correspondence should be addressed to Kiyon Chung; Chung.Kiyon@scrippshealth.org

Academic Editor: Giuseppe Murdaca

Cardiac disease is a well-known complication of antiphospholipid syndrome (APS), with many patients presenting with valvular thickening or vegetations, referred to as Libman–Sacks endocarditis (LSE). Because cases of APS with cardiac involvement are relatively rare, paucity of large clinical trials studying this complication has made management challenging. In the absence of acute heart failure and embolic events, a medical approach is usually selected, consisting of anticoagulation and possibly corticosteroids when another underlying autoimmune disease is present. However, the role of various anticoagulant classes and the duration of steroid therapy continue to be debated. Here, we present a 45-year-old woman who developed two vegetations in the setting of secondary APS while taking rivaroxaban before experiencing marked improvement with the use of enoxaparin and steroids.

1. Introduction

Antiphospholipid syndrome (APS) is an autoimmune disease characterized by the presence of various antiphospholipid antibodies that lead to inappropriate activation of platelets and the coagulation cascade. This ultimately manifests clinically with clotting in the venous and/or arterial systems. APS is often secondary to another autoimmune disease such as systemic lupus erythematosus (SLE), or may be a primary phenomenon in the absence of other immunological conditions. In order to make a diagnosis, clinical features must be accompanied by the presence of at least one of three antibodies: anticardiolipin, anti-β2 glycoprotein, or lupus anticoagulant.

In some cases, clotting can result in the formation of vegetations on cardiac valves, a form of nonbacterial thrombotic endocarditis (NBTE) called Libman–Sacks endocarditis (LSE). The disease is characterized pathologically by the presence of small, warty lesions of platelets and fibrin usually measuring about 1–5 mm, occurring mainly on the mitral valve, followed by the aortic valve in frequency

[1]. The disease ranges from being asymptomatic to presenting with life-threatening signs of systemic emboli or acute heart failure associated with valvular obstruction or regurgitation [2].

Treatment of LSE has been controversial, largely due to the lack of adequate randomized clinical trials. A surgical approach is typically used when criteria similar to those for infectious endocarditis (IE) are met [3–5]. When a medical approach is chosen, treatment depends on whether LSE occurs as a consequence of primary APS, or secondary APS associated with another underlying autoimmune condition. In the former, anticoagulation with warfarin is typically thought to be most effective, with the role of newer oral anticoagulants being less clear [6–8]. In the latter, anticoagulation along with steroid therapy are often used, although some observations have suggested that extended or recurrent use of steroids may actually worsen valvular function over time by leading to excessive scaring and fibrosis [9, 10].

Here, we describe a case of LSE occurring in the setting of secondary APS with SLE in which an abnormally large vegetation formed on the aortic valve concurrently with a smaller vegetation on the mitral valve.

2. Case Report

The patient is a 43-year-old female who presented with sharp, substernal, nonexertional chest pain, and shortness of breath. Her past medical history included secondary APS (lupus anticoagulant positive) in the setting of SLE, with multiple, recurrent deep venous thromboses of the lower extremities. She was diagnosed with myopericarditis during a hospitalization one year prior when she presented with similar symptoms and an elevated troponin, after which a coronary catheterization demonstrated no significant coronary artery disease. Examination revealed a 2/6 systolic ejection murmur, without any radiation, gallops, rubs, or jugular venous distension. Auscultation of the lungs revealed clear breath sounds.

An echocardiogram was ordered when she was found to have an elevated troponin level of 0.209 ng/ml without any evidence of acute ischemic pathology on her electrocardiogram. Subsequently, a 2 cm mass was seen on the aortic valve with evidence of obstructive pathology. A follow-up transesophageal echocardiogram redemonstrated this mass, along with a smaller mass on the mitral valve associated with mild mitral regurgitation (Figure 1). The aortic mass was consistent with fresh mobile thrombus, somewhat atypical for Libman–Sacks vegetations which usually have a more verrucous appearance. However, after blood cultures and an extensive workup for culture-negative endocarditis were negative, she was ultimately diagnosed with LSE and a recurrent flare of myopericarditis.

The patient's chest pain improved with colchicine, but her shortness of breath remained and was presumed to be from partial obstruction of the aortic valve by the large mass. After consultation with cardiothoracic surgery, medical therapy was initiated with a goal to avoid surgery if there were signs of improvement. She was already taking rivaroxaban when she originally presented, given that she had failed warfarin therapy in the past with persistently subtherapeutic INRs and recurrent DVTs, so she was started on therapeutic enoxaparin and aspirin. After a rheumatology consultation, hydroxychloroquine and prednisone were initiated as well. The patient remained stable with no new symptoms or signs of embolic events during her follow-up visits, and repeat transesophageal echocardiograms at 12 and 24 weeks demonstrated improvement in the size of both vegetations (Figure 2). Her prednisone was gradually tapered down over a period of 9 months.

3. Discussion

This case highlights many of the challenging aspects of managing patients with cardiac involvement in APS. The optimal treatment approach continues to be poorly defined, largely due to the fact that many recommendations regarding management originate from expert opinion and small observational case studies rather than randomized trials.

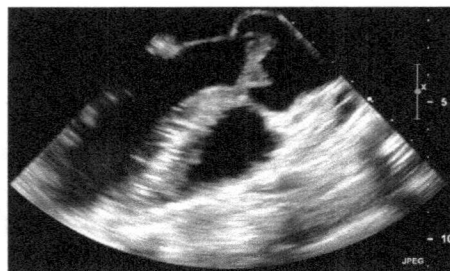

FIGURE 1: Initial echocardiogram showing a 2 cm mass on the right and noncoronary cusps of the aortic valve.

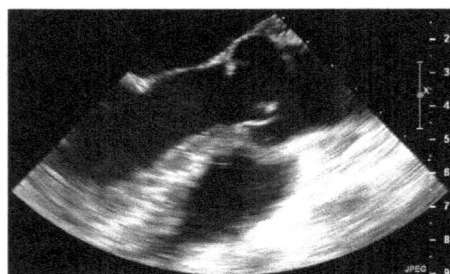

FIGURE 2: Follow-up transesophageal echocardiogram at 24 weeks showing a dramatic reduction in the size of the mass between the right and noncoronary cusps.

A treatment strategy begins with assessing the necessity of a surgical approach. Symptoms of acute heart failure, acute valvular regurgitation/stenosis, or recurrent embolization when recognized are considered to be relatively straightforward indications to consider surgical evaluation, in addition to patients who have failed medical management. Surgery is often offered to patients with mobile, left-sided vegetations greater than 1 cm for infective endocarditis, but this approach is not generalizable for cases of NBTE [4, 5]. Given the lack of embolization history, it seemed reasonable to proceed with an aggressive medical treatment plan before considering surgery.

After a commitment is made to a medical approach, a decision about the best form of anticoagulation is imperative. Warfarin with an INR goal of 2-3 has been considered the gold standard in patients with newly diagnosed APS presenting with their first thrombosis [6–8]. Given the relative ease of taking newer oral anticoagulants (NOACs), the role of these agents in APS has begun to be investigated. The RAPS trial compared the use of the direct oral anticoagulant, rivaroxaban, to moderate intensity anticoagulation with warfarin, demonstrating a noninferior anticoagulant ability with similar peak thrombin concentrations after 6 months, though the clinical implications of this finding were limited by insufficient power of the study despite showing no recurrent thromboses in the rivaroxaban group [11].

Additionally, the proper anticoagulant to use in the setting of warfarin failure continues to be perplexing. Various approaches include using high intensity anticoagulation with an INR goal of 3-4, the addition of aspirin or hydroxychloroquine to a moderate intensity anticoagulation regimen, or switching to a new anticoagulant class despite the lack of evidence to support any benefit of one class over vitamin K antagonists [12–14]. Given this patient's failure of warfarin and rivaroxaban, enoxaparin with aspirin seemed to be the most reasonable alternative. Ultimately a favorable response was seen, although it is unclear whether or not the patient's improvement was attributed to the change in anticoagulation or the addition of steroids.

When another underlying autoimmune process is present, steroids are frequently administered despite controversy over their benefits. Several case reports have demonstrated the ability of steroids to acutely decrease the amount of inflammation and disease activity, leading to rapid improvement in symptoms and imaging of the valves [15–17]. Despite these findings, hesitancy remains when deciding to initiate corticosteroid therapy, as several reports have noted that increases in hypertension, left ventricular hypertrophy, and accelerated atherosclerosis are more frequently seen in hearts treated with steroids making symptoms of heart failure more likely in the long term despite the initial acute improvement in symptoms [10, 18, 19]. The initial study that described these findings was done in 1975, and the duration of steroid treatment was unclear for the 36 patients described, so questions still remain about whether or not the benefits of a shorter course of steroids outweigh the potential long term deleterious effects on cardiac structure and function [9]. Additionally, there remains little evidence to support the use of steroids for primary APS.

4. Conclusion

This case demonstrates the challenges in managing a complicated presentation of Libman–Sacks endocarditis in the setting of warfarin and rivaroxaban failure. Anticoagulation with enoxaparin and aspirin in combination with prednisone ultimately lead to dramatic improvement, although questions still remain about whether or not this approach could be extrapolated to similar cases with reliable outcomes.

Conflicts of Interest

The authors declare that they have no conflicts of interest regarding the publication of this paper.

References

[1] J. L. Lee, S. M. Naguwa, G. S. Cheema, and M. E. Gershwin, "Revisiting Libman–Sacks endocarditis: a historical review and update," *Clinical Reviews in Allergy & Immunology*, vol. 36, no. 2-3, pp. 126–130, 2009.

[2] J. J. Miner and A. H. Kim, "Cardiac manifestations of systemic lupus erythematosus," *Rheumatic Disease Clinics of North America*, vol. 40, no. 1, pp. 51–60, 2014.

[3] D. Unic, M. Planinc, D. Baric et al., "Isolated tricuspid valve Libman-Sacks endocarditis in systemic lupus erythematosus with secondary antiphospholipid syndrome," *Texas Heart Institute Journal*, vol. 44, no. 2, pp. 147–149, 2017.

[4] A. Nakasu, T. Ishimine, H. Yasumoto, T. Tengan, and H. Mototake, "Mitral valve replacement for Libman-Sacks endocarditis in a patient with antiphospholipid syndrome

[5] A. A. Rabinstein, C. Giovanelli, J. G. Romano, S. Koch, A. M. Forteza, and M. Ricci, "Surgical treatment of non-bacterial thrombotic endocarditis presenting with stroke," *Journal of Neurology*, vol. 252, no. 3, pp. 352–355, 2005.

[6] G. Finazzi, R. Marchioli, V. Brancaccio et al., "A randomized clinical trial of high-intensity warfarin vs. conventional antithrombotic therapy for the prevention of recurrent thrombosis in patients with the antiphospholipid syndrome (WAPS)," *Journal of Thrombosis and Haemostasis*, vol. 3, no. 5, pp. 848–853, 2005.

[7] A. Holbrook, S. Schulman, D. M. Witt et al., "Evidence-based management of anticoagulant therapy: antithrombotic therapy and prevention of thrombosis, 9th ed: American College of Chest Physicians evidence-based clinical practice guidelines," *Chest*, vol. 141, no. 2, pp. e152S–e184S, 2012.

[8] G. Ruiz-Irastorza, M. J. Cuadrado, I. Ruiz-Arruza et al., "Evidence-based recommendations for the prevention and long-term management of thrombosis in antiphospholipid antibody-positive patients: report of a task force at the 13th International Congress on antiphospholipid antibodies," *Lupus*, vol. 20, no. 2, pp. 206–218, 2011.

[9] B. H. Bulkley and W. C. Roberts, "The heart in systemic lupus erythematosus and the changes induced in it by corticosteroid therapy. A study of 36 necropsy patients," *American Journal of Medicine*, vol. 58, no. 2, pp. 243–264, 1975.

[10] A. Doria, L. Iaccarino, P. Sarzi-Puttini, F. Atzeni, M. Turriel, and M. Petri, "Cardiac involvement in systemic lupus erythematosus," *Lupus*, vol. 14, no. 9, pp. 683–686, 2005.

[11] H. Cohen, B. J. Hunt, M. Efthymiou et al., "Rivaroxaban versus warfarin to treat patients with thrombotic antiphospholipid syndrome, with or without systemic lupus erythematosus (RAPS): a randomised, controlled, open-label, phase 2/3, non-inferiority trial," *Lancet Haematology*, no. 9, pp. e426–e436, 2016.

[12] M. A. Crowther, J. S. Ginsberg, J. Julian et al., "A comparison of two intensities of warfarin for the prevention of recurrent thrombosis in patients with the antiphospholipid antibody syndrome," *New England Journal of Medicine*, vol. 349, no. 12, pp. 1133–1138, 2003.

[13] H. Okuma, Y. Kitagawa, T. Yasuda, K. Tokuoka, and S. Takagi, "Comparison between single antiplatelet therapy and combination of antiplatelet and anticoagulation therapy for secondary prevention in ischemic stroke patients with antiphospholipid syndrome," *International Journal of Medical Sciences*, vol. 7, no. 1, pp. 15–18, 2010.

[14] S. Ahmed, A. Karim, D. Patel, R. Siddiqui, and J. Mattana, "Low-molecular weight heparin: treatment failure in a patient with primary antiphospholipid antibody syndrome," *American Journal of the Medical Sciences*, vol. 324, no. 5, pp. 279-280, 2002.

[15] A. M. Al-Moghairi, "Libman–Sacks endocarditis with an unusual presentation," *Journal of the Saudi Heart Association*, vol. 22, no. 3, pp. 143-144, 2010.

[16] S. Micallef and C. Mallia Azzopardi, "Antiphospholipid syndrome masquerading as a case of infective endocarditis," *BMJ Case Reports*, article pii: bcr-2018-224404, 2018.

[17] E. Ginanjar and Y. Yulianto, "Autoimmune disease with cardiac valves involvement: Libman-Sacks endocarditis," *Acta Medica Indonesiana*, no. 2, pp. 148–150, 2017.

[18] R. Hoffman, H. Lethen, U. Zunker, F. A. Schöndube, N. Maurin, and H. G. Sieberth, "Rapid appearance of severe mitral regurgitation under high-dosage corticosteroid therapy

33

Iatrogenic T-Cell Lymphoma with Associated Hemophagocytic Lymphohistiocyotsis in a Patient with Long-Standing Rheumatoid Arthritis

X. A. Andrade ⓘ,[1] H. E. Fuentes,[1] D. M. Oramas,[2] H. Mann,[1] and P. Kovarik[3]

[1]*Department of Medicine, John H. Stroger Jr. Hospital of Cook County, Chicago, IL, USA*
[2]*Division of Pathology, University of Illinois at Chicago, Chicago, IL, USA*
[3]*Department of Pathology, John H. Stroger Jr. Hospital of Cook County, Chicago, IL, USA*

Correspondence should be addressed to X. A. Andrade; xavier_ag18@hotmail.com

Academic Editor: Tatsuharu Ohno

Patients with rheumatoid arthritis are at increased risk of hematological malignancies, especially when exposed to immunosuppressive therapy. The mechanisms of lymphomagenesis remain poorly understood but factors implicated include high disease activity, exposure to antitumoral necrosis factor medications, and Epstein–Barr virus infection. Lymphoid malignancies of T-cell origin are uncommon in patients with rheumatoid arthirits. Clinical presentation with associated hemophagocytic lymphohistiocyotsis is rare and confers a poor prognosis. This case report illustrates a case of a patient with long-standing rheumatoid arthritis and an iatrogenic peripheral T-cell lymphoma with secondary hemophagocytic lymphohistiocytosis who achieved a complete response after intensive chemotherapy.

1. Introduction

Patients with rheumatoid arthritis (RA) have an increased risk of lymphoid malignancies compared to the general population. Several factors have been associated with increased risk of a secondary malignancy including chronic immunosuppressive treatment, anti-TNF medications, high disease activity, and long-standing disease. The mechanism of lymphomagenesis behind these factors and their implications in management and surveillance of lymphoid malignancies in patients with RA remain uncertain.

T-cell malignancies in patients with RA are uncommon, representing less than 10% of all lymphomas. Although secondary hemophagocytic lymphohistiocyotsis (HLH) is a rare presentation of T-cell lymphomas, it is an independent adverse prognostic factor. Recognition of T-cell lymphoma-associated HLH is key for a prompt diagnosis and treatment and improved outcomes.

We present a case of a patient with T-cell lymphoma-associated HLH and long-standing RA years after conventional immunosuppressive and biologic treatment.

2. Case Presentation

The patient is a 56-year-old woman with a history of rheumatoid arthritis diagnosed 11 years prior to admission. She was treated with methotrexate, hydroxychloroquine, and etanercept with good symptomatic control. Three years prior to admission, she developed etanercept-related scleromalacia perforans on her right eye and was switched to infliximab therapy.

The patient presented with a one-week history of fever, sore throat, and abdominal pain. Physical examination was relevant for jaundice, bilateral tonsillar enlargement, cervical and axillary lymphadenopathy (2 cm in diameter), and diffuse abdominal tenderness without guarding. Her neurological examination was unremarkable.

Laboratory testing showed altered liver function tests (AST 149 UI/L, ALT 69 UI/L, alkaline phosphatase 317 UI/L, gamma GT 305 UI/L, total bilirubin 9.9 mg/dl, and direct bilirubin 6.6 mg/dl), bicytopenia (WBC 8.2×10^9/L, neutrophils 58%, lymphocytes 7%, monocytes 15%, hemoglobin 10.6 g/dl, hematocrit 32%, and platelets 49.0×10^9/L), hyperferritinemia

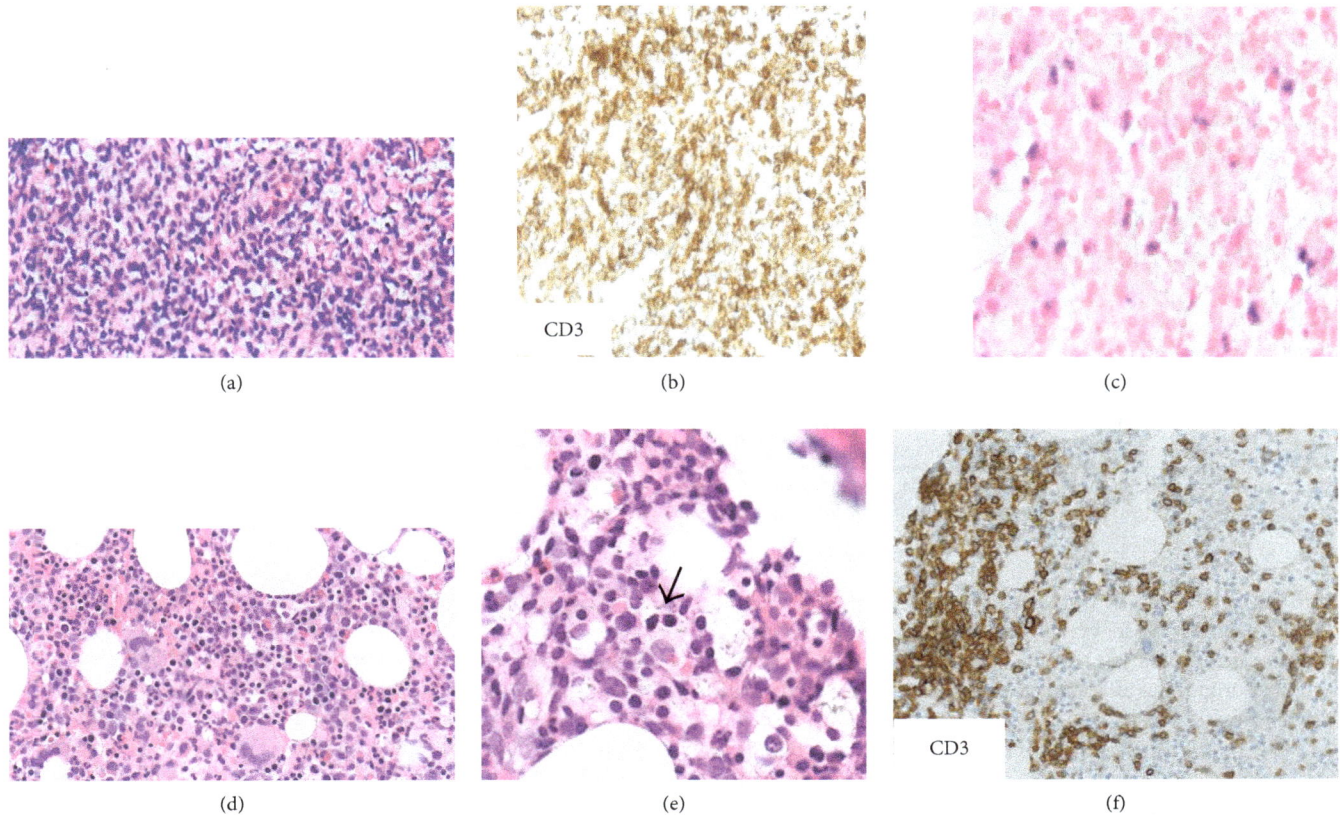

FIGURE 1: Lymph node biopsy shows small- to medium-sized atypical lymphocytes (a). In this infiltrate, immunohistochemistry is positive for CD3 (b) and in situ hybridization is positive for Epstein–Barr virus (c). Bone marrow biopsy shows clusters of atypical lymphocytes (d) and histiocytes with hemophagocytosis (e). Immunohistochemical staining for CD3 is positive (f).

(ferritin 4150 ng/ml), and hypertriglyceridemia (triglycerides 402 mg/dl). Thoracic, abdominal, and pelvic computerized tomography scans showed diffuse generalized lymphade-nopathy and splenomegaly with nodular hypodensities.

Due to the suspicion of a hematological malignancy, a bone marrow aspiration and a biopsy were performed which showed hypercellularity with a nodular and interstitial infiltration by small- to intermediate-sized atypical lymphocytes, macrophages with hemophagocytosis, and an inconclusive flow cytometry result for a lymphoproliferative disorder. The bone marrow karyotype was normal.

An axillary lymph node core biopsy was performed which showed a lymphoid infiltrate composed of small, intermediate, and large atypical lymphoid cells with foci of necrosis and angiocentric and angioinvasive features. Immunohistochemical stains were positive for CD3, CD5, and CD7, costained both CD4 and CD8 in atypical lymphoid cells, and displayed negative staining for CD10, CD20, CD30, and CD15. In situ hybridization for Epstein–Barr virus (EBV) was positive on atypical lymphoid cells coexpressing CD4 and CD8 (Figure 1). Karyotyping of lymph node tissues was not performed. Liver biopsy showed sinusoidal, lobular, and portal infiltrates of small- to intermediate-sized atypical lymphoid cells. Immunohistochemical stains showed that these cells were positive for CD3, CD5, CD7, and both CD4 and CD8 (Figure 1).

The patient was diagnosed with an iatrogenic immunodeficiency-related T-cell lymphoma and malignancy-associated hemophagocytic lymphohistiocyotsis. Immuno-suppressive therapy was discontinued at the time of diagnosis, and intravenous steroids were admistered on day 3 of admission. Ultimately, chemotherapy was started with CHOEP regimen (cyclophosphamide, doxorubicin, vincristine, eto-poside, and prednisone) every 21 days. After chemotherapy cycle 3, the patient showed significant improvement of cytopenias and liver function tests (Table 1).

The patient completed 6 cycles of chemotherapy without major complications. Positron emission computerized tomography imaging after the 6th cycle demonstrated a complete metabolic response. Currently, the patient remains in complete response two years after diagnosis and continues to receive medical care in our institution.

3. Discussion

Many descriptive studies have reported an increased incidence of lymphomas in patients with RA compared to the general population [1, 2]. Impaired T-cell function due to high disease activity [3] and chronic immunosuppressive therapy with methotrexate [4] have been implicated in lymphomagenesis; however, this association remains unclear as results from large descriptive studies have shown

TABLE 1: Clinical and laboratory findings through admission and during chemotherapy.

	Day 0	Day 3	Day 7	Cycle 1	Cycle 2	Cycle 3	Cycle 4	Cycle 5	Cycle 6
WBC ($\times 10^9$/L)	8.2	6.0	3.0	3.0	5.0	4.1	5.2	4.8	3.9
Hemoglobin (g/dl)	10.6	9.3	8.3	8.5	12.5	12.7	8.9	9.4	12.6
Platelets ($\times 10^9$/L)	41	62	129	110	97	147	170	68	181
Ferritin (ng/ml)	4150	—	—	—	—	—	—	—	—
Triglycerides (mg/dl)	400	—	—	—	—	—	—	—	155
AST (U/L)	149	213	111	94	68	40	27	18	16
ALT (U/L)	69	107	113	111	95	34	19	16	20
LDH (U/L)	979	1,093	540	529	427	299	287	154	136
Total bilirubin (mg/dl)	9.5	14	9.3	11.2	3.3	1.2	0.6	0.5	0.6
Direct bilirubin (mg/dl)	5.8	9.2	6.8	6.8	1.3	0.5	0.3	0.2	0.3
Temperature (°Fahrenheit)	102.2	98.2	98.7	97.8	—	—	—	—	—
Heart rate (bpm)	130	134	84	75	—	—	—	—	—

Methylprednisone dosed at 1 mg/kg IV was started on admission day 3; cycle 1 of R-CHOP was started on admission day 9; cycles 1 to 3 were administered with a 50% dose reduction of adriamycin and vincristine due to abnormal liver function tests; cycles 2 to 6 included etoposide 100 mg/m² IV on days 1 to 3.

conflicting results [5, 6]. More recently, anti-TNF medications received close attention due to several reports of lymphoid malignancies in patients with RA but a metanalysis by Bongartz et al. could not find convincing evidence for this association [7].

The relationship between Epstein–Barr virus (EBV) infections and lymphomagenesis is well established in patients with B-cell malignancies and chronic immunosuppression, but its role in T-cell malignancies is less known. There is a high prevalence of EBV infection in patients with T-cell lymphomas (TCLs) reaching around 25–58% [8, 9], but the mechanism of lymphomagenesis remains poorly understood. Even though there is heterogeneity in the methods of detection for EBV infection between retrospective studies, it has been consistently linked to worse overall and progression-free survival in patients with TCLs [8, 10].

Considering all lymphoid malignancies in patients with RA, TCLs represent less than 10% [4, 11]. Initial presentation as lymphoma-associated HLH (LAHLH) is more common on TCLs compared to those of B-cell origin [12]. However, the actual incidence of LAHLH in patients with RA and lymphoid malignancies is unclear and likely underreported due to the lack of standardized diagnostic criteria [13, 14].

There are no large prospective controlled studies to evaluate optimal therapy of TCLs and LAHLH. Most of the patients are treated with CHOP regimen (cyclophosphamide, adriamycin, vincristine, and prednisone), and etoposide is frequently added given its proven benefit on pediatric protocols for primary HLH [14] as in the case presented here.

TCLs with LAHLH have a significantly worse overall survival when compared with TCLs without LAHLH (2 months versus 45 months, resp.) as reported in retrospective studies [12, 15]. Multivariate analysis on a small retrospective study by Han et al. suggests that LAHLH is an independent prognostic factor associated with poor survival after adjustment for other known unfavorable features [12]. The benefit of a more intensive chemotherapy regimen and consolidation of response with bone marrow transplant is still uncertain and an open area of investigation.

4. Conclusion

LAHLH should be considered in patients with long-standing RA and unexplained fever, cytopenias, organomegaly, and lymphadenopathy, particularly if exposed to chronic immunosuppressive therapy and anti-TNF medications. When present, secondary HLH is an independent risk factor for poor prognosis. The benefit of a more intensive chemotherapy and consolidation with bone marrow transplant remains uncertain. Large trials with risk stratification and subgroup analysis may help elucidate this question.

The outcome of the patient presented in this case is exceptional. Arguably, early diagnosis and treatment with etoposide may have contributed to favorable outcomes.

Consent

Informed consent was obtained from the patient described in this report.

Conflicts of Interest

The authors declare that there are no conflicts of interest regarding the publication of this article.

References

[1] D. P. M. Symmons, "Lymphoma and rheumatoid arthritis-again," Rheumatology, vol. 46, no. 1, pp. 1-2, 2007.

[2] L. Mellemkjær, M. S. Linet, G. Gridley, M. Frisch, H. Møller, and J. H. Olsen, "Rheumatoid arthritis and cancer risk," European Journal of Cancer, vol. 32, no. 10, pp. 1753–1757, 1996.

[3] E. Baecklund, A. Iliadou, J. Askling et al., "Association of chronic inflammation, not its treatment, with increased lymphoma risk in rheumatoid arthritis," Arthritis & Rheumatism, vol. 54, no. 3, pp. 692–701, 2006.

[4] X. Mariette, D. Cazals-hatem, J. Warszawki, and N. Balandraud, "Lymphomas in rheumatoid arthritis patients treated with methotrexate : a 3-year prospective study in France," *Blood*, vol. 99, no. 11, pp. 3909–3915, 2002.

[5] D. P. Symmons and A. J. Silman, "Anti-tumor necrosis factor alpha therapy and the risk of lymphoma in rheumatoid arthritis: no clear answer," *Arthritis & Rheumatism*, vol. 50, no. 6, pp. 1703–1706, 2004.

[6] K. G. Moder, A. Tefferi, M. D. Cohen, D. M. Menke, and H. S. Luthra, "Hematologic malignancies and the use of methotrexate in rheumatoid arthritis: a retrospective study," *American Journal of Medicine*, vol. 99, no. 3, pp. 276–281, 1995.

[7] T. Bongartz, A. J. Sutton, M. J. Sweeting, I. Buchan, E. L Matteson, and V. Montori, "Anti-TNF antibody therapy in rheumatoid arthritis and the risk of serious infections and malignancies: systematic review and meta-analysis of rare harmful effects in randomized controlled trials," *JAMA*, vol. 295, no. 19, pp. 2275–2285, 2006.

[8] F. D'Amore, P. Johansen, A. Houmand, D. D. Weisenburger, and L. S. Mortensen, "Epstein-Barr virus genome in non-Hodgkin's lymphomas occurring in immunocompetent patients: highest prevalence in nonlymphoblastic T-cell lymphoma and correlation with a poor prognosis. Danish Lymphoma Study Group, LYFO," *Blood*, vol. 87, no. 3, pp. 1045–1055, 1996.

[9] X. G. Zhou, S. J. Hamilton-Dutoit, Q. H. Yan, and G. Pallesen, "High frequency of Epstein–Barr virus in Chinese peripheral T-cell lymphoma," *Histopathology*, vol. 24, no. 2, pp. 115–122, 1994.

[10] J. Dupuis, J. Emile, N. Mounier et al., "Prognostic significance of Epstein-Barr virus in nodal peripheral T-cell lymphoma, unspecified : a Groupe d ' Etude des Lymphomes de l ' Adulte (GELA) study," *Blood*, vol. 108, no. 13, pp. 4163–4169, 2013.

[11] E. Baecklund, C. Sundström, A. Ekbom et al., "Lymphoma subtypes in patients with rheumatoid arthritis: increased proportion of diffuse large B cell lymphoma," *Arthritis & Rheumatism*, vol. 48, no. 6, pp. 1543–1550, 2003.

[12] A.-R. Han, H. R. Lee, B.-B. Park et al., "Lymphoma-associated hemophagocytic syndrome: clinical features and treatment outcome," *Annals of Hematology*, vol. 86, no. 7, pp. 493–498, 2007.

[13] L. Fardet, L. Galicier, O. Lambotte et al., "Development and validation of the HScore, a score for the diagnosis of reactive hemophagocytic syndrome," *Arthritis & Rheumatology*, vol. 66, no. 9, pp. 2613–2620, 2014.

[14] J.-I. Henter, A. Horne, M. Aricó et al., "HLH-2004: diagnostic and therapeutic guidelines for hemophagocytic lymphohistiocytosis," *Pediatric Blood & Cancer*, vol. 48, no. 2, pp. 124–131, 2007.

[15] M. V. Shah, T. E. Witzig, M. O'Byrne et al., "Association of hemophagocytic lymphohistiocytosis (HLH) with poor outcomes in adults with NK- and T-cell lymphoma (NKTCL)," *Journal of Clinical Oncology*, vol. 33, 2015.

34

Cutaneous Vasculitis: An Unusual Presentation of a Biclonal Nodal Plasma Cell Dyscrasia

D. Swan,[1] M. Murphy,[2] and E. Elhassadi[1]

[1]*Haematology Department, University Hospital Waterford, Regional Cancer Center South East, University College Cork, Cork, Ireland*
[2]*Pathology Department, University Hospital Waterford, Regional Cancer Center South East, University College Cork, Cork, Ireland*

Correspondence should be addressed to D. Swan; dawnswan123@gmail.com

Academic Editor: Marie-Christine Kyrtsonis

We describe an unusual case of a biclonal nodal plasma cell dyscrasia, presenting with a vasculitic rash, end-organ damage, and cytopenias. Serum protein electrophoresis demonstrated a biclonal kappa-restricted paraprotein, with a negative skeletal survey and no bone marrow disease. Fluorodeoxyglucose-PET-CT (FDG-PET-CT) revealed nodal involvement, which was not appreciable clinically, and facilitated biopsy, confirming the diagnosis of a nodal plasmacytoma. Complete biochemical response and resolution of the vasculitic rash were achieved with bortezomib-based therapy.

1. Introduction

The incidence of multiple myeloma in the Republic of Ireland is around 5/100,000, with around 240 new cases presenting annually. Here, we discuss a challenging case of a biclonal nodal multiple myeloma, presenting with a vasculitic rash. Nodal and biclonal myelomas are individually extremely unusual, and the combination of both is vanishingly so. To date, and to the best of our knowledge, there have been no reported cases presenting with a vasculitic rash, a unique feature in our patient. This rare and unusual presentation of a condition seen commonly within the field of haematology required an individualised approach to care and necessitated modification of the routine investigational pathway recommended by the British Society of Haematology (BSH) [1].

2. Case Presentation

A 69-year-old lady was referred from the dermatology service in May 2016 for assessment of thrombocytopenia and rash. The rash was predominantly localised to the right leg and lower back and developed 3 weeks after ipsilateral total knee replacement surgery. She had normochromic, normocytic anaemia (Hb: 9.4 g/l), thrombocytopenia (105 × 10^9/l) with prominent rouleaux on peripheral blood film, and moderate

renal impairment without hypercalcaemia, with a normal erythrocyte sedimentation rate (ESR). Serum protein electrophoresis demonstrated a biclonal phenotype with a total IgG of 29.2 g/l, IgM of 0.44 g/l, and IgA of 33.8 g/l, with an IgA kappa band of 30.3 g/l and a small unquantifiable IgG kappa band. The absolute kappa free light chains were 259.08 mg/l, lambda free light chains were 48.72 mg/l, and the involved : uninvolved free light chain ratio was 5.32 (normal reference ranges: IgG 7–16 g/l, IgM 0.4–2.3 g/l, IgA 0.7–4.3 g/l, kappa free light chains 3.3–19.4 mg/l, lambda chain 5.71–26.3 mg/l, and ratio 0.26–1.65). Bence-Jones protein analysis was negative and beta-2-microglobulin was significantly elevated, at 10.48 mg/l. The X-ray skeletal survey was negative for lytic lesions.

Initial bone marrow examination demonstrated fewer than 10% plasma cells with no light chain restriction to suggest clonality. A repeat sample obtained from the contralateral iliac crest also contained fewer than 10% plasma cells, but these were kappa-restricted. Skin biopsy demonstrated changes consistent with the diagnosis of vasculitis. A fluorodeoxyglucose-PET-CT (FDG-PET-CT) was performed to localise the paraprotein-producing tumour, demonstrating bilateral FDG-avid cervical and axillary nodes, with a single mediastinal and portacaval node (Figures 1(a), 1(b), and 1(c)). The largest axillary node (7 mm) was biopsied revealing

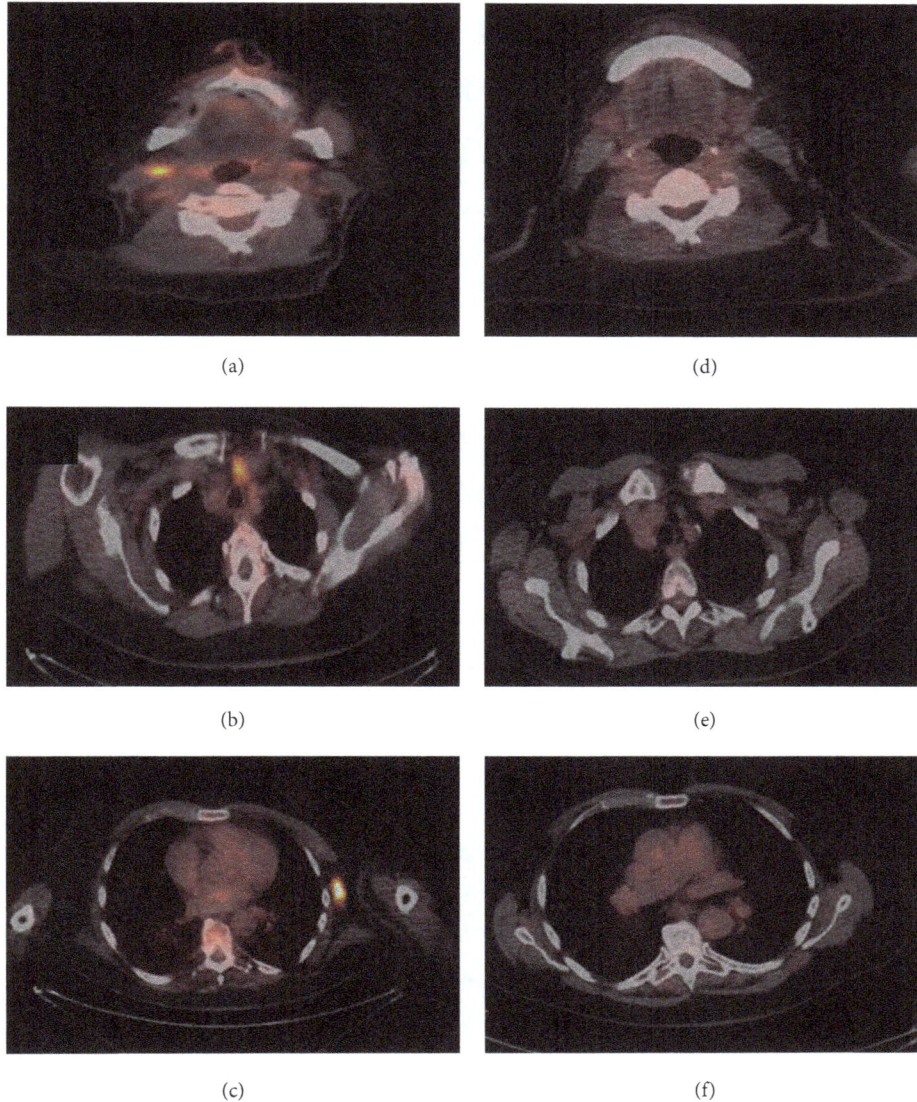

(a)

(d)

(b)

(e)

(c)

(f)

FIGURE 1: (a, b, c) Diagnostic axial FDG-PET images illustrate FDG-avid axillary, mediastinal, and cervical nodes, respectively. (c, d, f) Posttreatment axial PDG-PET images illustrate no FDG-avid evidence of residual disease at cervical, mediastinal, and axillary nodes, respectively.

replacement of the nodal architecture by a CD138 positive, kappa-restricted plasma cell infiltrate (Figure 2).

The patient was started on CyBorD chemotherapy (cyclophosphamide, bortezomib, and dexamethasone) with symptomatic improvement and resolution of the vasculitic rash. The paraprotein present in the beta region reduced to 7.2 g/l and the IgA kappa band became undetectable. Free light chain ratio normalised to 1.40 with an absolute kappa of 75.53 mg/l and lambda of 54.11 mg/l. Her anaemia significantly lessened, and thrombocytopenia resolved between chemotherapy cycles. A very good partial response (VGPR) was achieved according to the International Myeloma Working Group (IMWG) criteria. Moreover, repeat FDG-PET-CT following 4 cycles of treatment showed a complete response (Figures 1(d), 1(e), and 1(f)).

3. Discussion

This case is noteworthy in three regards: the presentation with a vasculitic rash, the biclonal phenotype of gammopathy, and the extramedullary lymph node presentation without significant bone marrow involvement. In addition to this, the emerging and developing role of PET-CT in the management of multiple myeloma has clear relevance to this case.

Paraneoplastic vasculitis is a well-documented but poorly understood phenomenon, which is known to be more common amongst patients with haematological malignancies. A recent study of 421 patients with cutaneous vasculitis identified malignancy in 3.8%, of which over half were haematological in origin [2]. The authors suggested factors that should prompt investigation for underlying neoplasm

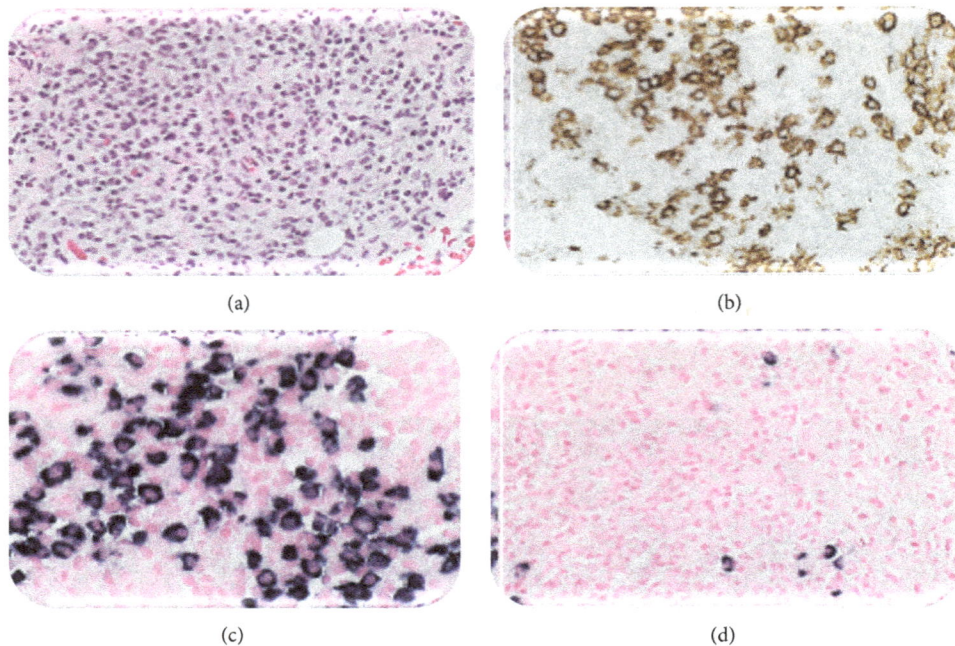

FIGURE 2: Left axillary lymph node biopsy. (a) Haematoxylin and eosin stain at ×40. (b) CD138 stain at ×40, strongly positive. (c) Kappa stain at ×40, strongly positive. (d) Lambda stain at ×40, negative demonstrating kappa light chain restriction.

including constitutional symptoms, abnormal circulating cells on peripheral blood smear, cytopenias, an elevated ESR, lymphadenopathy or organomegaly on clinical examination, and masses on imaging. Of the 9 patients in this study who were found to have a haematological malignancy, 100% were anaemic at the time of diagnosis, compared with 29% of patients with nonhaematological cancers and only 19% of those in whom a cancer diagnosis was not made. In this study, thrombocytopenia was reported in 12.5% of cases diagnosed with malignancy and <1% without. Our case presented with fatigue and investigations revealed bicytopenias and normal ESR; however, it should be noted that systemic corticosteroid therapy had been instigated by the dermatology team prior to our review, which could have mitigated this.

Biclonal multiple myeloma is a rare form of myeloma, with frequencies reported in the literature from 1 to 5%. A historical case series of 57 patients noted that 53% had an IgG and IgA band, and of 115 light chains reviewed, 70% were kappa [3]. Our case conformed to these observations. Recent work on the development of symptomatic myeloma from biclonal gammopathy of uncertain significance has not shown a greater risk of disease progression, or a poorer response to treatment in those that made progress [4], and there is no evidence to suggest that a different approach to therapy is warranted at the current time in those without evidence of organ damage or presence of high risk biomarkers. Development of a second clone following myeloma treatment does not also appear to impact outcome. Data on outcomes in those with symptomatic biclonal myeloma, such as our patient, is even more spare. Two cases of IgD/IgM myeloma have been reported, both with aggressive, chemotherapy-resistant behaviour [5], but to our knowledge, there is no robust evidence for those with symptomatic IgG/IgA disease.

Primary extramedullary plasmacytoma is also rare, accounting for only around 4% of plasma cell dyscrasias. There is some data suggesting that the risk of progression to multiple myeloma from a solitary primary lymph node plasmacytoma is less than for other extramedullary plasmacytomata and that recurrence posttreatment is rare [6], but evidence is limited to small case series and individual case reports. In contrast to this, patients with symptomatic extramedullary myeloma at diagnosis are more prone to high risk cytogenetic profiles, aggressive disease, and worsened outcomes [7, 8]. Optimal treatment is contentious, but there is some evidence that bortezomib-based therapies are efficacious in this setting and have been recommended by expert opinion [9, 10]. Our patient had constitutional symptoms, cytopenias, and renal impairment; hence, we felt that a bortezomib-based regime was an appropriate choice.

The role of FDG-PET-CT in the diagnosis and follow-up of myeloma is developing. At present, routine use of PET is not recommended in the most recent BSH guidelines due to insufficient evidence [11]. However, subsequent to our initial management of this case, in April 2017, the International Myeloma Working Group released a consensus statement on the role of FDG-PET in the diagnosis and management of multiple myeloma and other plasma cell disorders [12]. They recommend mandatory PET-CT to confirm suspected solitary plasmacytoma, if whole body MRI is unavailable, and to distinguish active from smouldering myeloma if skeletal survey is negative and whole body MRI is not possible. Here, we utilised PET-CT in order to localise the paraprotein-producing tumour and to facilitate confirmatory histological biopsy.

A meta-analysis of 14 studies found PET-CT to have superior specificity and sensitivity (96% and 77%, resp.) for the detection of sites of clonal plasma cells, particularly in extramedullary locations [13]. Mulligan and Badros reported that PET-CT is particularly useful for localisation of extramedullary disease, revealing additional lesions in around 30% diagnosed with a solitary plasmacytoma on MRI [14]. This feature benefited our case both diagnostically, as she lacked palpable nodes, masses, or size-significant lymphadenopathy by nonfunctional imaging modality criteria, and equally in terms of assessing response to treatment, for the same reasons. A lack of consensus currently exists regarding cut-off maximum standardised uptake values to distinguish positive from negative scans. In 2016, an Italian group proposed PET-CT criteria for use in myeloma at diagnosis and during treatment [15], which would include assessment of bone marrow uptake, osteolytic lesions, fractures, and extramedullary and paramedullary diseases. This may form the backbone of future reporting criteria.

The unusual nature of this case has meant that it has been both diagnostically and therapeutically challenging, with little robust evidence available to guide decision-making, as there are no randomised controlled studies focusing on patients with either biclonal myeloma or nodal disease. It highlights that the presence of a vasculitic rash should prompt consideration of underlying malignancy in certain patients, particularly those with anaemia or other cytopenias. Additionally, it demonstrates the emerging role of PET-CT in the management of plasma cell dyscrasias, with particular value in the setting of extramedullary disease.

Conflicts of Interest

The authors declare that they have no conflicts of interest.

Authors' Contributions

D. Swan wrote the paper, M. Murphy provided histology and reviewed the paper, and E. Elhassadi reviewed the paper.

References

[1] G. Pratt, M. Jenner, R. Owen et al., "Updates to the guidelines for the diagnosis and management of multiple myeloma," *British Journal of Haematology*, vol. 167, no. 1, pp. 131–133, 2014.

[2] J. Loricera, V. Calvo-Río, F. Ortiz-Sanjuán et al., "The spectrum of paraneoplastic cutaneous vasculitis in a defined population: incidence and clinical features," *Medicine (United States)*, vol. 92, no. 6, pp. 331–343, 2013.

[3] R. A. Kyle, R. A. Robinson, and J. A. Katzmann, "The clinical aspects of biclonal gammopathies. Review of 57 cases," *The American Journal of Medicine*, vol. 71, no. 6, pp. 999–1008, 1981.

[4] T. C. Mullikin, S. V. Rajkumar, A. Dispenzieri et al., "Clinical characteristics and outcomes in biclonal gammopathies," *American Journal of Hematology*, vol. 91, no. 5, pp. 473–475, 2016.

[5] Z. W. Chen, I. Kotsikogianni, J. S. Raval, C. G. Roth, and M. A. Rollins-Raval, "Biclonal IgD and IgM plasma cell myeloma: a report of two cases and a literature review," *Case Reports in Hematology*, vol. 2013, Article ID 293150, pp. 1–5, 2013.

[6] B. T.-Y. Lin and L. M. Weiss, "Primary plasmacytoma of lymph nodes," *Human Pathology*, vol. 28, no. 9, pp. 1083–1090, 1997.

[7] M. Varettoni, A. Corso, G. Pica, S. Mangiacavalli, C. Pascutto, and M. Lazzarino, "Incidence, presenting features and outcome of extramedullary disease in multiple myeloma: a longitudinal study on 1003 consecutive patients," *Annals of Oncology*, vol. 21, no. 2, pp. 325–330, 2010.

[8] S. Z. Usmani, C. Heuck, A. Mitchell et al., "Extramedullary disease portends poor prognosis in multiple myeloma and is over-represented in high-risk disease even in the era of novel agents," *Haematologica*, vol. 97, no. 11, pp. 1761–1767, 2012.

[9] L. Rosiñol, M. T. Cibeira, C. Uriburu et al., "Bortezomib: an effective agent in extramedullary disease in multiple myeloma," *European Journal of Haematology*, vol. 76, no. 5, pp. 405–408, 2006.

[10] T. Fukushima, T. Nakamura, M. Miki et al., "Complete response obtained by bortezomib plus dexamethasone in a patient with relapsed multiple myeloma with multiple plasmacytomas," *Anticancer Research*, vol. 30, no. 9, pp. 3791–3794, 2010.

[11] S. D'Sa, N. Abildgaard, J. Tighe, P. Shaw, and M. Hall-Craggs, "Guidelines for the use of imaging in the management of myeloma," *British Journal of Haematology*, vol. 137, no. 1, pp. 49–63, 2007.

[12] M. Cavo, E. Terpos, C. Nanni et al., "Role of 18 F-FDG PET/CT in the diagnosis and management of multiple myeloma and other plasma cell disorders: a consensus statement by the international myeloma working group," *The Lancet Oncology*, vol. 18, no. 4, pp. e206–e217, 2017.

[13] Y.-Y. Lu, J.-H. Chen, W.-Y. Lin et al., "FDG PET or PET/CT for detecting intramedullary and extramedullary lesions in multiple myeloma: a systematic review and meta-analysis," *Clinical Nuclear Medicine*, vol. 37, no. 9, pp. 833–837, 2012.

[14] M. E. Mulligan and A. Z. Badros, "PET/CT and MR imaging in myeloma," *Skeletal Radiology*, vol. 36, no. 1, pp. 5–16, 2007.

[15] C. Nanni, E. Zamagni, A. Versari et al., "Image interpretation criteria for FDG PET/CT in multiple myeloma: a new proposal from an Italian expert panel. IMPeTUs (Italian Myeloma criteria for PET USe)," *European Journal of Nuclear Medicine and Molecular Imaging*, vol. 43, no. 3, pp. 414–421, 2016.

35

A Case of Primary Refractory Immune Thrombocytopenia: Challenges in Choice of Therapies

Hanyin Wang [iD][1] **and Hande Tuncer**[2]

[1]*Department of Internal Medicine, Tufts Medical Center, 800 Washington St., Boston, MA 02111, USA*
[2]*Division of Hematology/Oncology, Tufts Medical Center, 800 Washington St, Boston, MA 02111, USA*

Correspondence should be addressed to Hanyin Wang; hwang@tuftsmedicalcenter.org

Academic Editor: Tomás J. González-López

The value of combination therapy for refractory ITP is not well defined. We present the case of a 29-year-old male with severe ITP refractory to initial standard therapy including steroids, IVIG, and subsequent splenectomy, who was treated with the combination therapy of rituximab, romiplostim, and mycophenolate and eventually developed thrombocytosis requiring platelet-pheresis. Our case highlights the importance of the need to understand predictors of response to standard upfront treatment of acute ITP.

1. Introduction

Immune thrombocytopenia (ITP) is an immune-mediated disorder characterized by isolated thrombocytopenia with peripheral blood platelet count less than 100×10^9/L [1]. An International Working Group (IWG) defined refractory ITP as cases that do not respond to or relapse after splenectomy while require treatment to reduce the risk of clinically significant bleeding [1]. Despite advances in the treatment of ITP in the past two decades, management of refractory ITP remains to be a challenge. The optimal sequence of treatment options is unknown. Furthermore, the role of combination therapy is not well defined.

We present the case of a 29-year-old male with pituitary apoplexy and severe ITP refractory to initial standard treatment including steroids and IVIG requiring further management including splenectomy, rituximab, romiplostim, and mycophenolate.

2. Case Presentation

A 29-year-old man with no significant past medical history presented to emergency department with 2 days of epistaxis and petechiae. The patient experienced upper respiratory infection symptoms 5 days prior to presentation. He was not taking any home medication. His family history was not significant. His vital signs were stable. Physical exam was notable for oral blisters and petechial rash over extremities. He was found to have a platelet count of 1×10^9/L. The rest of CBC was normal. Peripheral blood smear confirmed profound thrombocytopenia with normal platelet size and no platelet clumping. TSH, hepatitis C antibody, HIV antibody, *H. pylori* stool antigen, CMV PCR, and EBV PCR were all negative. Coagulation function and ADAMTS13 activity were normal. The respiratory viral panel was positive for rhinovirus. Bone marrow biopsy showed trilineage maturing hematopoiesis with markedly increased megakaryocytes. Bone marrow flow cytometry and cytogenetic analysis were unremarkable. He was diagnosed of ITP possibly triggered by rhinovirus infection.

After admission, the patient was immediately started on IV dexamethasone 40 mg daily for 4 days. IVIG 1 g/kg/day was administered on hospital days 4 and 5. The patient developed severe headache on hospital day 5. Head CT followed by sella MRI demonstrated a small focus of hemorrhage into a pituitary macroadenoma consistent with pituitary apoplexy. At this time, he was started on intravenous aminocaproic acid. He received daily platelet transfusion with no response in

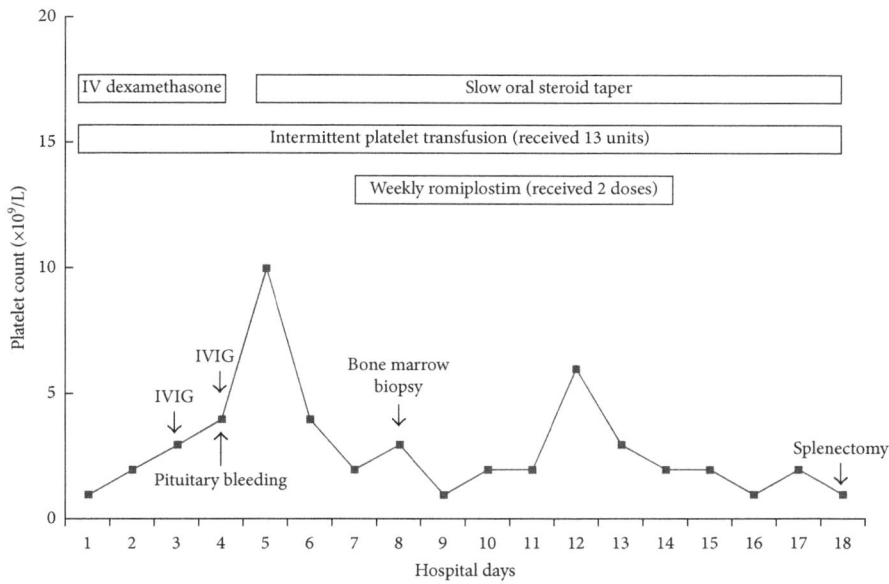

FIGURE 1: Platelet counts before splenectomy.

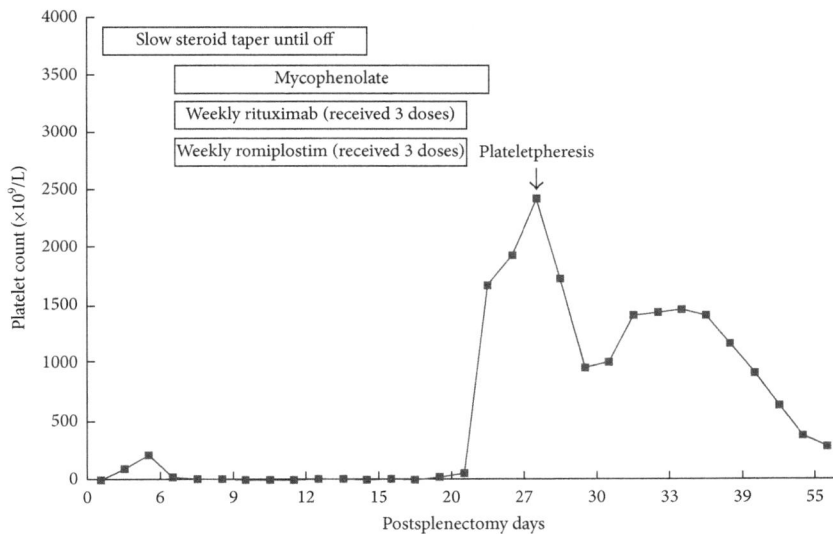

FIGURE 2: Platelet counts after splenectomy.

platelet count (Figure 1). Romiplostim was administered on hospital day 7 (6.5 μg/kg) and day 14 (10 μg/kg). Anti-D could not be used given his Rh-negative blood type. Dexamethasone was transitioned to prednisone 1 mg/kg/day and then gradually tapered down. His platelet count was refractory to all treatments above and remained at a single-digit level. Eventually, he underwent uncomplicated laparoscopic splenectomy on hospital day 18. He was discharged on postoperative day 2 with the maintenance dose of corticosteroids as his platelet count rose to 215×10^9/L.

On postoperative day 7, he was found to have a platelet count of 8×10^9/L during clinic follow-up. He was subsequently started on rituximab 375 mg/m² weekly, romiplostim 10 μg/kg weekly, and mycophenolate 500 mg twice daily. On postoperative day 20, his platelet count increased to 60×10^9/L. On postoperative day 27, he developed a mild headache, and his platelet count was found to be 2424×10^9/L (Figure 2). A head CT was done which showed no acute process but findings compatible with resolving pituitary apoplexy. He was admitted to hospital for urgent plateletpheresis given extreme thrombocytosis ($>1000 \times 10^9$/L) associated with headache and started on aspirin 81 mg q.d. for thromboprophylaxis. The plateletpheresis was performed with whole blood daily for three consecutive days. Platelet count immediately after last plateletpheresis was 1012×10^9/L. Platelet count remained elevated in the $1000–1400 \times 10^9$/L range for the first week after discharge before it started to normalize (Figure 2). All ITP treatments were discontinued. Platelet count was 288×10^9/L at postoperative week 8 and 477×10^9/L at postoperative week 39.

TABLE 1: Time to response of selected treatment options for adults with ITP [3, 10].

Treatment type	Initial response (days)	Peak response (days)
Splenectomy	1–56	7–56
Rituximab	7–56	14–180
Romiplostim	5–14	14–60
Mycophenolate mofetil	28–42	N/A

3. Discussion

There is little evidence to guide a sequence of treatments for patients with refractory ITP after an initial treatment course with corticosteroids (or IVIG or anti-D). Evolving therapies in the past 10 years, especially thrombopoietin receptor agonists (TPO-RAs) and rituximab, have decreased the rate of splenectomy as second-line treatment [2]. IWG recommended to defer splenectomy until the chronic phase of ITP (>6 months after diagnosis) in most cases [3]. However, splenectomy remains the treatment modality with the best response rates and the lower incidence of relapse [2]. In our case, splenectomy was adopted early because the patient developed critical pituitary apoplexy and had failed corticosteroids, IVIG, and romiplostim.

Compared to sequence single-agent therapy, the rationale for combination therapy is to target different pathways involved in platelet destruction with minimal overlapping toxicities. In our case, mycophenolate was added concurrently with romiplostim and rituximab when we failed to see an expected treatment response after splenectomy, and the platelet count again dropped to a critical level. Furthermore, the patient already failed romiplostim in the prior hospital course. The value of combination therapy for refractory ITP was not well defined. Immunosuppression therapies have been successfully added to rituximab [4] and TPO-RAs [5, 6], respectively. Since rituximab has a relatively long time to response (Table 1), TPO-RAs have been suggested as rational agents to combine with rituximab to induce a rapid increase in platelet counts. Based on the different mechanism of action of rituximab (reduces platelet destruction by depleting B cells) and TPO-RAs (stimulate platelet production in the bone marrow), synergistic effects of such a combination can be more than additive [7, 8]. Zhou et al. compared rituximab plus recombinant human thrombopoietin with rituximab alone for corticosteroid-resistant or relapsed ITP [9]. The combination group in this study has a significantly higher complete response rate and shorter time to response; however, there is no difference in long-term response [9].

The extreme thrombocytosis in our case appeared to be associated with combination therapy for ITP in the postsplenectomy setting, as discontinuation of ITP medications led to gradual improvement in platelet count. The most effective component(s) of our regimen that led to extreme thrombocytosis cannot be ascertained. Our patient developed thrombocytosis 3 weeks after initiation of the combination therapy. Based on the time to response (Table 1), both rituximab and romiplostim should have started to show effect, but mycophenolate has not reached its time to

response. Although postsplenectomy reactive thrombocytosis has an incidence rate of 75% [11, 12], it could not explain our patient's drop of platelet counts in the first week postoperatively. Thrombocytosis has been associated with both rituximab [13, 14] and romiplostim [15, 16] as single therapy, but in these cases, thrombocytosis never required plateletpheresis. In the largest trial assessing rituximab plus recombinant human thrombopoietin, the incidence of thrombocytosis was not reported, but the incidence of thrombosis was only 1.3% [9]. It is possible that the postsplenectomy status made our patient more susceptible to thrombocytosis. Severe postsplenectomy thrombocytosis requiring plateletpheresis has been reported in patients receiving romiplostim preoperatively [17, 18], but unlike our case, these patients suffered from thrombocytosis in the immediate postoperative period. When rituximab and romiplostim are used as single therapy, splenectomy does not influence their response rate [13, 19]. Although doses of the three medications in our case were well within the recommended range, it would be interesting to know if lower doses in the setting of combination therapy would decrease the rate of thrombocytosis.

In conclusion, we describe an unusual and challenging case of primary refractory ITP. The case highlights the need to understand predictors of response and relapse in this particular setting. Furthermore, the optimal choice and sequence of therapies remains poorly defined. Although there is some successful experience of adding rituximab to TPO-RAs, there is an inherit risk of thrombocytosis with possible synergistic effects from such a combination. The concurrent use of rituximab, mycophenolate, and TPO-RAs in the postsplenectomy period may further augment thrombocytosis risk in selected patients. Future studies are warranted to understand the predictors of response and to evaluate the safety and efficacy of combining rituximab, TPO-RAs, and immunosuppression therapy, especially in the postsplenectomy setting for patients with refractory ITP.

Conflicts of Interest

The authors declare that they have no conflicts of interest.

References

[1] F. Rodeghiero, R. Stasi, T. Gernsheimer et al., "Standardization of terminology, definitions and outcome criteria in immune thrombocytopenic purpura of adults and children: report from an international working group," *Blood*, vol. 113, no. 11, pp. 2386–2393, 2009.

[2] F. Palandri, N. Polverelli, D. Sollazzo et al., "Have splenectomy rate and main outcomes of ITP changed after the introduction of new treatments? A monocentric study in the outpatient setting during 35 years," *American Journal of Hematology*, vol. 91, no. 4, pp. E267–E272, 2016.

[3] D. Provan, R. Stasi, A. C. Newland et al., "International consensus report on the investigation and management of primary immune thrombocytopenia," *Blood*, vol. 115, no. 2, pp. 168–186, 2010.

[4] P. Y. Choi, F. Roncolato, X. Badoux, S. Ramanathan, S. J. Ho, and B. H. Chong, "A novel triple therapy for ITP using high-dose

dexamethasone, low-dose rituximab, and cyclosporine (TT4)," *Blood*, vol. 126, no. 4, pp. 500–503, 2015.

[5] A. Rashidi and M. A. Blinder, "Combination therapy in relapsed or refractory chronic immune thrombocytopenia: a case report and literature review," *Journal of Clinical Pharmacy and Therapeutics*, vol. 41, no. 5, pp. 453–458, 2016.

[6] F. Anwer, S. Yun, A. Nair, Y. Ahmad, R. Krishnadashan, and H. J. Deeg, "Severe refractory immune thrombocytopenia successfully treated with high-dose pulse cyclophosphamide and eltrombopag," *Case Reports in Hematology*, vol. 2015, Article ID 583451, 3 pages, 2015.

[7] Y. Li, Y. Y. Wang, H. R. Fei, L. Wang, and C. L. Yuan, "Efficacy of low-dose rituximab in combination with recombinant human thrombopoietin in treating ITP," *European Review for Medical and Pharmacological Sciences*, vol. 19, no. 9, pp. 1583–1588, 2015.

[8] D. Veneri, L. Soligo, G. Pizzolo, and A. Ambrosetti, "The association of rituximab and a thrombopoietin receptor agonist in high-risk refractory immune thrombocytopenic purpura," *Blood Transfusion*, vol. 13, no. 4, pp. 694-695, 2015.

[9] H. Zhou, M. Xu, P. Qin et al., "A multicenter randomized open-label study of rituximab plus rhTPO vs rituximab in corticosteroid-resistant or relapsed ITP," *Blood*, vol. 125, no. 10, pp. 1541–1547, 2015.

[10] C. Neunert, W. Lim, M. Crowther, A. Cohen, L. Solberg Jr., and M. A. Crowther, "The American Society of Hematology 2011 evidence-based practice guideline for immune thrombocytopenia," *Blood*, vol. 117, no. 16, pp. 4190–4207, 2011.

[11] P. N. Khan, R. J. Nair, J. Olivares, L. E. Tingle, and Z. Li, "Postsplenectomy reactive thrombocytosis," *Baylor University Medical Center Proceedings*, vol. 22, no. 1, pp. 9–12, 2009.

[12] M. A. Boxer, J. Braun, and L. Ellman, "Thromboembolic risk of postsplenectomy thrombocytosis," *Archives of Surgery*, vol. 113, no. 7, pp. 808-809, 1978.

[13] K. Alasfoor, M. Alrasheed, F. Alsayegh, and S. A. Mousa, "Rituximab in the treatment of idiopathic thrombocytopenic purpura (ITP)," *Annals of Hematology*, vol. 88, no. 3, pp. 239–243, 2009.

[14] A. A. Giagounidis, J. Anhuf, P. Schneider et al., "Treatment of relapsed idiopathic thrombocytopenic purpura with the anti-CD20 monoclonal antibody rituximab: a pilot study," *European Journal of Haematology*, vol. 69, no. 2, pp. 95–100, 2002.

[15] M. Khellaf, M. Michel, P. Quittet et al., "Romiplostim safety and efficacy for immune thrombocytopenia in clinical practice: 2-year results of 72 adults in a romiplostim compassionate-use program," *Blood*, vol. 118, no. 16, pp. 4338–4345, 2011.

[16] D. B. Cines, T. Gernsheimer, J. Wasser et al., "Integrated analysis of long-term safety in patients with chronic immune thrombocytopaenia (ITP) treated with the thrombopoietin (TPO) receptor agonist romiplostim," *International Journal of Hematology*, vol. 102, no. 3, pp. 259–270, 2015.

[17] J. Zimmerman, K. J. Norsworthy, and R. Brodsky, "Balancing therapy with thrombopoietin receptor agonists and splenectomy in refractory immune thrombocytopenic purpura: a case of postsplenectomy thrombocytosis requiring plateletpheresis," *Case Reports in Hematology*, vol. 2016, Article ID 5403612, 4 pages, 2016.

[18] J. S. Raval, R. L. Redner, and J. E. Kiss, "Plateletpheresis for postsplenectomy rebound thrombocytosis in a patient with chronic immune thrombocytopenic purpura on romiplostim," *Journal of Clinical Apheresis*, vol. 28, no. 4, pp. 321–324, 2013.

[19] D. J. Kuter, J. B. Bussel, R. M. Lyons et al., "Efficacy of romiplostim in patients with chronic immune thrombocytopenic purpura: a double-blind randomised controlled trial," *The Lancet*, vol. 371, no. 9610, pp. 395–403, 2008.

36

Bone Marrow-Liver-Spleen Type of Large B-Cell Lymphoma Associated with Hemophagocytic Syndrome: A Rare Aggressive Extranodal Lymphoma

Kirill A. Lyapichev,[1] Jennifer R. Chapman,[1] Oleksii Iakymenko,[1] Offiong F. Ikpatt,[1] Uygar Teomete,[2] Sandra Patricia Sanchez,[1] and Francisco Vega[1,3]

[1]Division of Hematopathology, Department of Pathology and Laboratory Medicine, University of Miami and Sylvester Comprehensive Cancer Center, Miami, FL, USA
[2]Department of Radiology, University of Miami and Sylvester Comprehensive Cancer Center, Miami, FL, USA
[3]Division of Hematology-Oncology, Department of Medicine, University of Miami and Sylvester Comprehensive Cancer Center, Miami, FL, USA

Correspondence should be addressed to Francisco Vega; fvega@med.miami.edu

Academic Editor: Kiyotaka Kawauchi

Recently, an unusual subtype of large B-cell lymphoma (LBCL) with distinctive clinicopathologic features has been recognized; it is characterized by involvement of bone marrow with or without liver and/or spleen, but no lymph node or other extranodal sites, usually associated with fever, anemia, and hemophagocytic lymphohistiocytosis (HLH). Because of this distinctive clinical presentation, it has been designated "bone marrow-liver-spleen" (BLS) type of LBCL. To date there is only one series of 11 cases of BLS type of LBCL with detailed clinical, pathologic, and cytogenetic data. Herein, we describe a case of BLS type LBCL presenting with associated HLH in a 73-year-old female. The bone marrow core biopsy showed cytologically atypical large lymphoma cells present in a scattered interstitial distribution and hemophagocytosis and infrequent large lymphoma cells were seen in the bone marrow aspirate smears. Circulating lymphoma cells were not seen in the peripheral blood smears. The patient underwent treatment with chemotherapy (R-CHOP) but unfortunately passed away 2 months after initial presentation. BLS type of LBCL is a very rare and clinically aggressive lymphoma whose identification may be delayed by clinicians and hematopathologists due to its unusual clinical presentation and pathologic features.

1. Introduction

Diffuse large B-cell lymphoma (DLBCL) is the most common non-Hodgkin lymphoma (NHL) accounting for almost 40% of cases [1]. DLBCL is an aggressive tumor that usually presents with rapidly enlarging lymph nodes or extranodal masses. Secondary bone marrow (BM) involvement occurs in approximately 10%–16% of patients with DLBCL, NOS; however BM is an unusual site to establish the initial diagnosis of DLBCL [2, 3]. In addition to stage IV DLBCL, NOS, subtypes of DLBCL with relatively frequent BM involvement include intravascular large B-cell lymphoma (IVLBCL),

splenic marginal zone lymphoma (splenic MZL), and T-cell/histiocyte-rich large B-cell lymphoma (THRLBCL) [1]. Recently a new subtype of DLBCL with frequent BM involvement and distinctive clinical and pathologic features has been recognized [4]. This lymphoma presents with BM involvement with or without involvement of the liver and/or spleen, often accompanied with severe anemia (100%), thrombocytopenia, hemophagocytic lymphohistiocytosis (HLH) (64%), and elevated lactate dehydrogenase (LDH) level in the absence of lymphadenopathy or other extranodal masses and with no prior history of lymphoma [4]. HLH is an uncommon a life-threatening disease of severe hyperinflammation caused by uncontrolled proliferation of activated lymphocytes and macrophages, characterized by proliferation of morphologically benign lymphocytes and macrophages that secrete high amounts of inflammatory cytokines. The current (2008) diagnostic criteria for HLH are a molecular diagnosis consistent with HLH (pathologic mutations of PRF1, UNC13D, or STX11) or fulfillment of five out of the eight criteria: (1) fever (>100.4°F, >38°C), (2) splenomegaly, (3) cytopenias (affecting at least two of three lineages in the peripheral blood: hemoglobin < 9 g/dL, platelets < 100 × 10^9/L, or Neutrophils < 1 × 10^9/L), (4) hypertriglyceridemia and/or hypofibrinogenemia (≤150 mg/100 ml), (5) ferritin ≥ 500 ng/ml, (6) hemophagocytosis in the bone marrow, spleen, or lymph nodes, (7) low or absent natural killer cell activity, and (8) soluble CD25 (soluble IL-2 receptor) >2400 U/ml (or per local reference laboratory) [5].

Because of its distinctive clinical presentation, this aggressive B-cell neoplasm has been named "bone marrow-liver-spleen" (BLS) type of LBCL (LBCL-BLS). Here, we present a case of LBCL-BLS associated with haemophagocytic syndrome in a 73-year-old female and compare it with previously published cases. Due to the limited availability of published accounts of this rare entity, we believe it is important to document our case in order to add to our understanding of this rare but clinically aggressive lymphoma.

2. Case Report

2.1. Clinical Presentation. A 73-year-old Hispanic female was admitted to our institution with weakness, fever, thrombocytopenia (70 × 10^9/L), neutropenia, elevated level of LDH (1010 U/L) and ferritin (>2000 ng/ml), and anemia (Hb 6.3 g/dL) of unclear etiology that required blood transfusions. She had no significant past medical history except for diabetes mellitus (DM).

Computed tomography (CT) scan at the time of admission revealed no evidence of mediastinal, hilar, or other systemic lymphadenopathy but showed marked enlargement of liver and spleen (Figure 1). The spleen showed numerous heterogeneous areas of hypoenhancement, ranging between 2 and 5 cms, consistent with a neoplasm and suspicious for lymphoma. The adrenal glands were grossly within normal limits. Lung windows demonstrated patency of the trachea and main bronchi. No definite discrete pulmonary nodules or masses were identified. Osseous windows showed no definite lytic, sclerotic, or destructive lesions.

2.2. Pathologic Findings. A BM biopsy was performed to investigate the etiology of the symptomatic anemia and thrombocytopenia. The BM core biopsy demonstrated a marrow cellularity of 60% with scattered large atypical lymphoid cells (Figure 2(a)). These cells were either scattered individually or formed loose clusters and represented approximately 10% of the total marrow cellularity (Figure 2(b)). Large clusters or sheets of lymphoma cells were not seen. Immunohistochemical studies showed that the tumor cells expressed pan-B-cell markers CD20 and CD79a and were negative for CD3, CD4, CD8, CD56, CD57, PD1, CD30, TdT, glycophorin, MPO, and CD117 (Figures 2(b) and 2(c)).

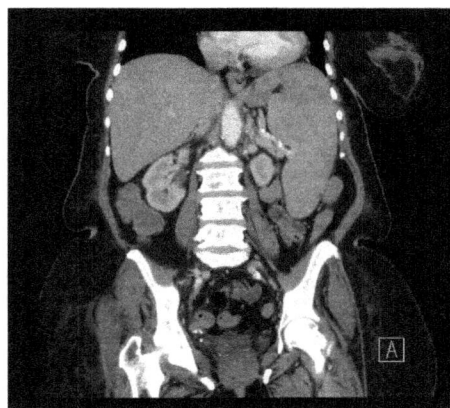

FIGURE 1: Abdominal and pelvic CT scan. Marked hepatomegaly and splenomegaly are identified. Spleen demonstrates numerous areas of heterogeneous hypoenhancement.

CD20 and CD79a highlighted the interstitial distribution of the tumor cells. Tumor cells inside the marrow sinusoids were not seen (Figure 2(b)). Similarly, a CD34 immunostain and dual PAX5 with CD34 immunostains failed to show tumor cells inside the vessels. The lack of intrasinusoidal and intravascular tumor excluded the diagnosis of IVLBCL (Figures 2(d) and 3(a) and Table 2). As per the Hans algorithm based on the expression of CD10, BCL6, and MUM1, our case was classified into the nongerminal center B-cell-like (non-GCB) subgroup. IHC showed CD10 reactivity in less than 30% of tumor cells and MUM1 reactivity in more than 30% of tumor cells (Figures 3(b) and 3(c)). Additionally, BM biopsy was stained for MYC and for BCL2 and showed a subset of positive tumor cells (Figures 4(a) and 4(b)). The lymphoma cells were negative for Epstein–Barr virus-encoded RNAs (EBER). Small reactive T-cells were distributed throughout the marrow and consisted of a mixed population of CD4 and CD8 positive T-cells. Importantly, nodules rich in T-cells associated with the lymphoma cells were not seen and therefore the diagnosis of THRLBCL was also excluded (Table 2).

Individual large, atypical lymphoid cells were also recognized on the aspirate smears (Figure 2(e)). In addition, there were numerous histiocytes demonstrating hemophagocytosis throughout the aspirate smears (Figure 2(f)). Mild trilineage dyspoiesis was seen. Some of the dyspoietic granulocytes had toxic changes. A peripheral blood smear showed no circulating lymphoma cells.

Flow cytometry immunophenotypic analysis was performed on BM specimen and was negative for the presence of monoclonal B cells or increased blasts. Conventional karyotyping was negative for any clonal abnormalities and showed a diploid female karyotype, 46;XX [6]. Immunoglobulin heavy chain (IgH) and kappa light chain PCR assays performed in BM aspirate material confirmed the presence of a monoclonal B-cell population. This discrepancy between flow cytometry results and molecular analysis could be explained by poor representation of the tumor cells during flow cytometry analysis and high sensitivity of PCR assay.

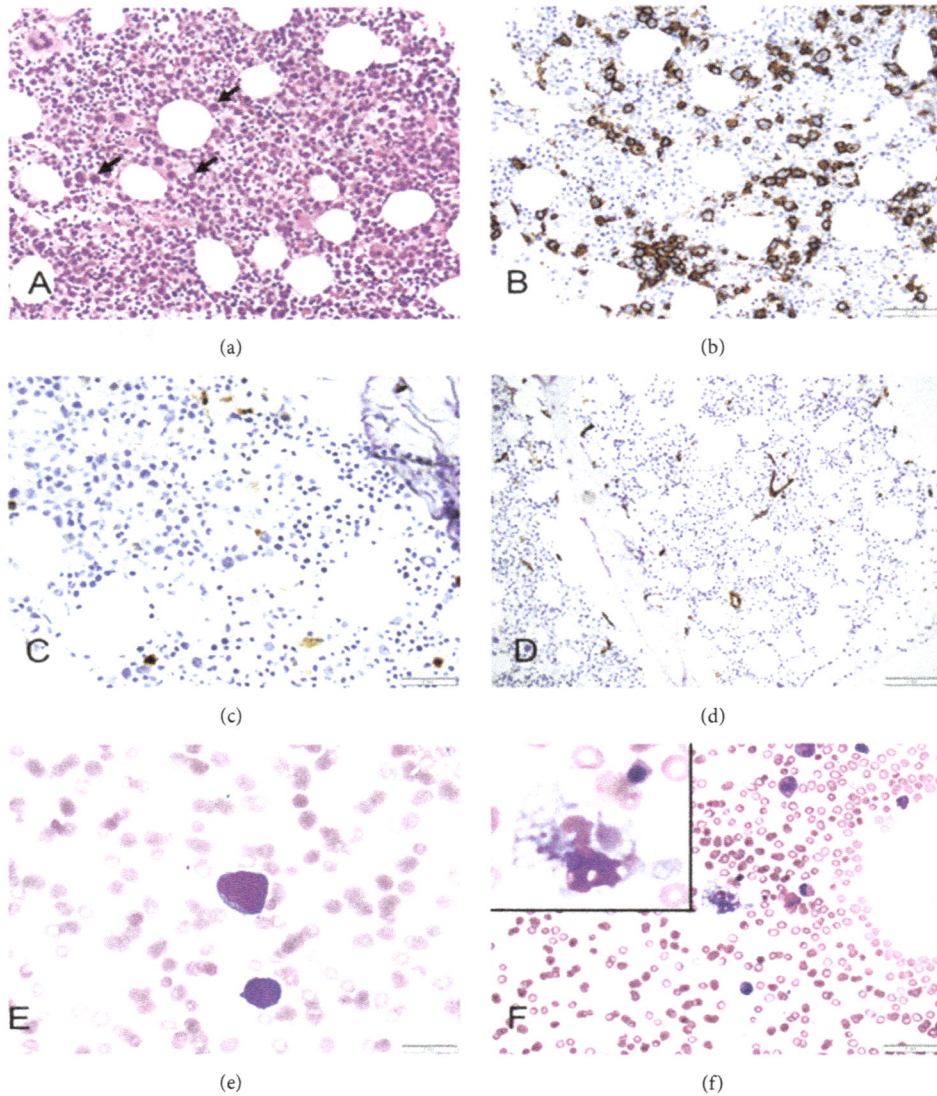

FIGURE 2: Histopathologic features. BM biopsy shows patchy interstitial infiltration of large lymphoma cells (arrows) without sinusoidal involvement (H&E; 400x) (a). By immunohistochemistry (IHC), the tumor cells are positive for CD20 (400x) (b) and negative for CD30 (400x) (c). CD34 highlights the capillary endothelial cells and confirms the lack of intravascular involvement by tumor cells (400x) (d). Lymphoma cells are large in size with large nuclei, high nuclear to cytoplasmic ratios, and open chromatin with one to several prominent nucleoli (Wright Geimsa; 100x) (e). BM aspirate smear shows histiocytic hemophagocytosis characterized by RBCs engulfing by histiocytes (Wright Geimsa; 100x) (f).

T-cell receptor (TCR) gamma PCR assay was negative for T-cell clonality.

Combining the pathologic findings with the clinical presentation, the patient was diagnosed with LBCL-BLS type. The neoplasm was associated with severe anemia, hepatosplenomegaly, and HLH syndrome. A biopsy of the spleen and the liver was not performed but based on the radiological studies both organs were considered involved by lymphoma.

2.3. Treatment and Clinical Course. After diagnosis, treatment with R-CHOP was immediately started. Approximately two months (51 days) after initiation of therapy the patient

developed septic shock due to chemotherapy induced neutropenia and passed away.

3. Discussion

LBCL-BLS type is distinctive aggressive LBCL with characteristic clinicopathological features and aggressive clinical behavior that has been relatively recently recognized [4]. Patients usually present with fever, anemia of unclear etiology, thrombocytopenia, and increased LDH. On imaging studies splenomegaly or hepatosplenomegaly is typical and many small (usually less than 3 cm) hypodense nodules can be identified. Bone marrow biopsy usually

(a)

(b)

(c)

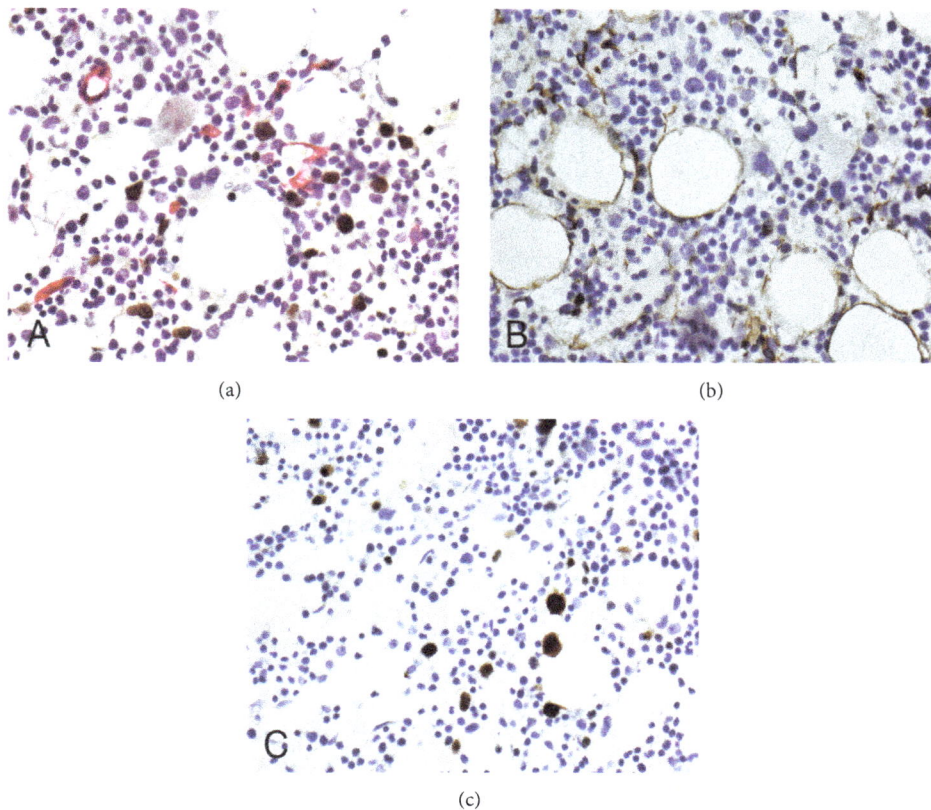

FIGURE 3: Histopathologic features. BM biopsy shows patchy interstitial infiltration of large, PAX5 positive lymphoma cells without sinusoidal (CD34 positive) involvement (400x) (a). By IHC, less than 30% of tumor cells are positive for CD10 (400x) (b) and more than 30% positive for MUM1 (400x) (c).

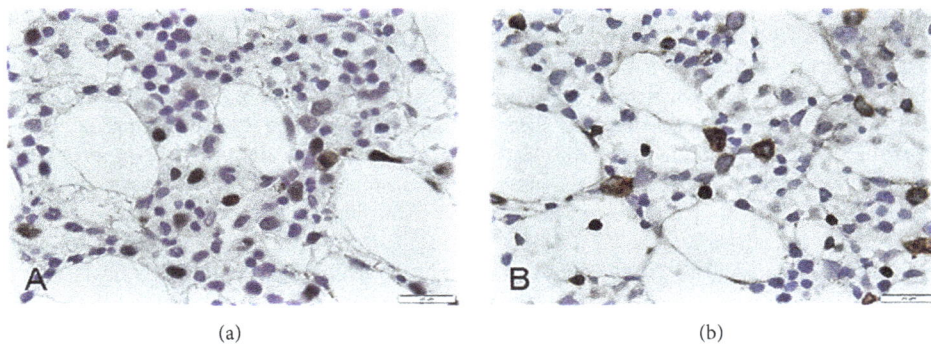

(a)

(b)

FIGURE 4: Histopathologic features. BM biopsy shows a subset of the tumor cells positive for MYC (100x) (a) and for BCL2 (100x) (b).

reveals hemophagocytosis and an interstitial distribution of large lymphoma cells with a mature B-cell phenotype. Importantly, the lymphoma cells are not involving vascular lumina or sinusoids, differentiating this presentation from that of intravascular large B-cell lymphoma. To date, there are no specific genetic abnormalities and viral associations identified.

Nonnodal, primary LBCL involving BM with or without involvement of liver and/or spleen and no other extranodal involvement has been variably published in the literature [7–16]. However, given that this type of LBCL is not currently defined in the WHO classification, previous studies which included different types of lymphomas have been inconsistent in their reports of pathologic features and clinical outcomes. These previous reports seem to describe clinically similar lymphomas presenting with marrow involvement with separation into different categories based on additional site of involvement (BM only, spleen and BM or spleen, liver and BM).

To find previously reported cases of LBCL-BLS similar to ours, during the literature search we selected only studies of LBCL with initial manifestation in the BM, liver, and/or spleen (BLS type) that lacked any lymph node or other extranodal involvement and included genetic and survival information. Additionally, to make our search more specific we excluded diagnoses of IVLBCL, splenic marginal cell lymphoma with transformation, primary bone LBCL, and THRLBCL and used "Large B-cell lymphoma, bone marrow, liver, and spleen" as the keywords during literature search by PubMed. Using these criteria, we found only two publications that seemed similar to the case of LBCL-BLS that we describe [4, 14].

One of these, a study by Iioka et al. [14], describes 10 cases of DLBCL confined to BM, spleen, and liver, as evidenced by the uniformly increased uptake of fluorodeoxyglucose (FDG) on positron emission tomography combined with computed tomography (PET/CT). They retrospectively reviewed the clinical records of patients with aggressive B-cell lymphoma who were diagnosed and treated in their institution between 2011 and 2015. The inclusion criteria were as follows: patients whose clinical stage was determined on the basis of a FDG-PET/CT imaging study; patients whose disease showed the uniformly increased uptake of the tracer in the BM with or without diffuse uptake in the spleen and/or liver, but lacked uptake in the lymph nodes; and patients in whom a BM examination was performed for the diagnosis. Burkitt lymphoma, mantle cell lymphoma, the transformation of low-grade B-cell lymphomas, and any leukemia/lymphoma entity known to arise primarily in the BM were excluded. This study might represent 10 cases of LBCL-BLS but the authors do not specifically discriminate it from IVLBCL [14].

The BM biopsies were available in 9 out of 10 cases. Histology revealed lymphoma cells that were large with a moderate amount of cytoplasm, large vesicular nuclei, and one or more prominent nucleoli. Immunohistochemistry showed that lymphoma cells were positive for CD20 and CD79a. CD5 was positive in two cases showing the intrasinusoidal infiltration pattern; CD5 positivity was confirmed by flow cytometry. BCL2 was positive in eight cases. Per the Hans algorithm based upon the expression of CD10, BCL6, and MUM1, all cases were classified into the nongerminal center B-cell-like (non-GCB) subgroup. But they did not discriminate their cases from IVLBCL (did not perform CD34 IHC, to see intrasinusoidal involvement). Additionally, authors agreed that they will need to perform comparative studies incorporating histopathology and findings on FDG-PET/CT due to distinguish LBCL-BLS from IVLBCL. A different study by Yeh et al. reported detailed clinical, pathologic, and cytogenetic data in a series of LBCL-BLS whose clinical and histopathologic features were similar to those of our case [4]. In looking at the histopathologic features and clinical outcomes of the patients in the Yeh et al. series and our own, LBCL-BLS type seems to be a distinct clinicopathologic type of LBCL which has an aggressive clinical course and poor survival (Table 1). These lymphomas are characterized by variable age at presentation: 26–80 years, predominantly male population (M : F, 8 : 4), fever (100%), anemia (100%), thrombocytopenia (83%), increased LDH level (92%), bone marrow involvement (100%) with HLH syndrome (67%), nongerminal center phenotype (83%, as established by Hans algorithm), splenomegaly (100%), and hepatomegaly (25%)

in the absence of lymphadenopathy and with no prior history of lymphoma. Additionally, it seems that the patient's survival rate depends at least in part on rapid lymphoma diagnosis and adequate and prompt treatment. Five patients (42%) in the previously reported series died in the first two and a half weeks after diagnosis (from 3 to 17 days); the patient we present died of lymphoma-related sepsis after only 51 days despite rapid lymphoma diagnosis and treatment initiation.

In Table 2 we compare LBCL-BLS as defined in this manuscript (LBCL involving BM, liver, and/or spleen but lacking intravascular or sinusoidal involvement and lacking nodal or other extranodal disease) with intravascular large B-cell lymphomas (Western and Asian types) and THRLBCL [1]. The lymphoma most similar to LBCL-BLS that is currently WHO-defined is IVLBCL, at least from the clinical perspective. Splenic MZL and THRLBCL might have similar clinical presentation too but usually they are very different pathohistologically and missing HLH. The lymphoma cells in splenic MZL are smaller and usually infiltrate BM with mixed pattern: combining nodular, paratrabecular, or diffuse with a distinctive intrasinusoidal component. Chromosomal translocation involving CDK6 gene at 7q21 as well as allelic loss of 7q31-32 is seen in a significant subset of the splenic MZL cases; NOTCH 2 and KLF2 mutations also might be present [17]. THRLBCL commonly involves liver, spleen, and bone marrow in addition to lymph node. In bone marrow, THRLBLC is characterized by multinodular aggregates rich in T-cells often associated with histiocytes and scattered large atypical lymphoid cells.

IVLBCL is a rare type of extranodal LBCL characterized by the selective growth of lymphoma cells within the lumina of capillaries and small/medium sized vessels. There are two IVLBCL subtypes: Western type characterized by symptoms related to the main organ involvement, predominantly central nervous system (CNS) or skin, and an Asian type in which the patients present with multiorgan failure, hepatosplenomegaly, pancytopenia, fever, B symptoms, and HLH. The second type (Asian type) of IVLBCL is closer in clinical presentation (pancytopenia, HLH, and skin and central nervous system involvements are uncommon) to LBCL-BLS with the pathologic difference being that lymphoma cells have a striking intravascular and intrasinusoidal distribution in Asian type IVLBCL. B symptoms are very common (55–76%) and lymphoma cells are more often of activated B-cell type in both types of IVLBCL as well as in LBCL-BLS [1]. Polymerase chain reaction (PCR) studies in both entities show negative results for Epstein–Barr virus (EBV) and human herpesviruses 6 and 8 (HHV6 and HHV8) infections in vast majority of cases. It is unclear at this time whether IVLBCL, particularly Asian type, and LBCL-BLS type, as reported herein, are variants of the same high-grade form of LBCL. A high incidence of HLH is also an important and characteristic feature of both IVLBCL and LBCL-BLS type. Although the precise mechanism underlying this lymphoma-associated HLH syndrome remains unclear, overproduction of TNF-α, INF-γ, IL-1a, IL-6, IL-10, and other cytokines by nonfunctional cytotoxic T/NK-cells as well as macrophage hyperactivation is thought to play a crucial role [18–20].

TABLE 1: Clinical features of patients with large B cell lymphoma initially manifesting in the bone marrow. Patients N1–N9 are from National Cheng Kung University Hospital; patients M1 and M2 are from University of Texas M.D. Anderson Cancer Center; and patient UM1 is from University of Miami. H/S: hepatomegaly/splenomegaly; HS: haemophagocytic syndrome; IPI: international prognostic index; C/T: chemotherapy; CHOP: cyclophosphamide, doxorubicin, vincristine, and prednisolone (E, epirubicin); R-ESHAP: rituximab, etoposide, methylprednisolone, cytarabine, and cisplatin; CVAD: Cyclophosphamide, vincristine, doxorubicin hydrochloride (Adriamycin), and dexamethasone; PBSCT: peripheral blood stem cell transplantation; F: female; M: male [4].

Case	Age/sex	Fever	H/S	Cytopenia	LDH	HS	Radiological splenic mass (>3 cm)	Treatment	IPI	Outcome (days)
N1	26/F	+	−/+	Leukopenia and anemia	293	−	—	C/T (CHOP*3, R-ESHAP), PBSCT	2	Alive (1560)
N2	73/F	+	−/+	Anaemia and thrombocytopenia	293	+	Many small hypodense nodules	C/T (CHOP*1, R-CHOP*5)	3	Dead (784)
N3	44/M	+	−/+	Anaemia and thrombocytopenia	745	−	Many small hypodense nodules	C/T (CEOP*1, R-CEOP*5, R-ESHAP*4), PBSCT	2	Dead (551)
N4	54/M	+	−/+	Pancytopenia	727	+	—	C/T (CHOP*6)	2	Dead (285)
N5	80/M	+	−/+	Anaemia and thrombocytopenia	319	−	Wedge-shaped hypodense infarct	—	4	Dead (17)
N6	72/F	+	−/+	Anaemia and thrombocytopenia	1255	+	—	—	4	Dead (8)
N7	76/M	+	−/+	Anaemia and thrombocytopenia	426	+	—	—	4	Dead (6)
N8	61/M	+	−/+	Anaemia and thrombocytopenia	160	+	—	—	3	Dead (4)
N9	75/M	+	−/+	Anaemia and thrombocytopenia	4464	+	Many small hypodense nodules	—	4	Dead (4)
M1	69/M	+	−/+	Anemia	482	−	—	C/T (R-CVAD*6)	4	Dead (84)
M2	60/M	+	+/+	Anaemia and thrombocytopenia	2266	+	Many small hypodense nodules	C/T (R-CVAD*6)	4	Dead (224)
UM1	73/F	+	+/+	Thrombocytopenia, neutropenia and anemia	1010	+	Numerous heterogeneous areas (2 to 5 cm)	C/T (R-CHOP with steroids)	4	Dead (51)

TABLE 2: Differential diagnosis of LBCL-BLS and subtypes of IVLBCL and TCHRLBCL.

	LBCL-BLS	IVLBCL (Western type)	IVLBCL (Asian type)	TCHRLBCL
CD20	+	+	+	+
CD79a	+	+	+	+
CD3	−	−	−	Background T cells
CD5	−	38%+	38% +	Background T cells
EBV	−	−	−	+
HLH	+	+/−	+	−
Peripheral lymph node involvement	−	−	−	+
Involvement of vascular lumina by lymphoma cells	−	+	+	−
Specific Alterations	None	None	19q13 and 8p21	−
Organ of involvement	BM, liver and/or spleen	CNS or skin	BM	Liver, spleen, BM
T cell rich lymphoid nodules	−	−	−	+
HCV infection association	−	−	−	−
Bone marrow, rich in T cell nodules	−	−	−	+

In addition to the difference in lymphoma cell distribution (intravascular versus BM interstitial), the Asian type of IVLBCL and LBCL-BLS type have also not yet shown overlapping molecular genetic features, supporting that these two lymphoma types are different. Specifically, Asian type IVLBCL has been associated with abnormalities of 19q13 and 8p21, which have not been found in LBCL-BLS type thus far [4, 6, 21]. LBCL-BLS type, alternatively, has shown multiple chromosomal defects including t(8;14)(q24;q32), dup(14)(q24;q32), inv(14)(q32), t(3;6), trisomy 18, add(19)(p13), del(8)(p22), del(3)(q21), and add(7)(p22) [4, 22, 23]. However, given the limited number of available cases in the literature at this time, additional studies are needed with specific comparisons of these two lymphoma types to determine their relatedness, or lack thereof. Finally, lack of CD29 (β-1 integrin) and CD54 (ICAM-1) in IVLBCL may be potentially useful diagnostic feature. Defects (downregulation) in these protein receptors on the lymphoma cells might prevent the neoplasm from invasion through vascular wall and contribute to the intravascular location.

4. Conclusion

We describe an unusual and clinically aggressive extranodal large B-cell lymphoma involving the BM, spleen, and liver (LBCL-BSL). This lymphoma appears to be a distinct but rare and controversial entity that may be a specific type of extranodal DLBCL, NOS [1]. However, aside from lymphoma cell distribution within vascular spaces and marrow sinusoids, this lymphoma has clinical features similar to those of Asian type IVLBCL. Importantly, the clinical presentation and disease course are particularly severe with rapid disease progression and high mortality rate during first weeks to months after initial symptoms. Overlapping clinical and morphological features can make it challenging to differentiate LBCL-BLS from more common lymphomas including splenic marginal zone lymphoma with large cell or

prolymphocytic transformation, THRLBCL and, particularly, IVLBCL (Asian type). Gene expression profiling studies comparing these entities may help in developing an understanding of the biology of these lymphomas and their relatedness as well as in predicting effective treatment protocols.

Conflicts of Interest

The authors declare that there are no conflicts of interest regarding the publication of this paper.

References

[1] N. L. J. Harris, S. A. Pileri, H. Stein, J. Thiele, and J. W. Vardiman, "WHO classification of tumours of haematopoietic and lymphoid tissues," Vol. 2. 2008.

[2] L. H. Sehn, D. W. Scott, M. Chhanabhai et al., "Impact of concordant and discordant bone marrow involvement on outcome in diffuse large B-cell lymphoma treated with R-CHOP," *Journal of Clinical Oncology*, vol. 29, no. 11, pp. 1452–1457, 2011.

[3] R. Chung, R. Lai, P. Wei et al., "Concordant but not discordant bone marrow involvement in diffuse large B-cell lymphoma predicts a poor clinical outcome independent of the International Prognostic Index," *Blood*, vol. 110, no. 4, pp. 1278–1282, 2007.

[4] Y.-M. Yeh, K.-C. Chang, Y.-P. Chen et al., "Large B cell lymphoma presenting initially in bone marrow, liver and spleen: An aggressive entity associated frequently with haemophagocytic syndrome," *Histopathology*, vol. 57, no. 6, pp. 785–795, 2010.

[5] J.-I. Henter, A. Horne, M. Aricó et al., "HLH-2004: diagnostic and therapeutic guidelines for hemophagocytic lymphohistiocytosis," *Pediatric Blood & Cancer*, vol. 48, no. 2, pp. 124–131, 2007.

[6] T. Murase, S. Nakamura, K. Kawauchi et al., "An Asian variant of intravascular large B-cell lymphoma: clinical, pathological and cytogenetic approaches to diffuse large B-cell lymphoma associated with haemophagocytic syndrome," *British Journal of Haematology*, vol. 111, no. 3, pp. 826–834, 2000.

[7] C. G. Roth and K. K. Reichard, "Subtle bone marrow involvement by large B-cell lymphoma with pronormoblast-like morphology and prominent but not exclusive sinusoidal distribution," *American Journal of Blood Research*, vol. 2, no. 2, pp. 113–118, 2012.

[8] D. Kajiura, Y. Yamashita, and N. Mori, "Diffuse large B-cell lymphoma initially manifesting in the bone marrow," *American Journal of Clinical Pathology*, vol. 127, no. 5, pp. 762–769, 2007.

[9] C. L. Alvares, E. Matutes, M. A. Scully et al., "Isolated bone marrow involvement in diffuse large B cell lymphoma: A report of three cases with review of morphological, immunophenotypic and cytogenetic findings," *Leukemia and Lymphoma*, vol. 45, no. 4, pp. 769–775, 2004.

[10] P. Bhagat, M. U. S. Sachdeva, P. Sharma et al., "Primary bone marrow lymphoma is a rare neoplasm with poor outcome: Case series from single tertiary care centre and review of literature," *Hematological Oncology*, vol. 34, no. 1, pp. 42–48, 2016.

[11] Y. Yamashita, D. Kajiura, L. Tang et al., "XCR1 expression and biased VH gene usage are distinct features of diffuse large B-cell lymphoma initially manifesting in the bone marrow," *American Journal of Clinical Pathology*, vol. 135, no. 4, pp. 556–564, 2011.

[12] W. G. Morice, F. J. Rodriguez, J. D. Hoyer, and P. J. Kurtin, "Diffuse large B-cell lymphoma with distinctive patterns of splenic and bone marrow involvement: Clinicopathologic features of two cases," *Modern Pathology*, vol. 18, no. 4, pp. 495–502, 2005.

[13] A. Martinez, M. Ponzoni, C. Agostinelli et al., "Primary bone marrow lymphoma: An uncommon extranodal presentation of aggressive non-hodgkin lymphomas," *American Journal of Surgical Pathology*, vol. 36, no. 2, pp. 296–304, 2012.

[14] F. Iioka, G. Honjo, T. Misaki et al., "A unique subtype of diffuse large B-cell lymphoma primarily involving the bone marrow, spleen, and liver, defined by fluorodeoxyglucose-positron emission tomography combined with computed tomography," *Leukemia and Lymphoma*, vol. 57, no. 11, pp. 2593–2602, 2016.

[15] H. Chang, Y.-S. Hung, T.-L. Lin et al., "Primary bone marrow diffuse large B cell lymphoma: A case series and review," *Annals of Hematology*, vol. 90, no. 7, pp. 791–796, 2011.

[16] J. A. Strauchen, "Primary bone marrow B-cell Lymphoma: report of four cases," *Mount Sinai Journal of Medicine*, vol. 70, no. 2, pp. 133–138, 2003.

[17] N. Martínez, C. Almaraz, J. P. Vaqué et al., "Whole-exome sequencing in splenic marginal zone lymphoma reveals mutations in genes involved in marginal zone differentiation," *Leukemia*, vol. 28, no. 6, pp. 1334–1340, 2014.

[18] J.-D. Lay, C.-J. Tsao, J.-Y. Chen, M. E. Kadin, and I.-J. Su, "Upregulation of tumor necrosis factor-α gene by Epstein-Barr virus and activation of macrophages in Epstein-Barr virus-infected T cells in the pathogenesis of hemophagocytic syndrome," *Journal of Clinical Investigation*, vol. 100, no. 8, pp. 1969–1979, 1997.

[19] B. J. Chen, B. Chapuy, J. Ouyang et al., "PD-L1 expression is characteristic of a subset of aggressive B-cell lymphomas and virus-associated malignancies," *Clinical Cancer Research*, vol. 19, no. 13, pp. 3462–3473, 2013.

[20] K. Devitt, J. Cerny, B. Switzer et al., "Hemophagocytic lymphohistiocytosis secondary to T-cell/histiocyte-rich large B-cell lymphoma," *Leukemia Research Reports*, vol. 3, no. 2, pp. 42–45, 2015.

[21] C. Shimazaki, T. Inaba, K. Shimura et al., "B-cell lymphoma associated with haemophagocytic syndrome: A clinical, immunological and cytogenetic study," *British Journal of Haematology*, vol. 104, no. 4, pp. 672–679, 1999.

[22] H. Geyer, N. Karlin, B. Palen, and R. Mesa, "Asian-variant intravascular lymphoma in the African race," *Rare Tumors*, vol. 4, no. 1, pp. 26–29, 2012.

[23] H. Khoury, V. S. Lestou, R. D. Gascoyne et al., "Multicolor karyotyping and clinicopathological analysis of three intravascular lymphoma cases," *Modern Pathology*, vol. 16, no. 7, pp. 716–724, 2003.

37

Extensive Intracardiac and Deep Venous Thromboses in a Young Woman with Heparin-Induced Thrombocytopenia and May-Thurner Syndrome

Yekaterina Kim,[1] Daniel C. Choi,[1] and Ali N. Zaidi[2]

[1]*Montefiore Medical Center, Albert Einstein College of Medicine, Bronx, NY, USA*
[2]*Montefiore Heart & Vascular Care Center, Albert Einstein College of Medicine, Bronx, NY, USA*

Correspondence should be addressed to Yekaterina Kim; yekim@montefiore.org

Academic Editor: Simon Davidson

A 38-year-old woman with a history of recurrent deep venous thromboses (DVTs) on chronic anticoagulation presented with acute left leg swelling. The patient was diagnosed with an acute left lower extremity (LLE) DVT in the setting of May-Thurner syndrome for which treatment with unfractionated heparin was started. Her hospital course was complicated by a new diagnosis of heparin-induced thrombocytopenia (HIT), with an incidental discovery of a large tricuspid valve mobile mass on a transthoracic echocardiogram (TTE). Subsequent imaging confirmed multiple right atrial thrombi along with LLE venous stent thrombosis and a new right LE acute DVT. Anticoagulation with argatroban for HIT thrombosis was started. She underwent a right atrial percutaneous thrombectomy and bilateral lower extremity thrombectomy with directed angioplasty and stent placement. This presentation is a rare manifestation of HIT with extensive intracardiac and deep venous thrombi, with successful staged interventions.

1. Introduction

HIT is an adverse immune reaction to heparin characterized by systemic platelet consumption and paradoxical thrombotic complications. HIT is mediated by immunoglobulins directed against platelet factor 4 (PF4) bound to heparin, which also activate platelets leading to thrombosis [1]. The incidence of HIT in hospitalized patients is estimated at 0.2% [2]. Thrombosis secondary to HIT can rarely precipitate severe complications, from intracranial thrombi to skin necrosis and limb artery thrombosis [3]. Intracardiac thrombosis is an onerous manifestation of HIT that has received increasing attention in the current case literature. We report a case of multiple large atrial thrombi associated with HIT in a patient with May-Thurner syndrome and acute bilateral deep venous thromboses (DVTs).

2. Case Report

A 38-year-old woman with a history of recurrent LLE DVTs in the setting of pregnancy and travel presented with new left leg swelling. She had a negative hypercoagulable workup and was previously treated with rivaroxaban. She had previous exposure to unfractionated heparin with no complications. Heparin infusion was started for her new LLE DVT. CT imaging revealed effacement of the left common iliac vein by the right common iliac artery suggestive of May-Thurner syndrome. Subsequent venogram revealed complete occlusion of the left external iliac vein and left common femoral vein for which thrombolysis with tissue plasminogen activator (tPA) was administered, followed by angiography with stent placement.

The patient's hospital course was complicated by a 44% decline in platelet count on day 6 of heparin therapy (baseline: 237K/μL to 133K/μL). Platelets continued to decline on heparin to a nadir of 52K/μL on hospital day 9 (Figure 1). At that time, her anticoagulation was switched to argatroban and testing revealed positive heparin/PF4 antibody by IgG ELISA (OD 2.502, Quest Diagnostics) and positive serotonin release assay (100% release at UFH 0.1 IU/mL and 0.5 IU/mL, Quest Diagnostics). The patient was asymptomatic until a

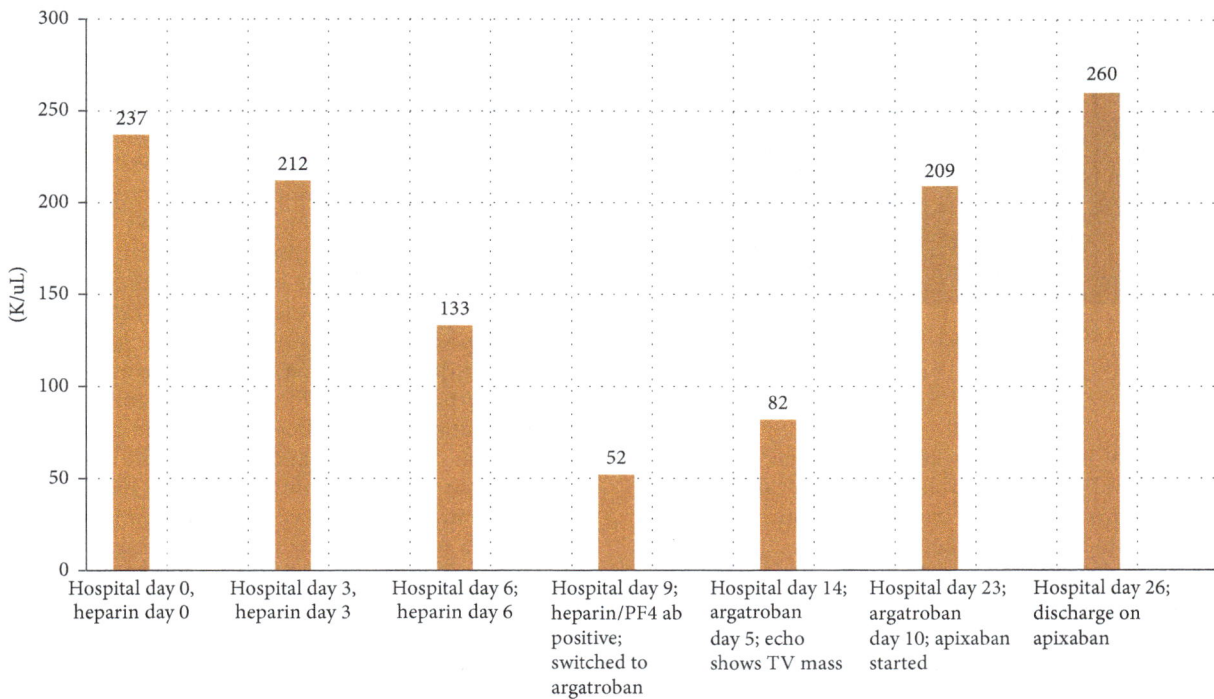

FIGURE 1: Timeline of platelet counts.

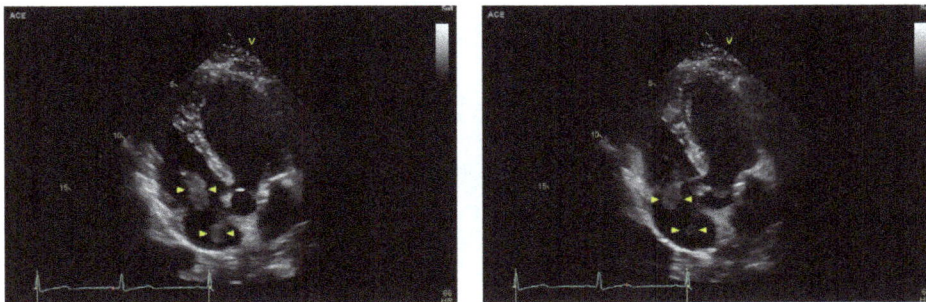

FIGURE 2: TTE showing the mobile right atrial mass that was traversing the tricuspid valve.

presyncopal episode on hospital day 14. TTE revealed a large mobile mass adherent to the tricuspid valve (Figure 2). A cardiac MRI revealed multiple right atrial thrombi (Figure 3). She was also noted to have LLE stent occlusion and an acute right lower extremity DVT. The patient was transferred to the cardiac intensive care unit (CICU) where she remained hemodynamically stable and asymptomatic. The patient subsequently underwent right atrial thrombectomy via AngioVac, revealing organizing thrombi on surgical pathology, with resolution of her clot burden on follow-up TTE. Her bilateral DVTs were treated with bilateral ultrasound-enhanced tPA thrombolysis followed by mechanical thrombectomy, angioplasty, and stent placement. After procedure, venogram showed significantly improved venous

flow through both lower extremities. She was started on apixaban and discharged home without complications.

3. Discussion

Heparin-induced thrombocytopenia is a rare but serious complication of heparin therapy, with incidence of HIT being 3% to 5% with unfractionated heparin and less than 1% with low-molecular-weight heparins [4]. While bleeding is justifiably the complication of foremost concern to clinicians in the setting of heparin use, thrombotic complications can be equally fatal and must also be considered. The patient in our case was found to have extensive HIT thrombosis with multiple large intracardiac thrombi and acute bilateral

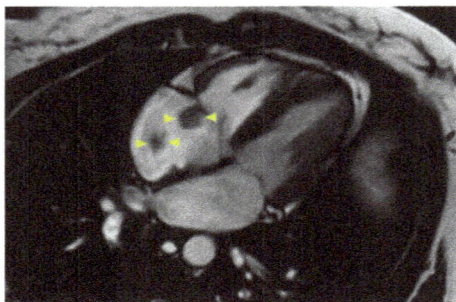

FIGURE 3: Cardiac MRI image showing multiple right atrial thrombi.

lower extremity DVTs. Given her clot burden, she was at high risk of pulmonary embolism and cardiopulmonary compromise, therefore requiring prompt interventions to reduce her morbidity and mortality risk.

HIT encompasses multiple clinical syndromes and can include nonimmune etiologies of thrombocytopenia as well. However, the activation of platelets by immunoglobulins (usually IgG) against PF4/heparin complexes is the pathophysiologic mechanism of greatest clinical concern [5]. Platelet-activating PF4/heparin IgG complexes typically form within 5–15 days of exposure to heparin and are associated with a 20–50% risk of thromboembolic events and a mortality rate of 20% [5]. Previous reports of intracardiac thrombi in the setting of HIT have described critically ill patients, often with cardiogenic shock or arrhythmias, which themselves can predispose to the formation of intracardiac thrombi [6, 7]. Remarkably in this case, the patient remained hemodynamically stable and asymptomatic, with no sign of cardiopulmonary compromise. Her case serves to reinforce the importance of a low threshold to discontinue heparin for alternative therapeutic anticoagulation in the setting of thrombocytopenia regardless of the patient's overt clinical state.

The use of novel oral anticoagulants (NOAC) in the management of HIT is an emerging subject of study. Clinical experience, though as yet limited, has shown good platelet count responses and tolerability in patients with HIT transitioned to NOAC, both directly after heparin discontinuation and after argatroban therapy [8, 9]. Our patient received a total of 10 days of argatroban therapy while hospitalized; her platelet count had recovered to $209K/\mu L$ when apixaban was started for lifelong anticoagulation given her risk for recurrent DVT. She received a loading dose of 10 mg twice daily for 7 days, transitioned as an outpatient to a maintenance dose of 5 mg twice daily. She remained without evidence of recurrent thrombosis at her 2-week and 3-month follow-ups.

This patient was incidentally found to have an anatomic predisposition to venous thrombi when CT revealed evidence of left common iliac vein compression against her fifth vertebral body by her right common iliac artery. This finding is suggestive of May-Thurner syndrome, a pathologic condition characterized by LLE venous insufficiency secondary to left iliac vein compression. As the compression is usually physiologic, May-Thurner syndrome is rarely considered

during the workup of recurrent DVTs; indeed the syndrome presents as DVT in only 2-3% of cases [10]. However, retrospective analysis of CT scans suggests prevalence of up to 24% [11], so May-Thurner syndrome remains an important consideration in young patients with recurrent DVTs without other localizing predispositions to thrombosis.

Studies suggest that endovascular correction of pathologic insufficiency via venous stenting may improve symptoms [12, 13]. Preexisting thrombi and thrombophilia can affect the technical success and outcomes of endovascular venous stenting. Our case illustrates the failure of an initial venous stenting intervention in the setting of active HIT, followed by the success of a staged endovascular intervention, where preexisting HIT-induced thrombi were treated by atrial thrombectomy before ultrasound-enhanced tPA thrombolysis, angioplasty, and stenting were completed.

HIT is an important consideration in patients hospitalized for thrombotic events with the delayed onset of thrombocytopenia while on heparin therapy. Despite the onerous potential consequences of HIT in this patient with extensive thrombosis in the setting of an anatomical predisposition to DVT, her relatively young age and excellent baseline functional capacity facilitated successful staged endovascular management of both her intracardiac thrombi and her acute DVTs.

Abbreviations

CICU: Cardiac intensive care unit
CT: Computed tomography
DVT: Deep venous thrombosis
HIT: Heparin-induced thrombocytopenia
Ig: Immunoglobulin
LLE: Left lower extremity
NOAC: Novel oral anticoagulants
PF4:   Platelet factor 4
SRA: Serotonin release assay
tPA: Tissue plasminogen activator
TTE: Transthoracic echocardiogram
UFH: Unfractionated heparin.

Consent

Written informed consent for this case report was obtained from patient.

Conflicts of Interest

The authors declare that there are no conflicts of interest regarding the publication of this paper.

References

[1] N. G. Kounis, G. D. Soufras, D. Lianas, and N. Patsouras, "Heparin-induced thrombocytopenia, allergy to heparins, heart failure, thrombi, and the Kounis syndrome," *International Journal of Cardiology*, vol. 214, pp. 508–509, 2016.

[2] M. A. Smythe, J. M. Koerber, and J. C. Mattson, "The incidence of recognized heparin-induced thrombocytopenia in a large,

tertiary care teaching hospital," *Chest*, vol. 131, no. 6, pp. 1644–1649, 2007.

[3] B. Nazliel, H. Z. B. Caglayan, I. Yildirim Capraz, C. Irkec, M. Yagci, and T. Gesoglu, "Heparin-induced thrombocytopenia leading to stroke, lower extremity arterial occlusive disease, and skin necrosis: a case report," *Platelets*, vol. 25, no. 2, pp. 129–131, 2014.

[4] S. Campisi, J.-F. Fuzellier, M. Vola, and J.-P. Favre, "Giant left ventricular thrombus formation associated with heparin-induced thrombocytopenia," *Annals of Thoracic Surgery*, vol. 98, no. 6, pp. e143–e145, 2014.

[5] T. E. Warkentin, "Think of HIT," *Hematology*, vol. 2006, pp. 408–414, 2006.

[6] A. Ahmed, H. AL-Mondhiry, T. J. Milling Jr., and D. Campbell, "Heparin-induced thrombocytopenia associated with massive intracardiac thrombosis: a case report," *Case Reports in Hematology*, vol. 2012, Article ID 257023, 4 pages, 2012.

[7] U. Aksu, O. Gulcu, and S. Topcu, "Left atrial thrombosis due to heparin-induced thrombocytopenia," *International Journal of Cardiology*, vol. 198, pp. 22–23, 2015.

[8] J. W. Skelley, J. A. Kyle, and R. A. Roberts, "Novel oral anticoagulants for heparin-induced thrombocytopenia," *Journal of Thrombosis and Thrombolysis*, vol. 42, no. 2, pp. 172–178, 2016.

[9] S. Y. Ong, Y. A. Chin, H. Than et al., "Rivaroxaban for heparin-induced thrombocytopenia: adding to the evidence," *Annals of Hematology*, vol. 96, no. 3, pp. 525–527, 2017.

[10] S. Kalu, P. Shah, A. Natarajan, N. Nwankwo, U. Mustafa, and N. Hussain, "May-Thurner syndrome: a case report and review of the literature," *Case Reports in Vascular Medicine*, vol. 2013, Article ID 740182, 5 pages, 2013.

[11] M. Peters, R. K. Syed, M. Katz et al., "May-Thurner syndrome: a not so uncommon cause of a common condition," *Proceedings (Baylor University. Medical Center)*, vol. 25, no. 3, pp. 231–233, 2012.

[12] R. E. Goldman, V. A. Arendt, N. Kothary et al., "Endovascular management of may-thurner syndrome in adolescents: a single-center experience," *Journal of Vascular and Interventional Radiology*, vol. 28, no. 1, pp. 71–77, 2017.

[13] Z. Liu, N. Gao, L. Shen et al., "Endovascular treatment for symptomatic iliac vein compression syndrome: a prospective consecutive series of 48 patients," *Annals of Vascular Surgery*, vol. 28, no. 3, pp. 695–704, 2014.

38

Sequential Kinase Inhibition (Idelalisib/Ibrutinib) Induces Clinical Remission in B-Cell Prolymphocytic Leukemia Harboring a 17p Deletion

H. Coelho, M. Badior, and T. Melo

Serviço de Hematologia, Centro Hospitalar de Vila Nova de Gaia/Espinho, Vila Nova Gaia, Portugal

Correspondence should be addressed to H. Coelho; henrique.coelho@chvng.min-saude.pt

Academic Editor: Tatsuharu Ohno

B-cell prolymphocytic leukemia (B-PLL) is a rare lymphoid neoplasm with an aggressive clinical course. Treatment strategies for B-PLL remain to be established, and, until recently, alemtuzumab was the only effective therapeutic option in patients harboring 17p deletions. Herein, we describe, for the first time, a case of B-cell prolymphocytic leukemia harboring a 17p deletion in a 48-year-old man that was successfully treated sequentially with idelalisib-rituximab/ibrutinib followed by allogeneic hematopoietic stem cell transplant (allo-HSCT). After 5 months of therapy with idelalisib-rituximab, clinical remission was achieved, but the development of severe diarrhea led to its discontinuation. Subsequently, the patient was treated for 2 months with ibrutinib and the quality of the response was maintained with no severe adverse effects reported. A reduced-intensity conditioning allo-HSCT from a HLA-matched unrelated donor was performed, and, thereafter, the patient has been in complete remission for 10 months now. In conclusion, given the poor prognosis of B-PLL and the lack of effective treatment modalities, the findings here suggest that both ibrutinib and idelalisib should be considered as upfront therapy of B-PLL and as a bridge to allo-HSCT.

1. Introduction

B-cell prolymphocytic leukemia (B-PLL) is a rare lymphoid neoplasm constituting approximately 1% of all cases of lymphocytic leukemia [1]. The median age at diagnosis of B-PLL is 69 years, and the condition has a similar distribution pattern among male and female patients, who typically present with B symptoms, marked lymphocytosis, massive splenomegaly, and minimal lymphadenopathy [2]. The diagnosis requires the presence of prolymphocytes, exceeding 55% of lymphoid cells in the peripheral blood [3]. However, distinguishing between B-PLL and chronic lymphocytic leukemia (CLL)—which has increased number of prolymphocytes and the blastoid variants of mantle cell lymphoma—solely on the basis of morphological assessments may be difficult, necessitating usage of immunophenotypic studies [3, 4]. B-PLL cells strongly express the surface immunoglobulins, IgM+/−IgD, and various B-cell antigens (CD19, CD20, CD22, CD79a and CD79b, and FMC7). Positive CD5 and CD23 expressions are seen in only 20–30% and 10–20% of the cases, respectively [2].

Treatment strategies for B-PLL remain to be established. The largest clinical trial of B-PLL included only 14 patients treated with pentostatin, and all other studies are limited to case reports or series with lesser than 10 patients [5]. Therefore, in the absence of clinical trials, clinicians typically employ a CLL-like treatment approach. Combinations of rituximab with fludarabine or bendamustine together with an anthracycline (mitoxantrone or epirubicin) have been reported to show significant activity in B-PLL [6–8]. However, resistance to purine analog/alkylator based therapy is high among B-PLL patients, as more than half of these patients have *TP53* abnormalities including del(17p) [3, 9, 10]. Until recently, alemtuzumab was the only effective therapeutic option for these patients, despite being associated with high rates of infections and short-lived responses [11, 12]. Lately, ibrutinib or idelalisib combined with rituximab has shown the best treatment outcome (response rates,

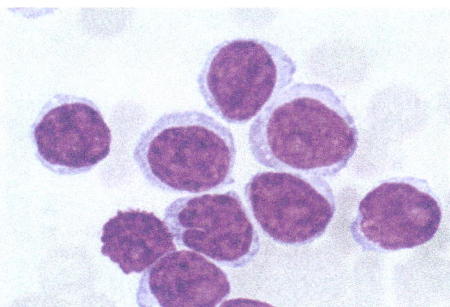

FIGURE 1: Peripheral blood smear. The lymphoid cells are of intermediate to large size with a prominent nucleolus and cytoplasm protrusions (Wright-Giemsa, ×1000).

progression-free survival, and overall survival) in *TP53*-disrupted CLL patients [13, 14]. Nevertheless, little is known about the treatment outcome of these new drugs in B-PLL, as very few patients have received either ibrutinib or idelalisib-rituximab [15, 16].

Herein, we report, for the first time, the efficacy of sequential kinase inhibition therapy (idelalisib-rituximab/ibrutinib) followed by allo-HSCT, in a patient diagnosed with B-PLL.

2. Case Presentation

A 48-year-old man was admitted in July 2015 with complains of abdominal discomfort, progressive night sweats, and a 10-kg weight loss over a period of 6 months. A full blood count showed the following findings: white blood cell count, 622×10^9/L; hemoglobin (Hb) concentration, 80 g/L; platelet count, 83×10^9/L; and LDH, 378 IU/L. A peripheral blood film demonstrated marked lymphocytosis with variably sized lymphocytes having clumped chromatin and central nucleoli (Figure 1). Peripheral blood immunophenotyping demonstrated that the lymphocyte population was composed almost exclusively of monoclonal B cells (95% of the lymphoid cells) with the following immunophenotype: $CD19^+$, $CD20^+$, $CD79b^+$, $CD5^+$, $FMC7^+$, $CD23^{+/-}$, and $CD10^-$. Fluorescent in situ hybridization (FISH) showed positive findings for del(17p) in 86% of the cells and negative findings for deletion of 11q, 13q, trisomy 12, and t(11; 14). A bone marrow biopsy revealed that B-PLL accounted for 80% of the cellularity in a markedly hypercellular marrow. The bone marrow was diffusely infiltrated with lymphoid cells expressing CD5, CD20, and CD79a, whereas CD10-, CD21-, CD23-, BCL6-, Cyclin D1-, and SOX11-positive cells were absent. A computed tomography scan of the chest, abdomen, and pelvis showed the presence of hepatomegaly and splenomegaly (craniocaudal height, 23 cm).

The patient started receiving idelalisib (150 mg twice daily) and rituximab (375 mg/m²; every two weeks for five doses and then every four weeks for 3 doses). The first two administration instances of rituximab were omitted due to a high tumor burden. Treatment with idelalisib-rituximab led to a rapid resolution (within 2 months) of the lymphocytosis (3.8×10^9/L), accompanied by normalization of the Hb

concentration (130 g/L) and platelet count (174×10^9/L) and resolution of the hepatosplenomegaly on CT (Figure 2). After 5 months of therapy, the patient developed grade 3 diarrhea (National Cancer Institute Common Terminology Criteria for Adverse Events v4.0) that resolved after treatment with prednisone (1 mg/kg id) along with discontinuation of idelalisib for 1 month. Thereafter, idelalisib was restarted at a low dose (150 mg daily), but recurrence of the diarrhea during the first week of treatment led to a definitive suspension and a change in therapy. Ibrutinib (420 mg daily) was commenced 2 weeks after idelalisib interruption, and, within the first 2 weeks, the patient developed a transient mild lymphocytosis (15×10^9/L). However, no significant side effects or clinical signs of B-PLL progression were noted, and, after a period of 2 months with ibrutinib, the Hb concentration (156 g/L), lymphocytes (4×10^9/L), and platelets (222×10^9/L) were found to be within the normal range, with no spleen enlargement on physical examination. The patient was treated with ibrutinib until admission for bone marrow transplantation. A reduced-intensity conditioning (RIC) allo-HSCT from a 10/10 HLA-matched unrelated donor was performed. The conditioning regimen included fludarabine (30 mg/m² for 6 consecutive days; days −10 to −5), oral busulfan (4 mg/kg/d for 2 consecutive days; days −6 to −5), and anti-T-lymphocyte globulin (10 mg/kg/d for 4 consecutive days; days −4 to −1) as well as prophylaxis against graft-versus-host disease (GvHD) with mycophenolate mofetil and tacrolimus tapered over 7 months. The regimen was well-tolerated with very mild toxicity and no major transplant-related complications. Six months after the transplant, counts of the lymphocytes, the neutrophils, and platelets and also the Hb concentration were within the normal range and no enlarged organs were detected on CT (Figure 2). In addition, flow cytometry and immunohistochemistry revealed that the bone marrow was free of clonal lymphoid cells. Furthermore, the FISH test carried out to detect leukemic cells harboring a 17p deletion yielded negative results. The patient has been well and in complete remission for 10 months now.

3. Discussion

B-PLL treatment modalities remain to be well-established and little is known about the efficacy of ibrutinib or idelalisib-rituximab for this disease. Recently, 5 patients with B-PLL carrying a genetic disruption of *TP53* were treated with idelalisib, and sustained remissions (6–10.5 months) were observed in 3 of these patients [15]. Adverse events were noted, namely, grade 2-3 transaminitis (3 patients) and CMV reactivation (1 patient), leading to temporary treatment interruption [15]. Ibrutinib was administered to 2 patients with B-PLL harboring complex cytogenetic abnormalities with aberrations in the *TP53* gene. Disease control was achieved with lymphocytosis resolution, accompanied by an improvement in Hb level, platelet count, and splenomegaly. Contrary to CLL, an increase in lymphocytosis was not observed following administration of ibrutinib [16].

Because of the availability of new promising alternative drugs, allogeneic hematopoietic stem cell transplantation

(a)

(b)

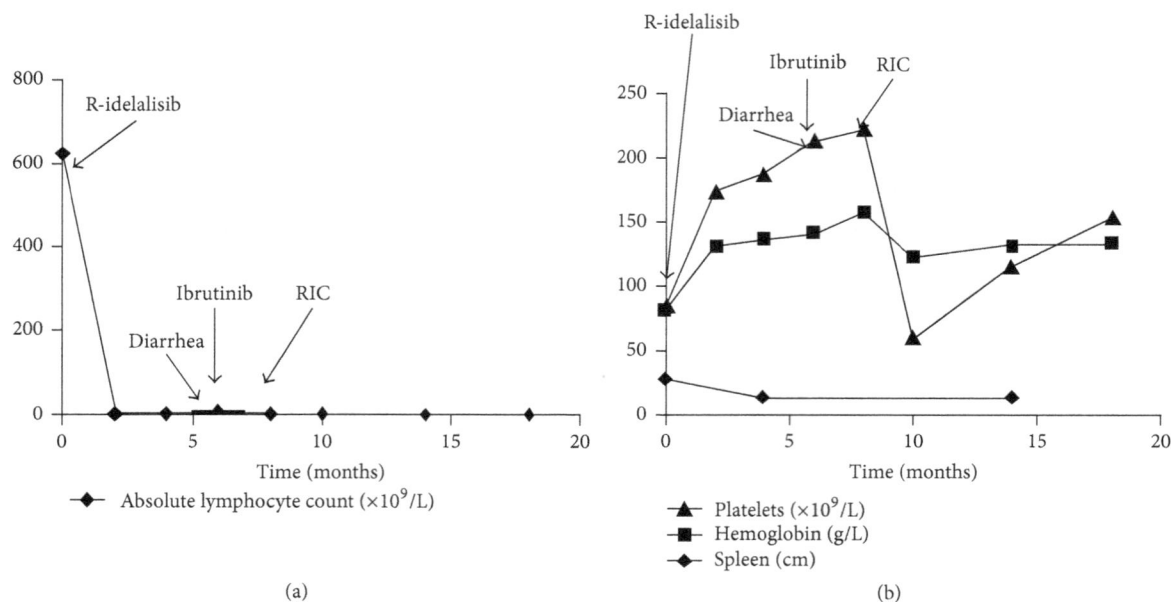

FIGURE 2: Response to idelalisib-rituximab started on day 0, ibrutinib started in month 6, and reduced-intensity conditioning allo-HSCT was performed in month 8. (a) Absolute lymphocyte count. (b) Platelet count, hemoglobin concentration, and spleen size (measured by CT scan/longest diameter).

(allo-HSCT), regarded as the only curative option for CLL, is now frequently deferred [17]. However, as B-PLL is often characterized by high-risk genetic abnormalities, which partly explains the poor outcomes and short survival times associated with conventional chemoimmunotherapy, suitable patient candidates should be considered for allo-HSCT on first remission.

In the present case, a rapid and meaningful response was observed in *TP53*-disrupted B-PLL treated sequentially with idelalisib-rituximab and ibrutinib. The response with idelalisib-rituximab was relatively robust and a toxicity profile similar to that already described in CLL was observed. As infusion-related reactions can be markedly decreased if the tumor load is first reduced with an initial course of rituximab-free chemotherapy, 2 cycles of rituximab were omitted [18]. Severe diarrhea, which developed in our patient, is one of the most common adverse events associated with idelalisib (7% of the patients) that prompts dose reduction (34%) and treatment discontinuation (20%) [19]. The clinical presentation of grade 3 diarrhea, after 5 months of therapy with idelalisib, as well as the time to its resolution (interruption of idelalisib and initiation of corticosteroid treatment) was as expected, concurring with another published report [19]. After having suspended idelalisib treatment, our patient started receiving ibrutinib. The disease remained in remission and no adverse events were registered. Ibrutinib is known to promote high response rates, leading to durable remissions in all genetic subsets of CLL patients, and discontinuation of ibrutinib is rarely due to adverse events related to the drug [20, 21]. Interestingly, we have observed an increase in lymphocytosis following the administration of ibrutinib, similar to that seen in CLL. The lymphocytosis, however, does not appear to be

associated with an increased risk of progression; nonetheless, these circulating cells may go back to tissue, and disease may become more aggressive following discontinuation of ibrutinib [21].

4. Conclusion

In conclusion, given the poor prognosis of B-PLL and the lack of effective treatment modalities, the findings presented here suggest that both ibrutinib and idelalisib should be considered as upfront therapeutic options for B-PLL and as a bridge to allo-HSCT in eligible patients.

Consent

Written informed consent was obtained from the patient for publication of this case report and any accompanying images.

Conflicts of Interest

The authors declare that they have no conflicts of interest.

Authors' Contributions

H. Coelho, M. Badior, and T. Melo jointly wrote and critically reviewed the manuscript.

References

[1] J. F. Yamamoto and M. T. Goodman, "Patterns of leukemia incidence in the United States by subtype and demographic

characteristics, 1997-2002," *Cancer Causes and Control*, vol. 19, no. 4, pp. 379–390, 2008.

[2] S. H. Swerdlow, E. Campo, and N. Harris, *World Health Organization Classification of Tumours of Haematopoietic and Lymphoid Tissues*, International Agency for Research on Cancer, Lyon, France, 2008.

[3] C. Dearden, "How I treat prolymphocytic leukemia," *Blood*, vol. 120, no. 3, pp. 538–551, 2012.

[4] F. Ravandi and S. O'Brien, "Chronic lymphoid leukemias other than chronic lymphocytic leukemia: Diagnosis and treatment," *Mayo Clinic Proceedings*, vol. 80, no. 12, pp. 1660–1674, 2005.

[5] H. Döhner, H. o. AD, J. Thaler et al., "Pentostatin in prolymphocytic leukemia: phase II trial of the european organization for research and treatment of cancer leukemia cooperative study group," *Natl Cancer Inst*, vol. 85, no. 8, pp. 658–662, 1993.

[6] A. Tempescul, J. Feuerbach, J.-C. Ianotto et al., "A combination therapy with fludarabine, mitoxantrone and rituximab induces complete immunophenotypical remission in B-cell prolymphocytic leukaemia," *Annals of Hematology*, vol. 88, no. 1, pp. 85–88, 2009.

[7] K. U. Chow, S. Z. Kim, and N. von Neuhoff, "Clinical efficacy of immunochemotherapy with fludarabine, epirubicin and rituximab in the treatment for chronic lymphocytic leukaemia and prolymphocytic leukaemia," *European Journal of Haematology*, vol. 5, pp. 426–433, 87.

[8] R. Weide, A. Pandorf, J. Heymanns, and H. Köppler, "Bendamustine/Mitoxantrone/Rituximab (BMR): A very effective, well tolerated outpatient chemoimmunotherapy for relapsed and refractory CD20-positive indolent malignancies. Final results of a pilot study," *Leukemia and Lymphoma*, vol. 45, no. 12, pp. 2445–2449, 2004.

[9] I. Del Giudice, Z. Davis, E. Matutes et al., "IgVH genes mutation and usage, ZAP-70 and CD38 expression provide new insights on B-cell prolymphocytic leukemia (B-PLL)," *Leukemia*, vol. 20, no. 7, pp. 1231–1237, 2006.

[10] P. Shindiapina, J. R. Brown, and A. V. Danilov, "A new hope: Novel therapeutic approaches to treatment of chronic lymphocytic leukaemia with defects in TP53," *British Journal of Haematology*, vol. 167, no. 2, pp. 149–161, 2014.

[11] S. L. McCune, J. P. Gockerman, and J. O. Moore, "Alemtuzumab in relapsed or refractory chronic lymphocytic leukemia and prolymphocytic leukemia," *Leuk Lymphoma*, vol. 43, no. 5, pp. 1007-11, 2002.

[12] B. T. Chaar and P. J. Petruska, "Complete response to alemtuzumab in a patient with B prolymphocytic leukemia," *American Journal of Hematology*, vol. 82, no. 5, p. 417, 2007.

[13] A. Wiestner, "The role of b-cell receptor inhibitors in the treatment of patients with chronic lymphocytic leukemia," *Haematologica*, vol. 100, no. 12, pp. 1495–1507, 2015.

[14] P. Jain, MJ. Keating, and W. Wierda, "Long term follow up of treatment with ibrutinib and rituximab (IR) in patients with high-risk Chronic Lymphocytic Leukemia (CLL)," *Clinical Cancer Research*, vol. 23, no. 9, pp. 2154–2158, 2017.

[15] T. A. Eyre, C. P. Fox, and P. Shankara, "Idelalisib-Rituximab induces clinical remissions in patients with TP53 disrupted B cell prolymphocytic leukaemia," *Br J Haematol*, vol. 177, no. 3, pp. 486-91, 2017.

[16] M. J. Gordon, P. W. Raess, and K. Young, "Ibrutinib is an effective treatment for B-cell prolymphocytic leukaemia," *British Journal of Haematology*, 2016.

[17] F. McClanahan and J. Gribben, "New insights into hematopoietic stem cell transplantation for chronic lymphocytic leukemia: a 2015 perspective," *Clinical Advances in Hematology & Oncology*, vol. 13, no. 9, pp. 586–594, 2015.

[18] P. J. Bugelski, R. Achuthanandam, and R. J. Capocasale, "Monoclonal antibody- induced cytokine-release syndrome," *Expert Review of Clinical Immunology*, vol. 5, no. 5, pp. 499–521, 2009.

[19] S. E. Coutré, J. C. Barrientos, and J. R. Brown, "Management of adverse events associated with idelalisib treatment: expert panel opinion," *Leuk Lymphoma*, vol. 56, no. 10, pp. 2779–2786, 2015.

[20] S. Molica, "The clinical safety of ibrutinib in chronic lymphocytic leukemia," *Expert Opinion on Drug Safety*, vol. 14, no. 10, pp. 1621–1629, 2015.

[21] F. Forconi, "Three years of ibrutinib in CLL," *Blood*, vol. 125, no. 16, pp. 2455-2456, 2015.

39

Pure Red Cell Aplasia Associated with Thymolipoma: Complete Anaemia Resolution following Thymectomy

David Ferreira ⓘ,[1,2] **Royston Ponraj,**[2] **Adrian Yeung,**[3] **and Jillian de Malmanche**[4]

[1]*Conjoint Associate Lecturer, University of New South Wales, Sydney, Australia*
[2]*Medical Department, Medical Registrar, Liverpool Hospital, Elizabeth St., Liverpool, NSW 2170, Australia*
[3]*Haematology Department, Haematology Advanced Trainee, Liverpool Hospital, Elizabeth St., Liverpool, NSW 2170, Australia*
[4]*Haematology Department, Haematology Staff Specialist, John Hunter Hospital, Lookout Rd., New Lambton Heights, NSW 2305, Australia*

Correspondence should be addressed to David Ferreira; dave_7@live.com.au

Academic Editor: Sergio Storti

Pure red cell aplasia is an uncommon cause of anaemia rarely associated with thymoma. A combination of immunosuppressive therapy and thymectomy offers a potential cure. Thymectomy alone rarely results in anaemia resolution. A seventy-three-year-old male with Klinefelter syndrome presented with progressively increasing shortness of breath and anaemia. Serological testing supported primary bone marrow pathology, and a bone marrow biopsy was performed. A pure red cell aplasia was seen on bone marrow examination, and computed tomography of the chest demonstrated a thymoma. Thymectomy was performed, and histology revealed a thymolipoma. Complete anaemia resolution was achieved following thymectomy alone. This suggests that thymomas may directly mediate immune dysregulation resulting in erythroid precursor destruction.

1. Introduction

Pure red cell aplasia (PRCA) is a rare cytopenia characterised by a marked reduction of erythroid precursors in the bone marrow. While most cases are idiopathic, there are a number of possible secondary causes. These include lymphoid and myeloid malignancies, autoimmune disease, viral infection, drugs, and thymoma [1].

Thymomas accounts for less than ten percent of all pure red cell aplasia [1, 2]. The mechanism by which they cause PRCA is incompletely understood. Anaemia is thought to result from a paraneoplastic immune mediated destruction of erythroid precursors [2]. Thymic histological findings are variable and can include medullary thymoma, spindle thymoma, epithelial thymoma, lymphocytic thymoma, thymic carcinoma, and thymolipoma [3, 4]. Treatment involves surgical resection in combination with immunosuppressive therapy, as surgery alone is generally ineffective

[3, 5]. The authors present a case of pure red cell aplasia secondary to thymolipoma with complete resolution of anaemia following surgical excision alone.

2. Case Report

A seventy-three-year-old gentleman presented with progressive shortness of breath over a two-month period. His medical history was significant for Klinefelter syndrome, heart failure with reduced ejection fraction, obstructive sleep apnoea, hypogonadism, haemochromatosis, and secondary polycythaemia requiring 6–12 monthly venesections. Clinical examination was unremarkable. On presentation, he had a normochromic normocytic anaemia with a haemoglobin of 82 g/L, a reticulocyte count of 2×10^9/L, and an elevated haptoglobin (Table 1). Vitamin B12, folate, and thyroid-stimulating hormone studies were normal, and serum ferritin was increased (Table 2). These

TABLE 1: Full blood count comparison.

	Normal range	6 months prior	Admission	3 months after thymectomy
White cells (10^9/L)	4.0–11.0	7.5	6.4	7.0
Red cells (10^{12}/L)	4.5–6.5	5.95	2.94	4.97
Haemoglobin (g/L)	130–180	160	81	150
Haematocrit (L/L)	0.38–0.52	0.498	0.243	0.466
Mean cell volume (fl)	80–100	79	83	94
Platelets (10^9/L)	150–400	264	354	252
Neutrophils (10^9/L)	2.0–8.0	5.2	4.4	4.6
Lymphocytes (10^9/L)	1.0–4.0	1.2	0.9	1.4
Monocytes (10^9/L)	0.2–1.0	1.0	0.9	0.9
Eosinophils (10^9/L)	0–0.4	0.1	0.1	0.1

TABLE 2: Anaemia screen during hospitilisation.

	Normal range	Admission
Reticulocytes (10^9/L)	10–100	2
Vitamin B12 (pmol/L)	130–850	228
Folate (nmol/L)	7.0–46.4	26.7
Ferritin (ug/L)	30–300	1196
Iron (umol/L)	11–30	57
Transferrin (g/L)	1.6–3.4	2.4
Transferrin saturation (%)	15–45	90
TSH* (mIU/L)	0.4–5.0	1.65
LDH† (U/L)	120–250	236
Haptoglobin (g/L)	0.3–2.0	2.68

*Thyroid-stimulating hormone; †lactate dehydrogenase.

laboratory results, notably the markedly reduced reticulocyte count, were consistent with reduced production of red cells in the bone.

Bone marrow biopsy demonstrated a marked reduction in erythroid precursors (two percent of the differential) consistent with pure red cell aplasia (Figure 1). Normal granulopoiesis and megakaryopoiesis were evident. Autoimmune screening (ANA, ENA, dsDNA, RF, and anticardiolipin antibodies) and viral screening were negative (hepatitis B, hepatitis C, human immunodeficiency virus, and parvovirus B19). Serum protein electrophoresis and immunosubtraction were negative for monoclonal bands, and flow cytometry was normal. There were no recent medication changes. A chest computed tomography was performed revealing an anterior mediastinal mass consistent with thymoma (Figure 2). An elective thymectomy was arranged with a cardiothoracic surgeon, and intermittent blood transfusions were provided while awaiting surgery.

Thymectomy was performed via a median sternotomy. Histopathology demonstrated normal thymic tissue mixed with mature adipose tissue, diagnostic of thymolipoma. No inflammation, granulomata, or neoplasia was identified. Three weeks following thymectomy, the patients' haemoglobin normalised with a complete resolution of his symptoms. After a year of follow-up, the patients' haemoglobin remains normal, without immunosuppressive therapy or ongoing transfusions.

3. Discussion

Thymolipomas account for 2–9% of all thymic neoplasms [6]. There have been three previous reports of PRCA associated with thymolipoma [3, 7, 8]. In all three cases, patients received both surgical resection and immunosuppressive therapy prior to any improvement in haemoglobin. We present a case of pure red cell aplasia associated with thymolipoma that resolved following thymectomy alone. The mechanism behind anaemia associated with thymolipoma is not understood. Complete resolution following thymectomy suggests that thymolipomas may directly mediate erythroid precursor destruction. The underlying mechanism may be that of immune cell maturation dysregulation and subsequent autoimmune destruction [2]. Thymolipomas are associated with autoimmune diseases including myasthenia gravis, aplastic anaemia, Graves' disease, and lichen planus [9]. Moreover, patients with Klinefelter syndrome have an increased risk for autoimmune disease, associated with the XXY karyotype [10].

This case serves as a reminder that primary bone marrow pathology is differential for every patient presenting with anaemia. Simple serological screening tests provide pivotal information to guide the investigation and management of patients presenting with anaemia. While uncommon, every patient with a PRCA warrants a chest computed tomography to identify a thymoma, as thymectomy offers a potential cure.

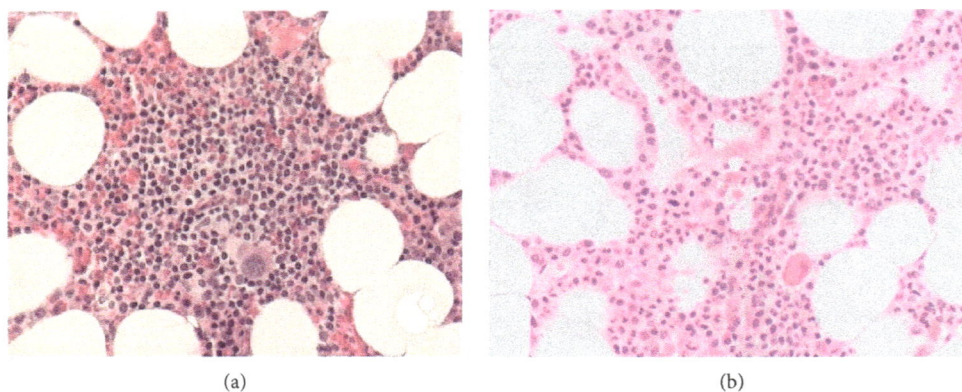

FIGURE 1: (a) Normal bone marrow biopsy demonstrating a predominance of erythroid precursors (note cells with round, dark nuclei). This image was originally published in ASH Image Bank. Peter Maslak. Normal adult bone marrow. ASH Image Bank. 2010; Trephine Biopsy-2. ©The American Society of Hematology. (b) Bone marrow biopsy taken from the patient, demonstrating marked reduction in erythroid precursors.

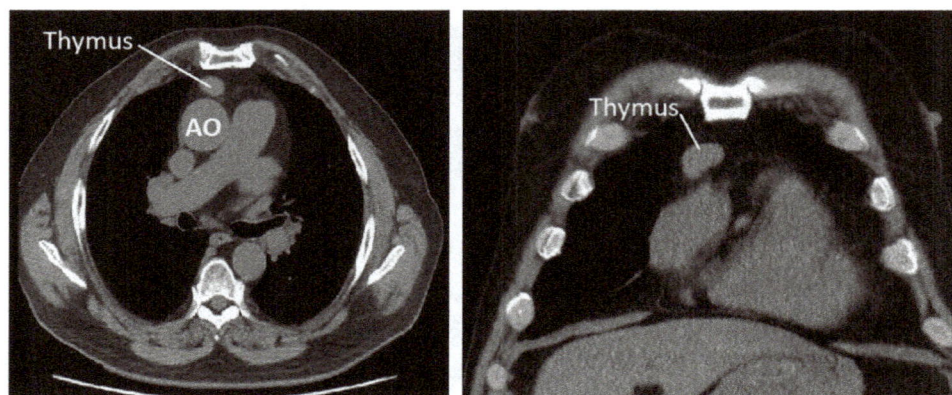

FIGURE 2: Thymoma on noncontrast chest computed tomography.

Consent

Verbal consent was provided by the patient with no risk of identification within the manuscript.

Conflicts of Interest

The authors have no conflicts of interest to declare.

Acknowledgments

We would like to acknowledge Russell Cox for his valuable assistance in procuring the histological slides.

References

[1] R. Charles, K. Sabo, P. Kidd, and J. Abkowitz, "The patho-physiology of pure red cell aplasia: implications for therapy," *Blood*, vol. 87, no. 11, pp. 4831–4838, 1996.

[2] M. Lacy, P. Kurtin, and A. Tefferi, "Pure red cell aplasia: association with large granular lymphocyte leukemia and the prognostic value of cytogenetic abnormalities," *Blood*, vol. 87, no. 7, pp. 3000–3006, 1996.

[3] C. A. Thompson and D. P. Steensma, "Pure red cell aplasia associated with thymoma: clinical insights from a 50-year single-institution experience," *British Journal of Haematology*, vol. 135, no. 3, pp. 405–407, 2006.

[4] K. F. Wong, K. F. Chau, J. K. Chan, Y. C. Chu, and C. S. Li, "Pure red cell aplasia associated with thymic lymphoid hyperplasia and secondary erythropoietin resistance," *American Journal of Clinical Pathology*, vol. 103, no. 3, pp. 346–347, 1995.

[5] C. Rosu, S. Cohen, C. Meunier, D. Ouellette, G. Beauchamp, and G. Rakovich, "Pure red cell aplasia and associated thymoma," *Clinics and Practice*, vol. 1, no. 1, p. 1, 2011.

[6] M. Nishino, S. K. Ashiku, O. N. Kocher, R. L. Thurer, P. M. Boiselle, and H. Hatabu, "The thymus: a comprehensive review-erratum," *RadioGraphics*, vol. 37, no. 3, p. 1004, 2017.

[7] K. G. McManus, M. S. Allen, V. F. Trastek, C. Deschamps, T. B. Crotty, and P. C. Pairolero, "Lipothymoma with red cell aplasia, hypogammaglobulinemia, and lichen planus," *Annals of Thoracic Surgery*, vol. 58, no. 5, pp. 1534–1536, 1994.

[8] E. Lebrun, F. Ajchenbaum, X. Troussard et al., "[Chronic lymphocytic leukemia, erythroblastopenia, thymolipoma]," *Nouvelle revue française d'hématologie*, vol. 27, no. 1, pp. 29–37, 1985.

[9] R. J. Rieker, P. Schirmacher, P. A. Schnabel et al., "Thymolipoma. A report of nine cases, with emphasis on its

40

Protracted Clonal Trajectory of a *JAK2* V617F-Positive Myeloproliferative Neoplasm Developing during Long-Term Remission from Acute Myeloid Leukemia

Stephen E. Langabeer[1], Karl Haslam[1], Maria Anne Smyth,[2] John Quinn,[2] and Philip T. Murphy[2]

[1]Cancer Molecular Diagnostics, St. James's Hospital, Dublin 8, Ireland
[2]Department of Haematology, Beaumont Hospital, Dublin 9, Ireland

Correspondence should be addressed to Stephen E. Langabeer; slangabeer@stjames.ie

Academic Editor: Sudhir Tauro

Although transformation of the myeloproliferative neoplasms (MPNs) to acute myeloid leukemia (AML) is well documented, development of an MPN in patients previously treated for, and in remission from, AML is exceedingly rare. A case is described in which a patient was successfully treated for AML and in whom a *JAK2* V617F-positive MPN was diagnosed after seven years in remission. Retrospective evaluation of the *JAK2* V617F detected a low allele burden at AML diagnosis and following one course of induction chemotherapy. This putative chemoresistant clone subsequently expanded over the intervening seven years, resulting in a hematologically overt MPN. As AML relapse has not occurred, the MPN may have arose in a separate initiating cell from that of the AML. Alternatively, both malignancies possibly evolved from a common precursor defined by a predisposition mutation with divergent evolution into MPN through acquisition of the *JAK2* V617F and AML through acquisition of different mutations. This case emphasizes the protracted time frame from acquisition of a disease-driving mutation to overt MPN and further underscores the clonal complexity in MPN evolution.

1. Introduction

The clonal evolution of a myeloproliferative neoplasm (MPN) into acute myeloid leukemia (AML) is complex: both the *JAK2* V617F and *CALR* exon nine mutations are absent in a significant number of MPN patients evolving to AML implicating the transformation of a common myeloid progenitor at a stage before acquisition of the MPN driver mutation or evolution from a distinct initiating precursor from that harboring the *JAK2* V617F or *CALR* mutation [1–3]. Furthermore, not only the type of additional mutations but also the order in which these mutations are acquired can influence clonal evolution and phenotype [4]. In contrast, the emergence of a *JAK2* V617F-positive MPN on the background of AML is exceedingly rare. Nearly all those cases reported have occurred in AML patients in long-term remission after chemotherapy or autologous stem cell transplantation and where retrospective genotyping of the AML presentation material was performed, demonstrating the absence of the *JAK2* V617F mutation [5–8]. Molecular investigation of another case suggested that the MPN may be secondary to the AML [9]. A case is described of a patient developing a *JAK2* V617F-positive MPN when in remission of AML for seven years and in whom retrospective molecular investigation was able to unravel the evolutionary trajectory of the MPN.

2. Case Report

A 64-year-old female presented in April 2010 with a two-week history of lethargy. A full blood count revealed a hemoglobin count of 8.6 g/dL, a platelet count of 48×10^9/L, and a white cell count of 96.4×10^9/L with a large population of blasts. On physical examination, there was no

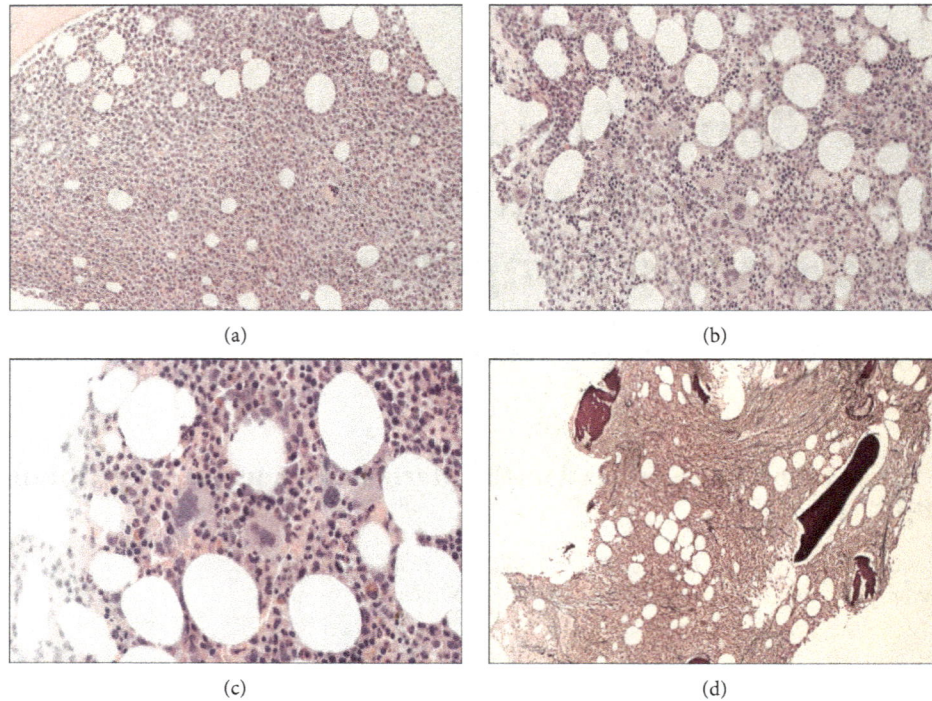

(a)

(b)

(c)

(d)

FIGURE 1: Bone marrow biopsy (a) at diagnosis of acute myeloid leukemia (AML) demonstrating infiltration by myeloblasts; (b) after one course of AML therapy showing atypical megakaryocyte morphology and focal clustering; (c) at diagnosis of myeloproliferative neoplasm (MPN) with myeloid hypercellularity and increased megakaryocytes; and (d) at diagnosis of MPN demonstrating increased reticulin deposition.

palpable liver or spleen. Peripheral blood immunophenotyping showed two blast populations: one population (20%) positive for HLA-DR, CD117, CD33, and CD13 and a second population (48%) positive for HLA-DR, CD33, CD13, CD14, and CD15. The bone marrow aspirate was hypercellular with the vast majority of cells either myeloblasts or monoblasts, all consistent with a diagnosis of acute myeloid leukemia (AML) of myelomonocytic type (Figure 1(a)). Cytogenetic analysis demonstrated a normal karyotype, and there was no evidence of an *FLT3* internal tandem duplication mutation. The patient achieved a morphological remission after one course of daunorubicin and cytarabine (3 + 10). The bone marrow trephine biopsy at this time showed no evidence of blasts but remained hypercellular with some abnormal megakaryocyte forms showing focal clustering (Figure 1(b)). The reticulin stain was normal. The patient completed three courses of consolidation chemotherapy ending in August 2010 with hemoglobin, hematocrit, red cell count, and platelets coming into normal range within two years of finishing AML treatment and remains in remission.

A mild neutrophilia (7.85×10^9/L) was noted in October 2013 and an eosinophilia (0.4×10^9/L) was noted in January 2017, slowly rising to 18.9×10^9/L neutrophils and 0.6×10^9/L eosinophils. Qualitative molecular analysis of peripheral blood in July 2017 showed no evidence of *BCR-ABL1* transcripts but detected the presence of the *JAK2* V617F mutation. Subsequent bone marrow aspirate and biopsy in August 2017 (seven years after completion of AML therapy) revealed hypercellularity with increased myelopoiesis undergoing normal maturation. Megakaryocytes were increased in number with some immature forms being seen and an increase in mature myeloid cells to erythroid cells (Figure 1(c)). Staining for reticulin demonstrated increased deposition (Figure 1(d)), resulting in a diagnosis of MPN unclassified. Currently, the patient is asymptomatic and is on no active therapy to control her white cell count.

Quantitative assessment of the *JAK2* V617F allele burden was performed on the archival material using an assay previously described with a sensitivity of 0.01% mutant alleles [10]. Quantitative PCR demonstrated bone marrow allele burdens of 0.2% at AML diagnosis (in independent duplicate samples), 5.7% after one course of AML therapy, and 72.7% at MPN diagnosis.

3. Discussion

Molecular analysis of AML derived from a *JAK2* V617F-positive MPN has demonstrated divergent pathways to transformation, highlighting the underlying clonal complexity of MPN evolution. In the case described herein, retrospective molecular investigation detected a low *JAK2* V617F allele burden at AML diagnosis that was further unmasked by the AML induction chemotherapy. As AML relapse has not occurred, the MPN may have arose in a separate initiating cell from that of the AML. Alternatively, both malignancies possibly evolved from a common precursor defined by a predisposition mutation with divergent evolution into MPN or AML through acquisition of

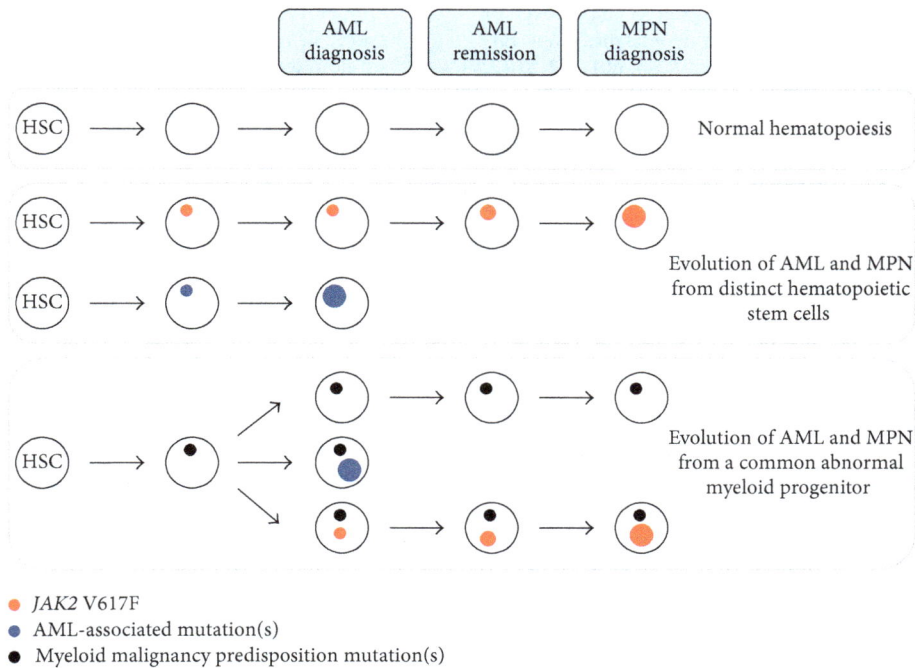

FIGURE 2: Possible divergent clonal trajectories of the *JAK2* V617F-positive myeloproliferative neoplasm and acute myeloid leukemia in tandem with normal hematopoiesis. AML: acute myeloid leukemia; MPN: myeloproliferative neoplasm; HSC: hematopoietic stem cell.

the *JAK2* V617F or AML-associated mutations, respectively (Figure 2). The chemoresistant *JAK2* V617F clone [11] remained clinically silent for seven years, although continually expanding, until hematological and morphological diagnosis of an MPN with a high *JAK2* V617F allele burden. The high *JAK2* V617F allele burden likely represents loss of heterozygosity in at least some mutant clones, analogous to that observed in the progression of polycythemia vera [12]. This phenomenon of a minor *JAK2* V617F clone at AML diagnosis has been described previously in a patient who developed polycythemia vera after five years in remission for AML treatment and in whom retrospective analysis revealed a *JAK2* V617F allele burden of 2.0% at the time of AML diagnosis [13]. Whole-exome sequencing and cluster analysis in a recently reported similar case suggest that preleukemic hematopoietic stem cells of AML can not only contribute to myeloid hematopoiesis during remission but may also give rise to another malignancy such as MPN [14]. Moreover, although de novo *JAK2* V617F-positive AML is uncommon, it can be associated with the *t*(8;21) and trisomy 8 cytogenetic abnormalities, with myelodysplastic changes, and a high allele burden [15, 16], features not observed in this case.

A protracted time course is clearly evident from acquisition of the initial *JAK2* V617F driver mutation to development of a hematologically and clinically overt MPN accentuating the different kinetics of development of MPN and AML and suggesting that initiation of the MPN may have been an earlier event relative to that of the AML. Studies have shown that this process may take several years and have attempted to quantify the annual increase in *JAK2* V617F allele burden [17]. A more recent study of long-term follow-up of blood donors who developed an MPN has shown a similar latency though individual variation does exist, which is possibly a reflection of both inherited and acquired genetic factors [18].

Finally, given the expanding focus in minimal residual disease-directed therapy for AML patients [19], caution is warranted in the interpretation of low-level mutations such as the *JAK2* V617F, as these may not represent residual disease but a latent, coexisting hematological malignancy.

Disclosure

Current address of Karl Haslam is Genomics Medicine Ireland, Cherrywood Business Park, Dublin 18, Ireland.

Conflicts of Interest

The authors declare that there are no conflicts of interest regarding the publication of this paper.

References

[1] P. J. Campbell, E. J. Baxter, P. A. Beer et al., "Mutation of JAK2 in the myeloproliferative disorders: timing, clonality studies, cytogenetic associations, and role in leukemic transformation," *Blood*, vol. 108, no. 10, pp. 3548–3555, 2006.

[2] A. Theocharides, M. Boissinot, F. Girodon et al., "Leukemic blasts in transformed JAK2 V617F-positive myeloproliferative disorders are frequently negative for the JAK2 V617F mutation," *Blood*, vol. 110, no. 1, pp. 375–379, 2007.

[3] S. E. Langabeer, K. Haslam, and E. Elhassadi, "The mutant CALR allele burden in essential thrombocythemia at transformation to acute myeloid leukemia," *Blood Cells, Molecules and Diseases*, vol. 65, pp. 66-67, 2017.

[4] C. A. Ortmann, D. G. Kent, J. Nangalia et al., "Effect of mutation order on myeloproliferative neoplasms," *New England Journal of Medicine*, vol. 372, no. 7, pp. 601–612, 2015.

[5] C. Chabannon, M. Bost, and D. Hollard, "A case of polycythemia vera occurring in a patient with acute non-lymphoblastic leukemia (ANLL) in long-term first complete remission," *Leukemia*, vol. 8, no. 7, pp. 1243-1244, 1994.

[6] A. R. Walker, P. G. Rothberg, and J. L. Liesveld, "A case of JAK2 positive essential thrombocythemia 16.5 years after autologous marrow transplantation for AML," *Bone Marrow Transplantation*, vol. 39, no. 11, pp. 725-726, 2007.

[7] E. Antonioli, P. Guglielmelli, G. Poli, V. Santini, A. Bosi, and A. M. Vannucchi, "Polycythemia vera following autologous transplantation for AML: insights on the kinetics of JAK2 V617F clonal dominance," *Blood*, vol. 110, no. 13, pp. 4620-4621, 2007.

[8] A. Belotti, E. Doni, E. Elli, V. Rossi, P. Pioltelli, and E. M. Pogliani, "Development of polycythemia vera after chemotherapy-induced remission of acute myeloid leukemia: a case report," *Acta Haematologica*, vol. 126, no. 1, pp. 52-53, 2011.

[9] S. Girsberger, A. Karow, P. Lundberg et al., "JAK2 V617F-mutated myeloproliferative neoplasia developing five years after wild-type JAK2 acute myeloid leukemia: a case report," *Acta Haematologica*, vol. 129, no. 1, pp. 23–25, 2013.

[10] K. Haslam, K. M. Molloy, E. Conneally, and S. E. Langabeer, "Evaluation of a JAK2 V617F quantitative PCR to monitor residual disease post-allogeneic hematopoietic stem cell transplantation for myeloproliferative neoplasms," *Clinical Chemistry and Laboratory Medicine*, vol. 52, no. 3, pp. e29–e31, 2014.

[11] E. Verger, E. Rattarittamrong, G. Letort, E. Raffoux, B. Cassinat, and J. J. Kiladjian, "Chemotherapy for post-myelofibrosis acute myeloid leukemia: eradication of the leukemic clone but not the MPN clone," *Leukemia and Lymphoma*, vol. 58, no. 3, pp. 749–751, 2017.

[12] A. M. Vannucchi, E. Antonioli, P. Guglielmelli, A. Pardanani, and A. Tefferi, "Clinical correlates of JAK2 V617F presence or allele burden in myeloproliferative neoplasms: a critical reappraisal," *Leukemia*, vol. 22, no. 7, pp. 1299–1307, 2008.

[13] C. A. Portell, M. A. Sekeres, H. J. Rogers, and R. V. Tiu, "De novo polycythemia vera arising 5 years following acute myeloid leukemia remission: suggestion of a chemotherapy resistant JAK2 clone," *British Journal of Haematology*, vol. 157, no. 2, pp. 266-267, 2012.

[14] S. Sato, H. Itonaga, M. Taguchi et al., "Clonal dynamics in a case of acute monoblastic leukemia that later developed myeloproliferative neoplasm," *International Journal of Hematology*, 2018, In press.

[15] S. Schnittger, U. Bacher, W. Kern, T. Haferlach, and C. Haferlach, "JAK2 V617F as a progression marker in CMPD and as a cooperative mutation in AML with trisomy 8 and t(8; 21): a comparative study on 1103 CMPD and 269 AML cases," *Leukemia*, vol. 21, no. 8, pp. 1843–1845, 2007.

[16] J. E. Hidlago-López, R. Kanagal-Shamanna, L. J. Medeiros et al., "Morphologic and molecular characteristics of de novo AML with JAK2 V617F mutation," *Journal of the National Comprehensive Cancer Network*, vol. 15, no. 6, pp. 790–796, 2017.

[17] C. Nielsen, S. E. Bojesen, B. G. Nordestgaard, K. F. Kofoed, and H. S. Birgens, "JAK2 V617F somatic mutation in the general population: myeloproliferative neoplasm development and progression rate," *Haematologica*, vol. 99, no. 9, pp. 1448–1455, 2014.

[18] T. McKerrell, N. Park, J. Chi et al., "JAK2 V617F hematopoietic clones are present several years prior to MPN diagnosis and follow different expansion kinetics," *Blood Advances*, vol. 1, no. 14, pp. 968–971, 2017.

[19] C. S. Hourigan, R. P. Gale, N. J. Gormley, G. J. Ossenkoppele, and R. B. Walter, "Measurable residual disease testing in acute myeloid leukemia," *Leukemia*, vol. 31, no. 7, pp. 1482–1490, 2017.

41

Myeloid Sarcoma of Orbits: Effectiveness of a Low-Dose Radiation Regimen

Shyam Ravisankar ⓘ,[1] Yair Levy,[2] and Maya Shah ⓘ[1]

[1]Division of Hematology and Oncology, Newark Beth Israel Medical Center, Newark, NJ, USA
[2]Department of Radiology, Newark Beth Israel Medical Center, Newark, NJ, USA

Correspondence should be addressed to Maya Shah; maya.shah@rwjbh.org

Academic Editor: Pier P. Piccaluga

Acute myeloid leukemia (AML) can present with extramedullary involvement known as myeloid sarcoma (MS). We present the case of a young woman who was diagnosed with AML and MS in bilateral orbits, brain, omentum, and retroperitoneum. She was treated with induction chemotherapy. Low-dose radiation was given to the orbits due to visual symptoms which resulted in complete response. The use of radiation therapy in orbital MS has not been studied extensively, and low dose may be adequate to achieve complete remission (CR) in selected patients.

1. Background

Acute myeloid leukemia (AML) can present with extramedullary (EM) involvement as granulocytic sarcoma also known as chloroma or myeloid sarcoma (MS). MS can present as an isolated extramedullary leukemic tumor, concurrently with or at relapse of acute myeloid leukemia. We present the case of a young female who had de novo AML with MS in bilateral orbits, brain, omentum, and retroperitoneum. The use of radiation therapy (RT) in orbital MS has not been studied extensively, and this presents a therapeutic dilemma.

2. Case Presentation

A 31-year-old African American female was found to have severe anemia on laboratory work performed by her gynecologist. The patient reported fatigue and dyspnea on exertion for about two months. She also had a two-week history of gum bleeding while brushing her teeth. She denied any other bleeding, weight loss, chills, or fevers. She had occasional blurry vision for about two weeks. Physical examination was unremarkable except for proptosis of the left eye. Visual fields and acuity were normal. A complete blood count showed a white blood cell count of 18×10^9/L with 50% blasts, hemoglobin of 5.7 g/dl, and a platelet count of 18×10^9/L. Bone marrow aspirate showed myeloblasts (64.2%) by flow cytometry. The myeloblasts were positive for CD13, CD33, CD34, MPO, and HLA-DR and negative for CD20 and CD19 on immunophenotyping. Fluorescent in situ hybridization (FISH) analysis revealed translocation t(8;21). Testing for FLT3 (Fms-like tyrosine kinase 3), CEBPA (CCAAT/enhancer-binding protein alpha) and NPM1 (nucleophosmin 1) was negative. Cerebrospinal fluid analysis was negative for involvement by leukemia. MRI of the brain demonstrated bilateral orbital masses measuring 2.6 cm on the right and 1.2 cm on the left (Figure 1). The left orbital mass spanned the intraconal and extraconal compartments and displaced the optic nerve superomedially. The right orbital mass was in the right orbital apex extending along the roof of the orbit. Both masses were separate from the optic nerve and the ocular globe. Both masses compressed the optic nerve at the apex. There was mild proptosis on the left and only minimal proptosis on the right. There was an enhancing dural-based lesion in the right posterior fossa measuring 11×3 mm (Figure 2). Nodules measuring around one centimeter were noted in the omentum, retroperitoneal

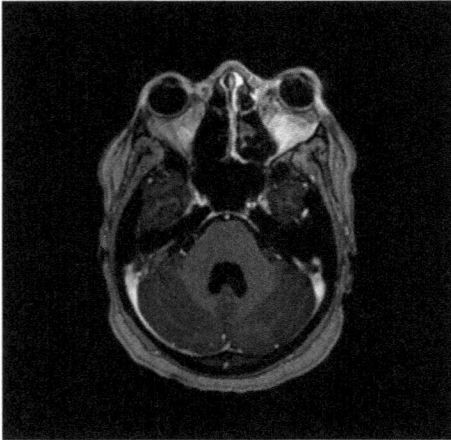

FIGURE 1

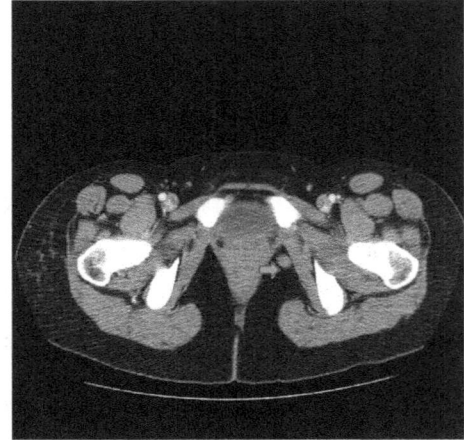

FIGURE 2

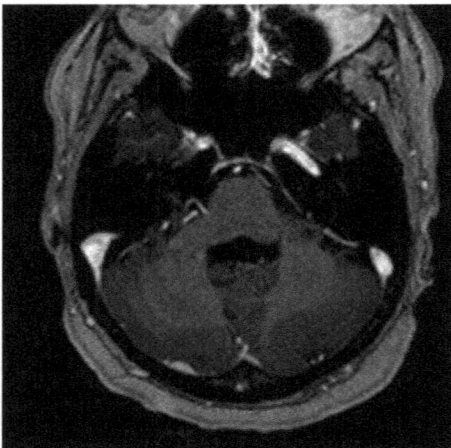

FIGURE 3

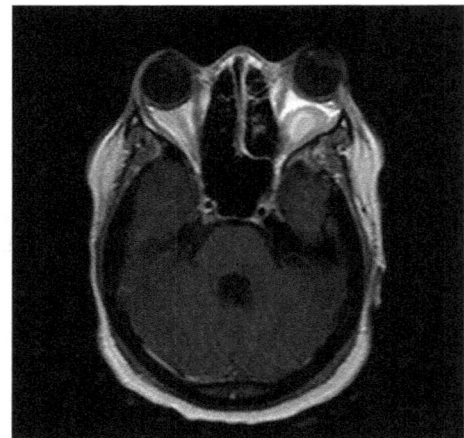

FIGURE 4

space, and the left ischiorectal fossa on computed tomography (CT) scan of the abdomen (Figure 3).

The patient was treated with cytarabine 200 mg/m² and daunorubicin 90 mg/m² (7 + 3 regimen) induction chemotherapy. Radiotherapy (RT) to the orbital MS was administered due to visual symptoms. The first treatment was on day 2 of chemotherapy. The treatment consisted of 50 cGy fractions using opposed lateral fields and half-beam blocks using 6 mV photons to both orbits. The planning was done in such a way that the lens was not in the radiation field, and the conus was included in the radiation field. Two days later, MRI of the brain showed interval resolution of the enhancing mass in the right orbital apex, decreased proptosis of the left eye secondary to decreased size, and enhancement of the orbital mass which had diminished in size to 1.5 × 1.0 cm compared to 2.6 × 1.9 cm on the prior scan (Figure 4). The dural-based mass in posterior fossa had nearly resolved. The patient had an improvement in blurry vision after two doses of RT. The patient received a total of 150 cGy to the right orbit and 200 cGy to the left orbit in four fractions over a week. The RT treatment details are shown in Table 1. There were no

TABLE 1

RT	Right orbit (cGy)	Left orbit (cGy)
Dose 1	50	50
Dose 2	50	50
Dose 3	50	50
Dose 4	0	50
Total dose	150	200

acute toxicities of RT. Complete hematologic and cytogenetic response was achieved on day 28 after the induction chemotherapy.

One month later, MRI of the brain showed a decrease in enhancement of the left orbital mass likely representing residual scar and complete resolution of MS in the right orbit and brain (Figure 5). Her visual symptoms and proptosis had resolved. There was also resolution of the dural-based posterior fossa lesion (Figure 6). CT scan of the abdomen and pelvis showed resolution of all the nodules in the abdomen and pelvis (Figure 7). She was evaluated for stem cell transplantation and was deemed to have low-risk disease. The patient proceeded to receive

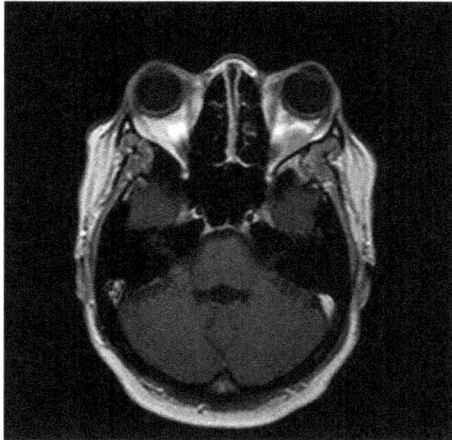

FIGURE 5

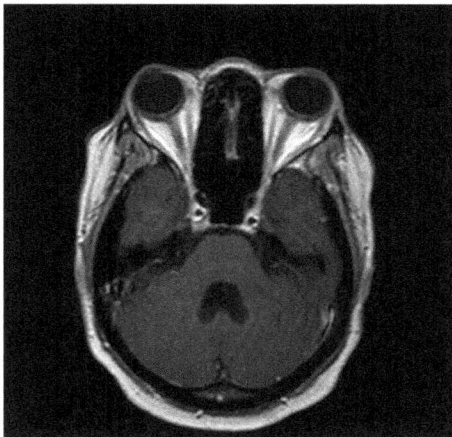

FIGURE 6

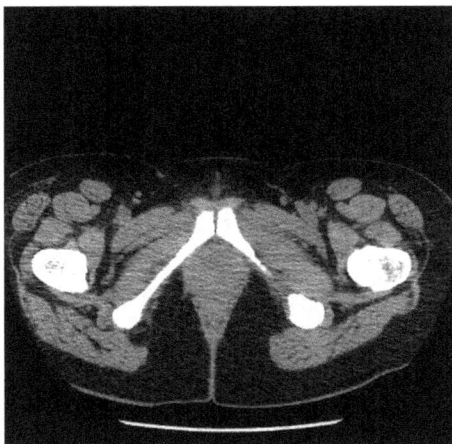

FIGURE 7

consolidation chemotherapy with high-dose cytarabine for four cycles. The patient remained in complete remission eighteen months since diagnosis. No chronic adverse effects of RT were reported.

3. Discussion

Myeloid sarcoma (MS) is a rare extramedullary (EM) tumor of immature myeloid cells, often referred to as chloroma because of its green color caused by the presence of myeloperoxidase (MPO) [1]. Primary MS may occur de novo in the absence of any past or current bone marrow involvement by acute myeloid leukemia (AML), myelodysplastic syndrome (MDS), or myeloproliferative disorder (MPD) [2]. The primary form of MS is relatively rare. On the other hand, secondary MS (associated with marrow involvement) occurs in approximately 1.4% to 9% of patients with AML [2, 3].

MS is most commonly reported in the skin, bone, and lymph nodes. It can however involve many other sites such as the central nervous system (CNS), oral and nasal mucosa, breast, genitourinary tract, chest wall, pleura, retroperitoneum, gastrointestinal tract, and testis [4, 5]. Orbital involvement is very rare in adults though commonly seen in children [6, 7]. The most common manifestation of MS is compressive symptoms involving the adjacent structures. It can also present with pain and bleeding. In the orbits, the most common symptom is proptosis. Other symptoms may include headache, photophobia, diplopia, and intermittent eye pain depending on the size of the lesions and the extent of involvement of other structures [8].

MS can be difficult to diagnose based on imaging alone especially in cases of primary MS. It can be mistaken for an abscess, hemorrhage, or even lymphoma. Imaging features, particularly of central nervous system MS, that help to distinguish these lesions from other common complications of leukemia include multiple enhancing solid masses occurring at different sites. One caveat is that a mass with an enhancing peripheral rim and a hypodense or hypointense center may be indistinguishable from an abscess. In such cases, aspiration biopsy is necessary for a definitive diagnosis. The imaging modalities commonly used are CT, magnetic resonance imaging (MRI), and FDG positron emission tomography (PET) scan. If there is bone marrow involvement, a biopsy may not be necessary for diagnosis of MS.

MS has been reported in association with a variety of chromosomal abnormalities. In particular, t(8;21)(q22;q22) has been identified in reported cases of MS occurring more commonly in childhood and/or at the orbital level [9, 10].

At initial presentation, patients with isolated MS without bone marrow involvement as well as those with AML should be treated with systemic chemotherapy. Radiation (RT) is used if there is residual disease after chemotherapy or as consolidation treatment. Surgical intervention can be considered if there is rapid enlargement of MS with significant impairment of function, especially in the CNS and orbits.

RT is typically used for CNS lesions. It can also be used for other sites if they are causing symptoms or do not resolve after systemic chemotherapy. RT was studied in a retrospective analysis of thirty eight patients who underwent treatment for MS at a single institution [11]. It should be noted that there were no patients with orbital MS in the study. It was found that RT resulted in excellent local disease control and palliation of symptoms without significant toxicity. The study authors recommended irradiating MS to at least 20 Gy and proposed 24 Gy in 12 fractions as an appropriate regimen.

In another single-institution study of twenty patients, clinicopathologic features and responses to RT of MS were studied which revealed that the CR rate was optimal using RT doses between 20 Gy and 30 Gy with conventional fractionation. 97% of the patients achieved good local control of MS. Younger age, BMT prior to RT, and AML had a higher rate of CR. It is important to note that CR rate was not statistically different between the patients who received RT dose less than 22 Gy versus greater than 22 Gy. There were no patients with orbital MS in this study as well. RT to the orbits can lead to both acute and chronic toxicities. Erythema, conjunctivitis, keratitis, corneal ulceration, iritis, and retinal edema are some of the acute adverse effects of RT. Tissue necrosis, decreased tear production, telangiectasia, scleral melting, neovascularization, retinopathy, and secondary cancers can occur as long-term sequelae of orbital RT.

In our patient with bilateral orbital MS, RT at a low dose of 200 cGy was adequate to achieve CR. MRI after the first dose of RT showed a good response with complete resolution of the right orbital lesion and a 50% reduction of the left orbital lesion. It should be noted that the patient was receiving systemic chemotherapy in addition to RT. Based on the rapid response to therapy, a short course of low-dose RT was planned to avoid potential adverse effects to the eyes. We propose that the RT dose in patients with orbital MS should be individualized based on the size and location of the lesions. It may be valuable to obtain MRI or CT scan depending on the location of MS after the first-dose RT to evaluate the response and tailor the RT treatment plan.

4. Conclusion

MS is a rare extramedullary manifestation of AML. Regardless of the location, it is considered a systemic disease and should be treated with systemic chemotherapy. Radiation therapy in addition to systemic chemotherapy has been used with success to control MS. Low dose and short course of RT may be sufficient to achieve CR in selected patients with symptomatic orbital involvement who received systemic chemotherapy.

Conflicts of Interest

The authors declare that there are no conflicts of interest regarding the publication of this paper.

References

[1] R. D. Brunnung, E. Matutes, and G. Flandrin, "Acute myeloid leukemias," in *Pathology and Genetics of Tumors of Haematopoietic and Lymphoid Tissue*, E. S. Jaffe, N. L. Harris, H. Stein, and J. W. Vardiman, Eds., pp. 77–105, World Health Organization Classification of Tumors, IARC Press, Lyon, France, 2001.

[2] A. M. Tsimberidou, H. M. Kantarjian, E. Estey et al., "Outcome in patients with nonleukemic granulocytic sarcoma treated with chemotherapy with or without radiotherapy," *Leukemia*, vol. 17, no. 6, pp. 1100–1103, 2003.

[3] R. S. Neiman, M. Barcos, C. Berard et al., "Granulocytic sarcoma: a clinicopathologic study of 61 biopsied cases," *Cancer*, vol. 48, no. 6, pp. 1426–1437, 1981.

[4] S. A. Pileri, S. Ascani, M. Cox et al., "Myeloid sarcoma: clinicopathologic, phenotypic and cytogenetic analysis of 92 adult patients," *Leukemia*, vol. 21, no. 2, pp. 340–350, 2007.

[5] H. Al-Khateeb, A. Badheeb, H. Haddad, L. Marei, and S. Abbasi, "Myeloid sarcoma: clinicopathologic, cytogenetic, and outcome analysis of 21 adult patients," *Leukemia Research and Treatment*, vol. 2011, Article ID 523168, 4 pages, 2011.

[6] V. Dinand, S. P. Yadav, A. K. Grover, S. Bhalla, and A. Sachdeva, "Orbital myeloid sarcoma presenting as massive proptosis," *Hematology/Oncology and Stem Cell Therapy*, vol. 6, no. 1, pp. 26–28, 2013.

[7] C. Payne, W. C. Olivero, B. Wang et al., "Myeloid sarcoma: a rare case of an orbital mass mimicking orbital pseudotumor requiring neurosurgical intervention," *Case Reports in Neurological Medicine*, vol. 2014, Article ID 395196, 4 pages, 2014.

[8] R. Schwyzer, G. G. Sherman, R. J. Cohn, J. E. Poole, and P. Willem, "Granulocytic sarcoma in children with acute myeloblastic leukemia and t(8;21)," *Medical and Pediatric Oncology*, vol. 31, no. 3, pp. 144–149, 1998.

[9] J. E. Rubnitz, S. C. Raimondi, A. R. Halbert et al., "Characteristics and outcome of t(8;21)-positive childhood acute myeloid leukemia: a single institution's experience," *Leukemia*, vol. 16, no. 10, pp. 2072–2077, 2002.

[10] R. Bakst, S. Wolden, and J. Yahalom, "Radiation therapy for chloroma (granulocytic sarcoma)," *International Journal of Radiation Oncology, Biology, Physics*, vol. 82, no. 5, pp. 1816–1822, 2012.

[11] W. Y. Chen, C. W. Wang, C. H. Chang et al., "Clinicopathologic features and responses to radiotherapy of myeloid sarcoma," *Radiation Oncology*, vol. 8, p. 245, 2013.

42

Dermatomyositis Associated with Myelofibrosis following Polycythemia Vera

Naomi Fei and Sarah Sofka

Department of Internal Medicine, West Virginia University Hospital, 1 Medical Center Dr., Morgantown, WV 26505, USA

Correspondence should be addressed to Naomi Fei; naomi.fei@gmail.com

Academic Editor: Eduardo Arellano-Rodrigo

Dermatomyositis (DM) is a unique inflammatory myopathy with clinical findings of proximal muscle weakness, characteristic rash, and elevated muscle enzymes. The association of DM and malignancy, most commonly adenocarcinoma, is well known. There have been few case reports of primary myelofibrosis associated with DM. We present the case of a 69-year-old male with a history of polycythemia vera (PV) who developed proximal muscle weakness, dysphagia, and rash. He was found to have elevated creatinine kinase and skin biopsy was consistent with DM. Due to persistent pancytopenia a bone marrow biopsy was performed and showed postpolycythemic myelofibrosis. To our knowledge, this is the first case reported of this unique association.

1. Introduction

Dermatomyositis (DM) is an autoimmune mediated inflammatory myopathy characterized by proximal muscle weakness and classic dermatologic findings including violaceous pigmentation (heliotrope sign) [1]. Though primarily idiopathic, DM has been associated with underlying malignancies in a paraneoplastic manner [1–4]. To our knowledge, this is the first case report with DM associated with secondary myelofibrosis following polycythemia vera.

2. Case Report

A 69-year-old male with a 15-year history of polycythemia vera (PV), JAK2 V617 positive, presented with a chief complaint of worsening weakness over 4 days. His bilateral upper and lower extremities became spontaneously weak without pain, and he reported difficulty ambulating. He also noted significant dysphagia and mild hoarseness, urinary retention, and constipation.

The patient's PV had previously been managed with hydroxyurea which was discontinued 2 months prior due to pancytopenia. Patient denied any fevers or night sweats; however, he did endorse weight loss and fatigue due to poor oral intake secondary to dysphagia.

On presentation, the patient was vitally stable. Physical exam was significant only for marked proximal, bilateral, upper, and lower extremity weakness. Splenomegaly was absent. Patient was also noted to have a violaceous rash across his forehead.

Initial complete blood cell count was significant for leukopenia with left shift (WBC 3.1 g/dL), normocytic anemia (Hgb 7.0 g/dL, MCV 89.9 fL), and a normal platelet count. Peripheral blood smear noted teardrop red blood cells and circulating nucleated red cells (Figure 1). ESR was mildly elevated (26) as was CRP (8.5) indicative of an inflammatory state. Labs supportive of myositis included elevated creatinine kinase (6201 U/L), aldolase (42 U/L), LDH (747 U/L), and myoglobin (2843 mcg/L).

MRI with contrast of the spine and brachial plexus were positive for edema of all visualized muscle groups compatible with myositis. Muscle biopsy was attempted but was nondiagnostic and open surgical biopsy was considered. Due to ongoing comorbid conditions, less invasive skin biopsy was performed instead. Pathology at the site of violaceous rash on forehead was consistent with dermatomyositis (Figures 2–4).

Given age and dysphagia at presentation, patient was at high risk for underlying neoplastic process and a malignancy screen was performed. Serum paraneoplastic antibody panel was positive only for striational antibody with titer

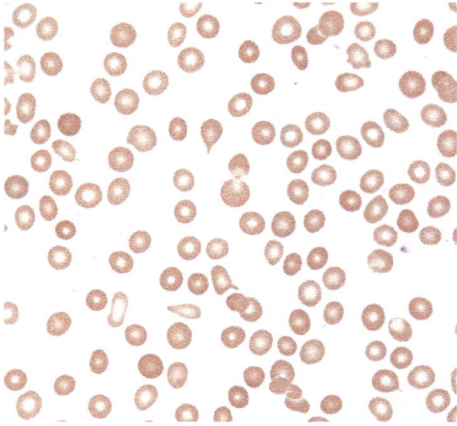

FIGURE 1: Peripheral blood smear with pancytopenia and teardrop red blood cells (Wright 400x).

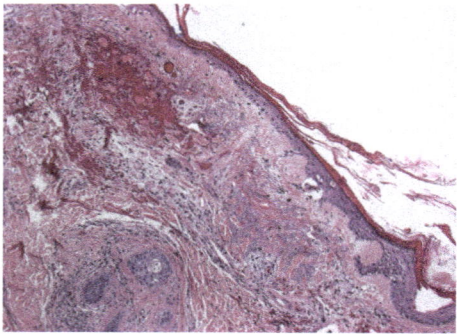

FIGURE 2: Epidermal atrophy with prominent basement membrane (H&E 100x). Dermal edema with blue mucin and mild perivascular mononuclear infiltrate (mainly lymphocytes).

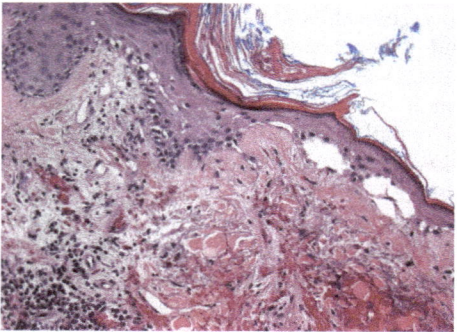

FIGURE 3: Vacuolar change due to basal cell degeneration (H&E 200x). Civatte bodies at the papillary dermis. Prominent perivascular lymphocytes at left lower corner.

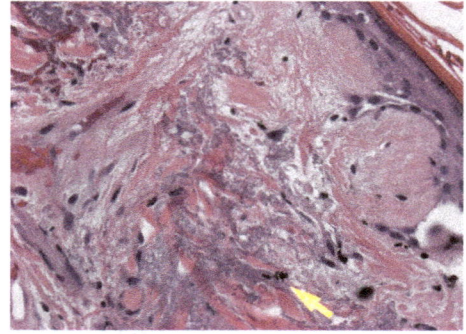

FIGURE 4: Melanin incontinence into dermis (yellow arrow) (H&E 400x).

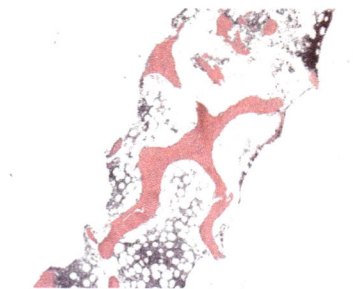

FIGURE 5: The bone is normocellular with megakaryocytic hyperplasia and moderate fibrosis (bone marrow, left posterior iliac crest, clot section, and trephine core biopsies, 100x).

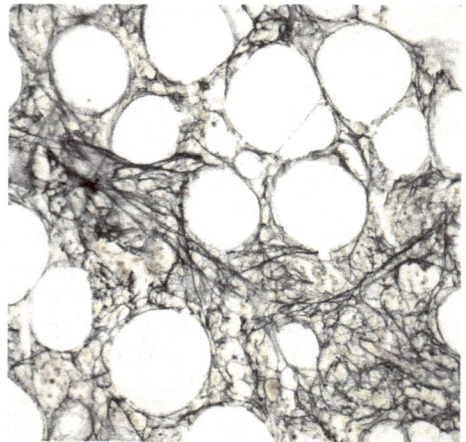

FIGURE 6: Marrow reticulin fibers moderately increased with storage iron present (bone marrow biopsy, left posterior iliac crest, and reticulin stain, 400x).

1:960. CSF paraneoplastic antibody was negative. CT with contrast of the chest, abdomen, and pelvis was negative for splenomegaly and masses.

Due to history of PV and declining blood counts, a bone marrow biopsy was performed. Immunohistochemical staining with CD34, CD71, Factor VIII, and MPO was performed. Pathologist review reported normocellular marrow with megakaryocyte hyperplasia, mild decrease in erythroid precursors, and moderate fibrosis (Figures 5-6). Results were consistent with postpolycythemic myelofibrosis (MF). Staging yielded IPSS 2 (INT-1) and DIPSS 3 (INT-2), high intermediate to high risk MF. Given the temporal relationship of symptom onset with conversion of PV to MF, the patient was considered to have dermatomyositis associated with secondary MF.

Original treatment included prednisone 40 mg daily and azathioprine 100 mg daily; however, symptoms progressed and pancytopenia worsened over 2 weeks. Azathioprine and prednisone were discontinued, and intravenous immunoglobulin (IVIG) was administered. 1 day after treatment, the patient developed shortness of breath and was found to have a pulmonary embolus with right peroneal deep vein thrombosis. IVIG was subsequently discontinued and the patient was treated with warfarin. Prednisone was restarted at an increase of 60 mg daily and azathioprine was restarted at 100 mg daily. The patient experienced gradual resolution of weakness but required G-tube placement for continued dysphagia.

At a six-month follow-up patient reported resolving weakness with regain of ambulation and swallowing capacity. At this time, prednisone is gradually being tapered. Post-polycythemic MF is currently managed with surveillance as patient is not transfusion dependent and is not a transplant candidate given poor performance status.

3. Discussion

Dermatomyositis (DM) is an autoimmune mediated inflammatory myopathy characterized by proximal muscle weakness and classic dermatologic findings including violaceous pigmentation (heliotrope sign). Definitive diagnosis of DM requires a skin or muscle biopsy in the setting of clinical disease [1].

While the majority of DM is idiopathic in etiology, 15–30% of adult onset DM is associated with malignancy [2, 3]. Risk factors of underlying malignancy in the setting of adult onset DM include older age at disease onset, dysphagia, evidence of capillary damage on muscle biopsy, and cutaneous leukocytoclastic vasculitis [5–7]. While ovarian and lung cancers are most frequently identified with DM, hematologic malignancies have also been associated, most commonly B-cell lymphoma, T-cell lymphoma, and myelodysplastic syndrome [8–11]. There have also been individual cases of primary myelofibrosis associated with DM [4, 12, 13]. To our knowledge, this is the first case of secondary myelofibrosis that has been associated with dermatomyositis.

Autoimmunity is a common theme of both DM and MF. DM is a known autoimmune inflammatory myopathy and MF is associated with increased autoantibody production and circulating immune complexes [4, 12]. Additionally, the association between autoimmune disorders and idiopathic MF has been reported in 10–14% of cases [14–17]. This case of postpolycythemic MF presents the possibility of an immune paraneoplastic mechanism associating secondary MF and DM. Regenerating muscle cells in myositis have been observed to express antigens similar to cancer tissue [1, 18]. In the setting of hematologic malignancy, a paraneoplastic immune response may inadvertently target muscle tissue leading to DM.

The differential diagnosis of this case includes hydroxyurea induced DM-like eruption. Prior case reports have shown development of DM while on hydroxyurea and resolution of DM after cessation of the medication [19, 20]. Given that this patient stopped hydroxyurea 2 months prior to the onset of DM, hydroxyurea induced DM is a less likely diagnosis.

Immunosuppression with concurrent treatment of the underlying malignancy is indicated in the setting of paraneoplastic DM. First-line immunosuppressive therapy often includes prednisone. Prior cases of primary myelofibrosis have shown response to azathioprine and prednisone regimens [12]. However, as seen in this case, neoplastic DM may demonstrate poorer response to treatment than DM in the absence of cancer [1]. High dose intravenous steroids have been documented as a potential second-line therapy [21]. IVIG has also been shown to be beneficial in resistant cases of DM [22, 23].

Prior case reports have documented resolution of DM after treatment of underlying neoplasm [24, 25]. Unfortunately, given the poor clinical condition many patients with paraneoplastic DM present with, surgical resection or chemotherapy may not be tolerated.

An alternative therapeutic target may be the Janus Kinase (JAK) 2 receptor with inhibitors such as ruxolitinib or tofacitinib. JAK2 activating mutations including V617F have been found in multiple myeloproliferative neoplasms such as PV, essential thrombocytopenia, and MF [26]. JAK kinase overactivity has also been noted in several autoimmune disorders including rheumatoid arthritis, systemic lupus erythematosus, and other autoantibody-driven diseases [27]. Given its activity in both autoimmune and myeloproliferative processes, JAK2 inhibition would be a reasonable target in paraneoplastic DM. Case reports documenting concurrent resolution of dermatomyositis and post-PV MF after use of ruxolitinib have been previously reported [28].

Conflicts of Interest

The authors declare that there are no conflicts of interest regarding the publication of this paper.

Acknowledgments

The authors acknowledge Ali Makki Aldawood, M.D., West Virginia University Hospital, Department of Pathology, 1 Medical Center Dr., Morgantown, WV 26505.

References

[1] M. Wolff, C. Mancuso et al., "Paraneoplastic Dermatomyositis with cutaneous and myopathic disease responsive to adrenocorticotropic hormone therapy," *The Journal of Clinical and Aesthetic Dermatology*, vol. 10, no. 1, pp. 57–62, 2017.

[2] J. P. Callen, J. F. Hyla, G. G. Bole, and D. R. Kay, "The Relationship of Dermatomyositis and Polymyositis to Internal Malignancy," *Archives of Dermatology*, vol. 116, no. 3, pp. 295–298, 1980.

[3] B. E. Barnes, "Dermatomyositis and malignancy: a review of the literature," *Annals of Internal Medicine*, vol. 84, no. 1, pp. 68–76, 1976.

[4] H. Taskapan, S. Gürsoy, M. Cetin, O. Oymak, and Ö. Özbakir, "Development of dermatomyositis in a patient with primary myelofibrosis," *Hematology*, vol. 6, no. 2, pp. 131–134, 2001.

[5] A. Urbano-Marquez, J. Casademont, and J. M. Grau, "Polymyositis/dermatomyositis: The current position," *Annals of the Rheumatic Diseases*, vol. 50, no. 3, pp. 191–195, 1991.

[6] R. E. Hunger, C. Dürr, and C. U. Brand, "Cutaneous leukocytoclastic vasculitis in dermatomyositis suggests malignancy," *Dermatology*, vol. 202, no. 2, pp. 123–126, 2001.

[7] J. Wang, G. Guo, G. Chen, B. Wu, L. Lu, and L. Bao, "Meta-analysis of the association of dermatomyositis and polymyositis with cancer," *British Journal of Dermatology*, vol. 169, no. 4, pp. 838–847, 2013.

[8] B. Sigurgeirsson, B. Lindelöf, O. Edhag, and E. Allander, "Risk of cancer in patients with dermatomyositis or polymyositis," *The New England Journal of Medicine*, vol. 326, no. 6, pp. 363–367, 1992.

[9] C. L. Hill, Y. Zhang, B. Sigurgeirsson et al., "Frequency of specific cancer types in dermatomyositis and polymyositis: a population-based study," *The Lancet*, vol. 357, no. 9250, pp. 96–100, 2001.

[10] I. Marie, L. Guillevin, J.-F. Menard et al., "Hematological malignancy associated with polymyositis and dermatomyositis," *Autoimmunity Reviews*, vol. 11, no. 9, pp. 615–620, 2012.

[11] G. Tsuji, S. Maekawa, K. Saigo et al., "Dermatomyositis and Myelodysplastic Syndrome with Myelofibrosis Responding to Methotrexate Therapy," *American Journal of Hematology*, vol. 74, no. 3, pp. 175–178, 2003.

[12] A. Ito, M. Umeda et al., "A case of dermatomyositis associated with chronic idiopathic myelofibrosis," *Rinsho Shinkeigaku*, vol. 46, no. 3, pp. 210–213, 2006.

[13] A. Muslimani, M. S. Ahluwalia, P. Palaparty, and H. A. Daw, "Idiopathic myelofibrosis associated with dermatomyositis," *American Journal of Hematology*, vol. 81, no. 7, pp. 559-560, 2006.

[14] H. Enright and W. Miller, "Autoimmune phenomena in patients with myelodysplastic syndromes," *Leukemia & Lymphoma*, vol. 24, no. 5-6, pp. 483–489, 1997.

[15] T. Okamoto, M. Okada, A. Mori, K. Sabeki et al., "Correlation between immunological abnormalities and prognosis in myelodysplastic syndrome patients," *The International Journal of Hematology*, vol. 66, pp. 345–351, 1997.

[16] L. I. Kornblihtt, P. S. Vassalllu, P. G. Heller, N. R. Lago, C. L. Alvarez, and F. C. Molinas, "Primary myelofibrosis in a patient who developed primary biliary cirrhosis, autoimmune hemolytic anemia and fibrillary glomerulonephritis," *Annals of Hematology*, vol. 87, no. 12, pp. 1019-1020, 2008.

[17] M. Camós, E. Arellano-Rodrigo, D. Abelló et al., "Idiopathic myelofibrosis associated with classic polyarteritis nodosa," *Leukemia and Lymphoma*, vol. 44, no. 3, pp. 539–541, 2003.

[18] L. Casciola-Rosen, K. Nagaraju, P. Plotz et al., "Enhanced autoantigen expression in regenerating muscle cells in idiopathic inflammatory myopathy," *Journal of Experimental Medicine*, vol. 201, no. 4, pp. 591–601, 2005.

[19] T. M. Zappala, K. Rodins, and J. Muir, "Hydroxyurea induced dermatomyositis-like eruption," *Australasian Journal of Dermatology*, vol. 53, no. 3, pp. e58–e60, 2012.

[20] B. de Unamuno-Bustos, R. Ballester-Sánchez, V. Sabater Marco, and J. Vilata-Corell, "Dermatomyositis-Like Eruption Associated With Hydroxyurea Therapy: A Premalignant Condition?" *Actas Dermo-Sifiliográficas (English Edition)*, vol. 105, no. 9, pp. 876–878, 2014.

[21] I. Arshad and D. Barton, "Dermatomyositis as a paraneoplastic phenomenon in ovarian cancer," *BMJ Case Reports*, vol. 2016, Article ID 215463, 2016.

[22] M. C. Dalakas, "Intravenous immunoglobulin in autoimmune neuromuscular diseases," *Journal of the American Medical Association*, vol. 291, no. 19, pp. 2367–2375, 2004.

[23] S. Aslanidis, A. Pyrpasopoulou, N. Kartali, and C. Zamboulis, "Successful treatment of refractory rash in paraneoplastic amyopathic dermatomyositis," *Clinical Rheumatology*, vol. 26, no. 7, pp. 1198–1200, 2007.

[24] H. Kamiyama, K. Niwa, S. Ishiyama et al., "Ascending Colon Cancer Associated with Dermatomyositis Which Was Cured after Colon Resection," *Case Reports in Gastroenterology*, vol. 10, no. 2, pp. 338–343, 2016.

[25] H. Yoshie, R. Nakazawa, W. Usuba et al., "Paraneoplastic Dermatomyositis Associated with Metastatic Seminoma," *Case Reports in Urology*, Article ID 7050981, 2016.

[26] A. Sanz, D. Ungureanu, T. Pekkala et al., "Analysis of jak2 catalytic function by peptide microarrays: The role of the JH2 domain and V617F mutation," *PLoS ONE*, vol. 6, no. 4, Article ID e18522, 2011.

[27] M. M. Seavey and P. Dobrzanski, "The many faces of Janus kinase," *Biochemical Pharmacology*, vol. 83, no. 9, pp. 1136–1145, 2012.

[28] T. Hornung, V. Janzen, and J. Wenzel, "Remission of recalcitrant dermatomyositis treated with ruxolitinib," *New England Journal of Medicine*, vol. 371, no. 26, pp. 2537-2538, 2014.

43

A Giant Right Heart Thrombus-in-Transit: The Challenge of Anticoagulation in Factor V Leiden Thrombophilia

Andrew Chu [ID],[1] **Thu Thu Aung,**[1] **Minni Shreya Arumugam,**[2] **Mauricio Danckers,**[1] **Mohi Mitiek,**[1] **and Jonathan Leslie**[1]

[1]*Internal Medicine Residency Department, Aventura Hospital and Medical Center, 20900 Biscayne Boulevard, Aventura, FL 33190, USA*
[2]*Internal Medicine Residency Department, SUNY Upstate Medical University, 750 East Adams Street, Syracuse, NY 13210, USA*

Correspondence should be addressed to Andrew Chu; andrewxu29@yahoo.com

Academic Editor: Tomás J. González-López

Factor V Leiden (FVL) is an autosomal dominant condition resulting in thrombophilia. Factor V normally acts as a cofactor for prothrombinase, helping cleave prothrombin to thrombin. A single point mutation in it disrupts factor V, making it unreceptive to protein C and increasing the risk of thrombosis. FVL mutation associated with right heart thrombus is a rare entity. Right heart thrombus or right heart thrombus-in-transit is associated with high mortality. We present a 51-year-old male with a past medical history of FVL homozygous mutation and recurrent blood clots, who has failed multiple different oral anticoagulants. He presented to the hospital with symptoms of shortness of breath and subsequently found to have a giant right heart thrombus. He was treated with surgical embolectomy. This case underscores the challenges faced by patients with FVL and recurrent blood clots.

1. Introduction

Right heart thrombus-in-transit (RHTT) is a rare occurrence and is associated with high mortality if left untreated. Increasing use of echocardiography has helped identify this disease early. RHTT associated with FVL thrombophilia proved to be a great challenge for clinicians due to the lack of strong medical evidence. No long-term anticoagulation is recommended in asymptomatic FVL homozygotes or heterozygotes [1]. For FVL patients, who have an active clot, long-term anticoagulation is recommended. The duration of treatment is decided on individual basis. We report a case of giant RHTT in a 51-year-old man with FVL mutation and recurrent blood clots who had been on multiple different oral anticoagulants. This case hopes to bring out the topic of RHTT and raises the challenges of anticoagulation in such individuals.

2. Case Presentation

A 51-year-old male was admitted to our hospital with a three-day history of shortness of breath. He mentioned of dry cough associated with chest discomfort. The pain was localized to the mid-sternum, nonradiating, exacerbated in supine position, and improved with sitting. He was taking aspirin at home for his symptoms. He denied history of sick contact, fever, chills, weight loss, night sweat, diaphoresis, palpitation, or dizziness.

He had an extensive past history including FVL homozygous mutation, recurrent lower extremity deep venous thrombosis (DVT) with inferior vena cava (IVC) filter placed, congestive heart failure requiring automatic implantable cardioverter-defibrillator (AICD) placement, and hypertension.

The patient was initially diagnosed with FVL mutation when he had his first episode of lower extremity DVT in 2002. At that time, he was placed on warfarin therapy with a goal international normalized ratio (INR) of 2-3. In 2007, he had a recurrent episode of lower extremity DVT and bilateral pulmonary embolism (PE) despite being compliant with warfarin and close INR monitoring. His INR on admission was 2.1. During admission, he had an IVC filter placed and his goal INR was increased to 2.5–3.5. In 2015, he had another recurrent lower extremity

DVT despite having a higher target INR of 3.2. Warfarin was switched to rivaroxaban 15 mg twice a day for 21 days followed by 20 mg once daily. He denied a family history of malignancy or thrombophilia. He did undergo computed tomography (CT) of the abdomen and pelvis in 2015 which did not show gross evidence of intra-abdominal or pelvic mass. CT of the chest did not show evidence of pulmonary nodule.

The patient was taking aspirin 81 mg daily, atorvastatin 40 mg daily at bedtime, carvedilol 3.125 mg twice daily, lisinopril 5 mg daily, furosemide 40 mg daily, and rivaroxaban 20 mg once daily. The vital signs on admission were 99.5°F, heart rate 130 beats per minute, blood pressure 120/75 mmHg, respiratory rate 18 breaths per minute, and oxygen saturation 94% on 32% fraction of inspired oxygen. Physical examination was remarkable for distend jugular vein and crackles at bilateral lung bases. The results of blood work including complete blood count and comprehensive metabolic panel were within normal limits. Blood urea nitrogen was 19 mg/dL and serum creatinine was 0.9 mg/dL. Work up for autoimmune diseases came back negative. His prothrombin time was 26.1 seconds, activated partial thromboplastin time was 31.9 seconds, and the international normalized ratio was 2.35. Anterior-posterior chest X-ray illustrated a normal pattern. Venous Doppler of lower extremities revealed acute non-occlusive extensive thrombosis involving the bilateral common femoral, femoral, and popliteal veins. CT of the chest with contrast showed absence of pulmonary embolism, questionable right ventricular mass, moderate-sized pericardial effusion, and reflux of iodine contrast into the IVC and hepatic veins, suggesting right heart strain (Figure 1). Transthoracic echocardiogram showed ejection fraction between 25 and 30%, moderate diffuse hypokinesis of the left ventricle, and dilated left atrium. There was a definite, large, echogenic, highly mobile mass measuring 5.29 cm × 8.61 cm, up to 9.1 cm in length. The mass extended from the right atrium to the right ventricle, moving back-and-forth across the tricuspid valve (Figure 2). Ultrasound of IVC showed patent IVC filter without clots. He was taken for emergent right atrial and ventricular embolectomy. The thrombus was found to be originating from the coronary sinus (Figure 3). There were a small amount of clots around the AICD wires which were removed. Repeat transthoracic echocardiogram showed no mass, but mildly dilated right atrium and ventricle with trace pericardial effusion. The patient was then started on unfractionated heparin drip.

On postoperative day 11, the patient underwent sternal wound re-exploration due to gradual downward trend of his hemoglobin. He had a sternal dehiscence during which an extensive clot was found despite being on anticoagulation with unfractionated heparin drip. Heparin-induced antibody was negative. He had the clot removed surgically. The patient continued to improve and transitioned from unfractionated heparin drip with target PTT 50–60 seconds to dabigatran 150 mg oral twice a day. He was subsequently discharged to cardiac rehab facility and has been doing well.

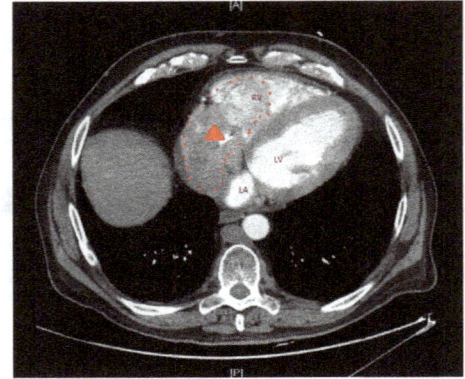

Figure 1: CT angiography of thorax displaying a suspected mass (dotted line) in the right side of the heart embedding the defibrillator wire (in red arrow head).

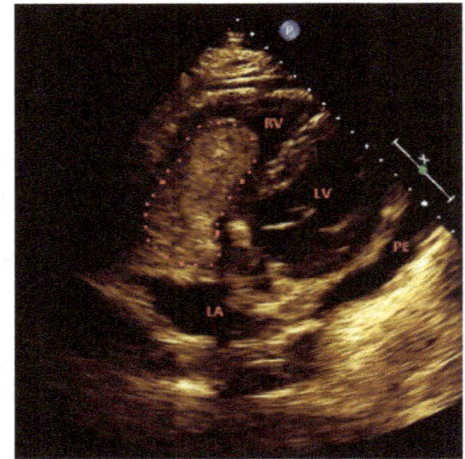

Figure 2: Transthoracic echocardiogram apical four chamber view showing the mobile mass (dotted line) within the right side of the heart. RV, right ventricle; LV, left ventricle; LA, left atrium; PE, pericardial effusion.

3. Discussion

Right heart thrombus-in-transit (RHTT) occurs in 4% of pulmonary embolism. It can originate and be dislodged from extremities DVT, form in situ due to structural heart disease, or sometimes be associated with hardware such as pacemakers and prosthetic valves. The overall mortality rate in patient with RHTT is 28% [2]. Management of RHTT includes anticoagulation, systemic thrombolysis, catheter-directed intervention, or surgical embolectomy. In the recent meta-analysis published by Athappan et al. [3], surgical embolectomy has the greatest mortality benefit compared to systemic thrombolysis or anticoagulation alone (13.9%, 18.3%, and 37.1%, respectively). Very limited medical literatures have been published regarding management of RHTT in patients with FVL mutation.

FVL mutation is the most common inherited hypercoagulable state. It occurs due to a single point mutation on chromosome one, a G-to-A substitution leading to an amino acid replacement. This mutation leads to the inability of

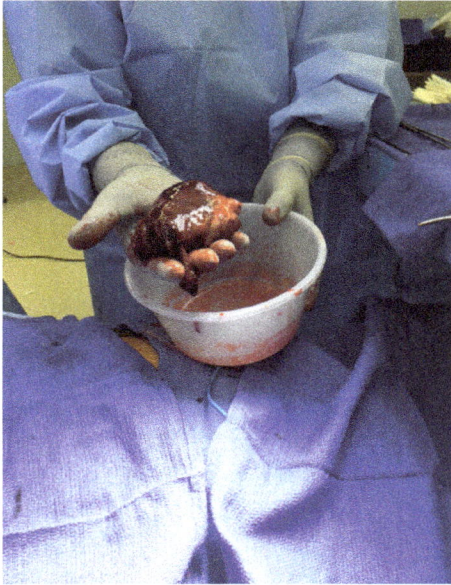

FIGURE 3: The giant right heart thrombus from surgical embolectomy.

protein C to cleave and degrade factor V, leading to increased tendency to form blood clots [4]. Individuals who are heterozygous for FVL mutation have three to eightfold increased risk of venous thrombosis. The risk increased to 18- to 80-fold in individuals who are homozygous for FVL mutation [5]. Hence, the probability of developing an intracardiac thrombus would be higher in patients with hypercoagulable disorders than the general population. In addition to inherited hypercoagulability, intracardiac foreign bodies such as pacemakers and prosthetic valves have been associated with right heart thrombus.

No treatment is warranted for asymptomatic patients with FVL. For individuals with first venous thromboembolic event, anticoagulation therapy is generally administered for 6 months [4]. The treatment for venous thromboembolism includes initial anticoagulation with intravenous unfractionated heparin or subcutaneous low-molecular-weight heparin followed by oral anticoagulation with warfarin (target INR between 2 and 3). Prolonged duration with anticoagulation may be considered for certain individuals with increased recurrence risk of venous thromboembolism and uncertain nature of the index of venous thromboembolism [6]. However, any decision regarding the ideal duration of therapy must take into account the risk of bleeding with prolonged anticoagulation. FVL heterozygosity or prothrombin G20210A should not influence decisions about duration of anticoagulation therapy [4]. For individuals who developed recurrent venous thromboembolism while on warfarin, and their INR was within the target range of 2 and 3, an increased target INR or switching to a different oral anticoagulant can be considered. This must be done after weighing the risks and benefits. However, there is no medical literature to support this practice as events of recurrent venous thromboembolism are rare in FVL. Most importantly, clinicians must ensure patients are compliant with oral anticoagulation therapy.

Newer oral anticoagulants such as direct thrombin inhibitor (dabigatran) and factor Xa inhibitors (rivaroxaban, apixaban, and edoxaban) can be considered for patients who developed recurrent venous thromboembolism despite being compliant with warfarin therapy. These medications do not require frequent blood monitoring or dose adjustment. They also have lower interaction with other medications. Currently, there are reversal agents for dabigatran and rivaroxaban, should there be a need of one. There are currently no available data regarding the role of these newer oral anticoagulants in FVL.

Our patient with FVL homozygosity had a history of multiple recurrent venous thromboembolic events despite being on warfarin therapy and good medication compliance. He presented once again with another recurrent venous thromboembolism despite being on rivaroxaban. Therefore, we decided to anticoagulate our patient with dabigatran which has different pharmacologic mechanisms from warfarin and rivaroxaban.

Several cases have been reported regarding inheritable hypercoagulable states and RHTT. Nagae et al. reported a right ventricular mass in a 14-year-old girl who subsequently diagnosed with familial heparin cofactor II deficiency [7]. Corre et al. reported a case of coronary sinus thrombosis due to FVL [8]. Hajsadeghi et al. reported a 36-year-old man presented with productive coughs and hemoptysis [9]. He was subsequently found to have a right ventricular thrombosis and diagnosed with FVL.

Our patient's right-sided intracardiac thrombus is the largest ever reported associated with FVL. Significant attention was brought to our treatment team on how much hemodynamic compensation our patient has developed despite the thrombus causing almost-total-occlusion of blood flow from the right atrium to the right ventricle. Hemodynamic compensation was largely due to hypermobility of the RHTT, preventing the total occlusion of blood flow through the tricuspid valve. Our patient also had acquired factors for thrombophilia including low blood flow state due to underlying cardiomyopathy and presence of AICD wires and IVC filter which were the nidus for thrombosis. We believe that the patient's underlying inherited thrombophilia played the greatest role in developing this massive RHTT. The choice of anticoagulation continues to be the challenge in our patient as he had failed on two different anticoagulants in the past.

4. Conclusion

We have known inherited thrombophilia for several decades. However, the role of anticoagulation and different anticoagulants continues to be mysterious as there are no clear guidelines. This becomes a more challenging subject when dealing with RHTT, a near fatal disease if not managed properly. More studies are required to define the roles of different anticoagulants in inherited thrombophilia.

Conflicts of Interest

The authors declare that they have no conflicts of interest.

References

[1] V. de Stefano, P. Chiusolo, K. Paciaroni, and G. Leone, "Epidemiology of factor V Leiden: clinical implications," *Seminars in Thrombosis and Hemostasis*, vol. 24, no. 4, pp. 367–379, 1998.

[2] J. L. Carson, M. A. Kelley, A. Duff et al., "The clinical course of pulmonary embolism," *New England Journal of Medicine*, vol. 326, no. 19, pp. 1240–1245, 1992.

[3] G. Athappan, P. Sengodan, P. Chacko, and S. Gandhi, "Comparative efficacy of different modalities for treatment of right heart thrombi in transit: a pooled analysis," *Vascular Medicine*, vol. 20, no. 2, pp. 131–138, 2015.

[4] J. L. Kujovich, "Factor V Leiden thrombophilia," *Genetics in Medicine*, vol. 13, no. 1, pp. 1–16, 2011.

[5] R. M. Bertina, B. P. Koeleman, T. Koster et al., "Mutation in blood coagulation factor V associated with resistance to activated protein C," *Nature*, vol. 369, no. 6475, pp. 64–67, 1994.

[6] S. R. Deitcher and M. C. P. Gomes, "Hypercoagulable States," in *Cleveland Clinic*, Cleveland Clinic, Cleveland, OH, USA, 2003.

[7] N. Nagae, T. Watanabe, M. Miura, T. Minowa, S. Hirooka, and M. Washio, "Right ventricular thrombosis due to familial heparin cofactor II deficiency," *Kyobu Geka. The Japanese Journal of Thoracic Surgery*, vol. 43, no. 10, pp. 830–834, 1990.

[8] O. Corre, G. Gueret, M. Gilard, J. F. Abgrall, and C. C. Arvieux, "Coronary thrombosis on patient with the factor V Leiden mutation," *Annales Francaises d'Anesthesie et de Reanimation*, vol. 21, no. 5, pp. 440–444, 2002.

[9] S. Hajsadeghi, R. Naghshin, M. Hejrati, and S. R. J. Kerman, "Right ventricular thrombus in a 36-year-old man with factor V Leiden," *Journal of Tehran University Heart Center*, vol. 10, no. 1, pp. 46–49, 2015.

44

Transformation of T-Cell Acute Lymphoblastic Lymphoma to Peripheral T-Cell Lymphoma

Michael Markow,[1] Abu-Sayeef Mirza (ID),[2] Lia Perez,[3] Haipeng Shao,[4] Pedro Horna,[5] Claudio Anasetti,[4] Lubomir Sokol,[4] and Mohammad O. Hussaini[4]

[1]Department of Pathology, Ohio State University, Columbus, OH, USA
[2]Department of Internal Medicine, University of South Florida, Tampa, FL, USA
[3]Bone Marrow Transplant Program, Moffitt Cancer Center, Tampa, FL, USA
[4]Moffitt Cancer Center, Tampa, FL, USA
[5]Mayo Clinic, Rochester, MN, USA

Correspondence should be addressed to Abu-Sayeef Mirza; mirzaa@mail.usf.edu

Academic Editor: Salah Aref

Nonhepatosplenic/noncutaneous $\gamma\delta$ peripheral T-cell lymphoma (NHNC$\gamma\delta$ PTCL) represents a miscellaneous group of unrelated T-cell lymphomas of which only isolated cases have been reported. We describe two cases of transformation from T-lymphoblastic leukemia/lymphoma to NHNC$\gamma\delta$ PTCL. Transformation into more aggressive disease is a rare event in T-cell lineage-derived hematologic malignancies compared to B-cell neoplasms. Nevertheless, both of our cases involved relapse as PTCL manifested with skin involvement and an overt shift from blastic morphology to large granular leukemia-like mature T cells. Among other notable molecular characteristics, expression of immature markers such as TdT was lost in both cases. Based on cytogenetics, phenotype, and morphology, both patients represent a novel phenomenon of clonal transformation from T-ALL to PTCL which has rarely been reported in the literature. Such transformation may carry important diagnostic and biological implications.

1. Introduction

Peripheral T-cell lymphomas (PTCLs) comprise a heterogeneous group of indolent and aggressive T-cell lymphomas that confer a variable prognosis [1]. T-cell receptor gamma-delta (TCR$\gamma\delta$) PTCLs are characterized based on their expression of $\gamma\delta$ glycoproteins within the TCR complex rather than more common alpha-beta ($\alpha\beta$) glycoproteins identified in normal T-cells and in most T-cell neoplasms [2]. $\gamma\delta$ T-cells are subdivided into Vδ1 and Vδ2 subtypes and have demonstrated capacity for cytotoxicity, memory, and antigen presentation [3]. Mature $\gamma\delta$ PTCLs have no clear etiology to date and can be divided into three categories based on location: hepatosplenic (HSTL$\gamma\delta$), cutaneous (PCTCL$\gamma\delta$), and nonhepatosplenic/noncutaneous (NHNC$\gamma\delta$ PTCL). HSTL$\gamma\delta$ and PCTCL$\gamma\delta$ both carry a similarly dismal prognosis [4].

NHNC$\gamma\delta$ PTCL represents a miscellaneous group of unrelated T-cell lymphomas of which only isolated cases have been reported; thus, characterization remains limited. Reported sites of involvement include lymph nodes and mucosal sites (nasopharynx and intestine), as well as the larynx, thyroid, lung, breast, and testis [5–8]. NHNC$\gamma\delta$ subtypes of PTCLs generally behave more aggressively compared to $\alpha\beta$ counterparts with an exception of $\gamma\delta$ variant of T-cell large granular lymphocyte (LGL) leukemia [9].

No cytogenetics findings unique to NHNC$\gamma\delta$ PTCL have been reported [10]. i7q, if detected, is not specific to $\gamma\delta$ PCTLs [11]. Gene sequencing of $\gamma\delta$ PCTLs has demonstrated conservation of *LGR4*, *C3AR1*, and *SCARF2* among all $\gamma\delta$ PTCLs [12]. Notably, the NHNC$\gamma\delta$ PTCLs had *CCL19*, *MMP9*, and *UBD* mutations, whereas HSTL$\gamma\delta$ PCTLs did not. These mutations were also strongly conserved in the $\alpha\beta$ PTCLs studied. Although there is evidence that some variants of $\gamma\delta$ PTCLs respond *in vitro* to aurora kinase inhibitors, among all PTCLs, those with TCR$\gamma\delta$ have the worst prognoses [13–15].

(a)

(b)

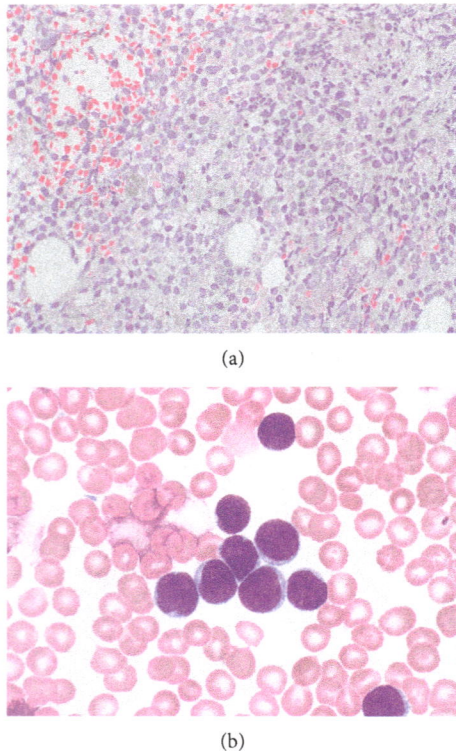

FIGURE 1: Patient 1, bone marrow with T-cell ALL: (a) H&E core biopsy, 500x; (b) aspirate cytology, 1000x.

As opposed to PTCL, the expression of $\gamma\delta$ TCR is relatively common in (up to 50%) in T-lymphoblastic leukemia/lymphoma (T-ALL). Clinical features are similar to those that express $\alpha\beta$ TCR, and outcomes are comparable [8]. Here, we describe a case of transformation from T-ALL to NHNC$\gamma\delta$ PTCL. Despite being rarely reported, we also report a second case of PTCL arising in a patient with prior T-ALL. Such transformation may carry important diagnostic and biological implications.

2. Case Presentations

2.1. Patient 1. Patient 1 is a 31-year-old gentleman diagnosed with T-cell ALL after presenting with diffuse petechial rash, cervical lymphadenopathy, abdominal pain, and a WBC of 121 K/μL with 40% blasts (Figure 1). Cytogenetics showed 46, XY,add(13) (p11.2)[3]/46,XY[17]. No BCR/ABL was detected by FISH; CSF was uninvolved. T-ALL was CD4+/CD8+, CD2+, CD3+, CD5+ (dim), CD7+, and TdT (dim). He was treated with vincristine, daunorubicin, pegylated L-asparaginase, and prednisolone achieving complete remission (CR). He was referred for hematopoietic stem cell transplant three months later which was delayed due to chemotherapy complications. During this period, he received leucovorin and glucarpidase. Prior to the transplant, a bone marrow biopsy was negative, but revealed clonal TCR β and γ gene rearrangements. In addition, CSF showed numerous LGL-like cells. The patient developed high grade fever and over one hundred erythematous plaques on his trunk, upper

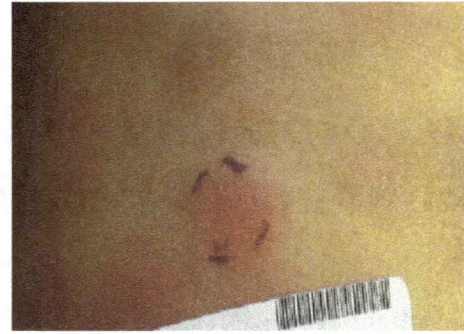

FIGURE 2: Patient 1, erythematous patches and plaques of PTCL distributed predominantly on torso and upper extremities.

extremities, and lower extremities (Figure 2). Skin biopsy showed NHNC$\gamma\delta$ PTCL (Figure 3) as did staging bone marrow biopsy (Figure 4). The malignant cells demonstrated mature chromatin, LGL-like morphology with prominent azurophilic granules resembling those seen in patient 2's PTCL (see below). They coexpressed CD4, CD8, CD56, cytotoxic markers, and γ- TCR. TdT was negative. Molecular studies of the PTCL demonstrated that both the T-ALL and PTCL shared identical clonal TCR rearrangement peaks for both TCR β and TCR γ (Table 1).

Six months after initial CR, the patient was initiated on ICE therapy and intra-Ommaya reservoir methotrexate (later switched to intrathecal cytarabine). The skin lesions and CSF involvement initially resolved; however, he developed fevers, new generalized skin $\delta\gamma$-PTCL, nodal/hepatic progression by radiology, and CSF recurrence consistent with progressive disease. Bone marrow transplant was deferred, and the patient was admitted for hyper-CVAD chemotherapy. However, the patient requested transfer despite the worsening condition. Current clinical status is unknown.

2.2. Patient 2. Patient 2, deceased, was a 63-year-old Caucasian female with a past medical history significant for stage III invasive ductal carcinoma, ER/PR/HER2 negative, with 1 of 9 axillary lymph nodes positive for carcinoma, diagnosed at age 52. She underwent a left segmental mastectomy (lumpectomy) procedure with axillary lymph node dissection, radiation treatment, and 4 cycles of doxorubicin and cyclophosphamide chemotherapy. Other medical problems included hypertension, hyperlipidemia, herpes zoster, childhood rheumatic fever, menopause, and hypersensitivity pneumonitis.

She initially presented with a mediastinal mass, dyspnea, and pericardial and recurrent right-sided pleural effusions. Biopsy of the mediastinal mass revealed blasts with cyCD3+, TdT+, CD4+/8+, CD7+ (Figure 5). TCR gamma gene rearrangement studies demonstrated clonal gene rearrangements. The peripheral blood and bone marrow were also involved.

She was treated with 18 cycles of hyper-CVAD followed by POMP maintenance for 18 months and remained in remission for nearly 4 years. Thereafter, she developed dyspnea, and radiographic imaging showed several simultaneous masses, including a 4.7 × 4.0 cm right atrial mass and a left flank mass, in addition to pleural effusions.

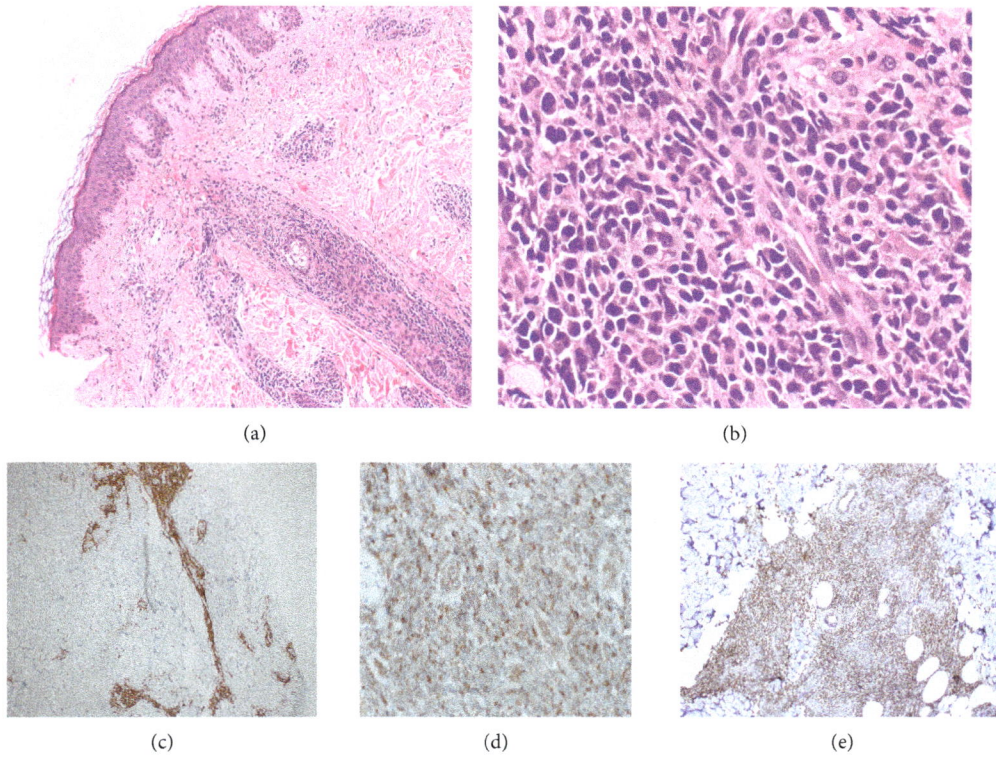

FIGURE 3: Patient 1, right flank skin with PTCL: (a) H&E, 100x; (b) H&E, 400x; (c) CD3, 100x; (d) TdT immunoperoxidase, 400x; (e) TCR gamma, 200x.

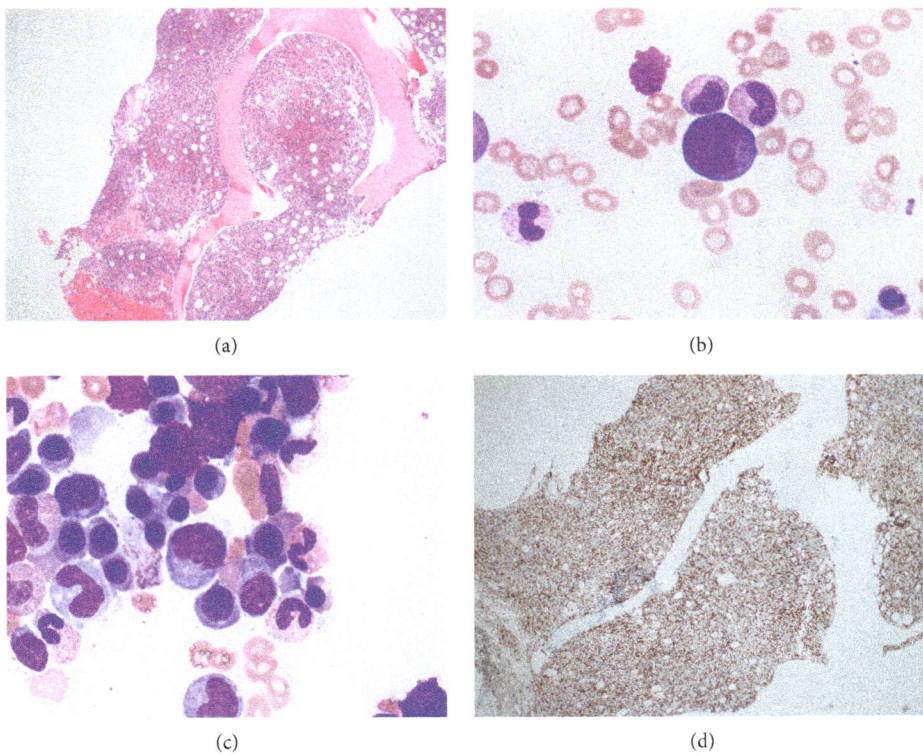

FIGURE 4: Patient 1, bone marrow with PTCL: (a) H&E, 40x; (b, c) aspirate cytology, 1000x; (d) CD3, 100x.

TABLE 1: Patient 1 pathological findings, by site.

Site (days from original diagnosis)	Diagnosis	Morphology	IHC (T-cell population of interest)	Flow (T-cell population of interest)	Gene rearrangements	Peripheral blood CBC with 100-cell differential count (%)*
Left iliac crest 0 days	T-cell ALL	Small- to medium-sized blast population comprising 95% of cells; marrow nearly 100% cellular	Positive: TdT, beta F1 Negative: TCRγ	Positive: CD3, CD4/CD8 dual positive, CD2, CD5 (d), CD7, and TDT (d) Negative: CD1a, CD34, CD117	TβA 257 TβB 269 TβC 182.9, 190.84 TγA 190.94, 214.3 TγB 172.9	WBC[a] 18.7 Hemoglobin[b] 10.5 MCV[c] 92.8 Platelets[a] 211 Lymphocytes 15 Atypical lymphocytes 0 Blasts 1
Left iliac crest 104 days	No evidence of malignancy	nc	np	nc	TβA 256 TβB 126, 263.8 TβC 190.63 TγA Germline TγB 172.4	WBC[a] 3.62 Hemoglobin[b] 10.8 MCV[c] 92.8 Platelets[a] 334 Lymphocytes 37 Atypical lymphocytes 0 Blasts 0
Cerebrospinal fluid 120 days	T-cell ALL	Large granular lymphocyte-like cells with condensed chromatin, inconspicuous nucleoli, eccentric nuclei, and moderate pale blue cytoplasm with prominent azurophilic granules	np	Positive: CD3c, CD7, CD8, CD45 (b), CD4 equivocal Negative: CD3, TdT, CD34	np	WBC[a] 2.44 Hemoglobin[b] 9.5 MCV[c] 88.3 Platelets[a] 104 Lymphocytes 34.4 Atypical lymphocytes 0 Blasts 0
Right iliac crest 124 days	γδ PTCL	Atypical lymphohistiocytic T-cell infiltrate with granulomas; large mononuclear lymphocytes with round to irregular nuclear contours and moderate eccentric light blue pale cytoplasm and cytoplasmic granules	Positive: CD2, CD3 (>50%), CD5, CD7 (f), CD8, CD56, perforin, TIA, CD4 (equivocal) Negative: TdT, CD117, CD68, CD34, CD1a, CD99, granzyme-B, CD30, CD57, CD25, ISH EBER	Positive: CD3, CD3c, CD5, CD7, CD4 (d), CD8 (d), CD45 Negative: TdT, CD34, CD56	TβA 275 TβB 126, 258, 263.8 TβC 182.92, 190.63 TγA 214.13 TγB 172.48	WBC[a] 2.56 Hemoglobin[b] 8.7 MCV[c] 88.1 Platelets[a] 76 Lymphocytes 28.9 Atypical lymphocytes 0 Blasts 0

TABLE 1: Continued.

Site (days from original diagnosis)	Diagnosis	Morphology	IHC (T-cell population of interest)	Flow (T-cell population of interest)	Gene rearrangements	Peripheral blood CBC with 100-cell differential count (%)*
				nd	np	WBC[a] 2.61 Hemoglobin[b] 9.8 MCV[c] 87.9 Platelets[a] 98 Lymphocytes 32.2 Atypical lymphocytes 0 Blasts 0
Skin, right arm 125 days	γδ PTCL	Atypical lymphoid cells	Positive: CD2, CD3, CD5, CD4, CD8, CD56, TIA, CD99 (d), granzyme-B, TCRγ Negative: CD7, TdT, CD34, CD1a			
Skin, right flank 189 days	γδ PTCL	Atypical lymphocytic infiltrate comprised of large pleomorphic with round to irregular nuclear contours and ample cytoplasm with prominent nucleoli and elevated N:C ratio	Positive: CD3, CD4, CD8, TCRγ, CD56 Negative: TdT, Beta F1, CD20	Positive: CD3, CD5, CD4/CD8 dual positive, CD45, CD56 Negative: CD7 (partial loss)	np	WBC[a] 9.1 Hemoglobin[b] 10.9 MCV[c] 95.8 Platelets[a] 58 Lymphocytes 8 Atypical lymphocytes 0 Blast 0

Note: (b) bright; (d) dim; (f) focal; (s) positive in subset. +/− equivocal; nc, noncontributory; nd, nondiagnostic due to insufficient specimen; np, not performed. [a]In k/μL; [b]in g/dL; [c]in fL. *Manual differential used when available; otherwise, automated impedance counts were utilized.

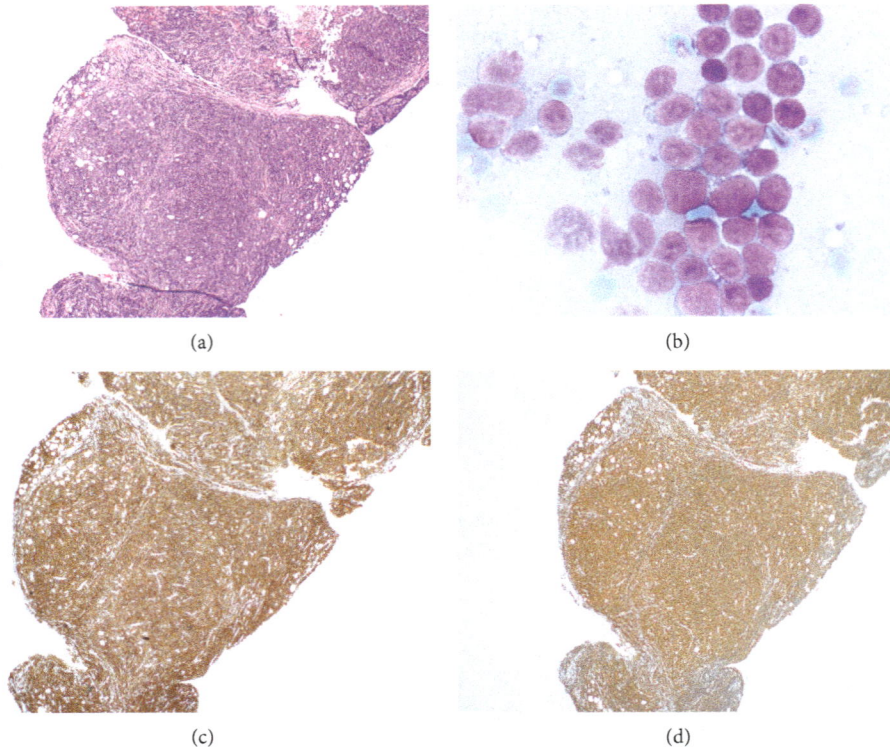

FIGURE 5: Patient 2; mediastinal mass with T-cell ALL: (a) H&E, 100x; (b) cytology, 1000x; (c) CD3, 100x; (d) TdT, 100x.

Biopsy of the atrial mass was nondiagnostic showing myocardial and fibrous tissue. The chest wall (flank) mass was biopsied showing involvement by PTCL (Figure 6). Pleural fluid analysis showed involvement by CD3+ large lymphoid cells with markedly irregular nuclear contours, cytoplasmic azurophilic granules, lacking TdT and CD7, and showing positivity for CD8. Clonal TCR β and γ gene rearrangements were detected. Staging bone marrow biopsy showed no evidence of T-ALL.

However, clonal TCR β and γ gene rearrangements were detected with a possible similar peak to that detected in the pleural effusion sample (Table 2). Shared identical clonal TCR peaks were not noted between T-ALL and PTCL specimens, but comparison is limited by the fact that TCR testing was performed in different labs and may have used disparate primer sets and analysis parameters. The patient later received 2 cycles of ESHAP resulting in partial response. However, PET scan showed SUV of 11 in the cardiac area. Romidepsin salvage chemotherapy was administered. The patient continued to have large pleural effusions with respiratory issues and eventually opted for hospice. She died 4 months after her presentation with PTCL and 50 months after her original diagnosis of T-cell ALL, at age 64.

3. Discussion

In both cases, there was relapse as PTCL manifested with skin involvement and an overt shift from blastic morphology to "LGL-like" mature T cells with ample cytoplasm and abundant azurophilic granules. Phenotypically, expression of immature markers such as TdT was lost in both cases. Both patients reasonably represent a novel phenomenon of clonal transformation from T-ALL to PTCL which has rarely been reported in the literature. In patient 1, there is clear evidence of a clonal relationship as demonstrated by identical monoclonal TCR peaks. Also, both PTCL and T-ALL cases demonstrated the relatively immature CD4+/CD8+ immunophenotype. HSTL$\gamma\delta$ are often CD4-/CD8-, recapitulating normal $\gamma\delta$ T cells, and less commonly C8+/CD4-is seen. In other $\gamma\delta$ PTCLs, CD4+/CD8− phenotype may be observed perhaps deriving from a subset of normal $\gamma\delta$ T cells that harbor this phenotype [8]. However, dual CD4+/CD8+ has not been typically reported and is difficult to explain [16]. A clonal relationship is less clear for patient 2. However, the genesis of an entirely new PTCL in a patient with established T-ALL would be unusual indeed. TCR gene rearrangements cannot be reliably compared between the original T-ALL and PTCL due to their performance in differing laboratories.

Morphologically, $\gamma\delta$ PTCLs are a heterogeneous group. However, in both our cases we find a "LGL-like" morphology with large cells with ample cytoplasm containing cytoplasmic granules further supporting the notion that a common phenomenon may be at play in these two cases. Furthermore, SNP microarray performed on patient 2's PTCL showed clonal alterations in 95% of the cells, but clonal evolution was seen in 41–55% of the cells suggesting further that this represents a type of transformation. Furthermore, homozygous interstitial deletion 14q32.2 was detected which houses *BCL11B*. *BCL11B* encodes a transcription factor

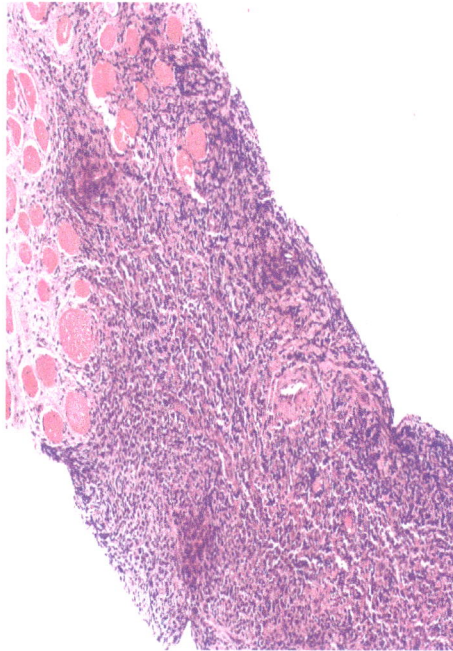

(a)

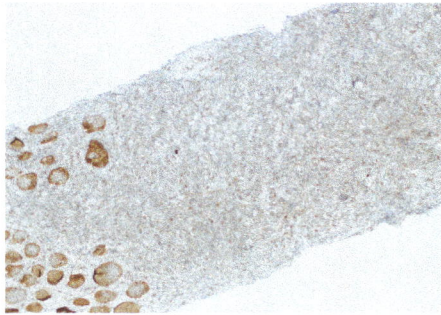

(b)

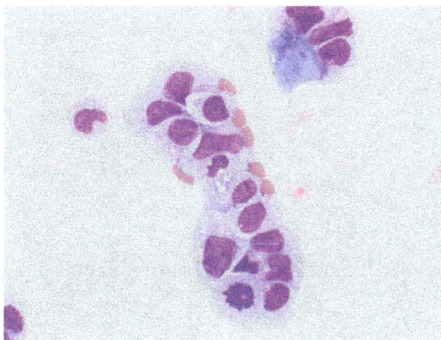

(c)

FIGURE 6: Patient 2: (a) flank mass with PTCL, H&E, 100x; (b) flank mass, TdT immunoperoxidase, 200x; (c) pleural fluid cytospin cytology, 500x.

necessary for normal T-cell development and has been implicated in T-ALL pathogenesis [17]. Another line of evidence that supports the idea that these cases may represent a novel phenomenon is the detection of aberrations occurring at similar genetic loci in both cases. In patient 1, karyotype showed 46,XY,add (13) (p11.2) [3]/46,XY[17] in the original T-ALL. In patient 2, SNP array performed on PTCL containing pleural fluid showed aberration at a similar locus: 13p11.1q24.21(34,474,059–115,670,586)x1-2.

If this truly represents transformation, we must consider the pathophysiology of such conversion. It may be postulated that chemotherapy may have forced the original T-ALL cells to undergo some degree of maturation. However, the disparate chemotherapy regimens in both cases, lack of similar conversions in other patients treated with these typical chemotherapy regimens, and temporal distance of relapse in patient 2 (3-4 years) do not support this speculation. More likely, acquisition of additional mutations in T-cell differentiation genes may have created a genetic context to allow for such transdifferentiation. This is supported by SNP array analysis performed on patient 2's PTCL showing clonal evolution. Another possibility is that malignant clones of T-ALL and PTCL developed separately from a common precursor sharing an initial transforming event. Subsequently, T-cell ALL and PTCL could evolve secondary to additional and separate transforming events.

The transformation into more aggressive disease is a rare event in T-cell lineage-derived hematologic malignancies compared to B-cell neoplasms. A patient with $\gamma\delta$-variant of LGL leukemia who developed aggressive ALL-like disorder after about 20 years of an indolent course has previously been reported [16]. Interestingly, cytology of leukemic cells during aggressive phase of disease did not differ significantly from LGLs assessed during indolent phase of disease. However, LGLs of the aggressive leukemia revealed very high Ki-67 proliferation index of 80%, and SNP array showed multiple genetic abnormalities most probably implicated in the transformation. This report supports our hypothesis that transformation in T-cell lymphomas/leukemia is a very rare event and that multiple acquired somatic mutations secondary to therapeutic or environmental factors likely facilitated the transformed phenotype.

Besides the pathophysiology, the clinical and biological nature of these transformed PTCLs can be considered challenging. Should these cases be considered "ALL-like" disorders given their putative clonal derivation from T-ALL or do they represent a new entity with unique biology? The second case was considered to be a new entity with unique biology, hence the aggressive, chemotherapy refractory course that resulted.

In summary, we report two cases of NHNC PTCL arising in patients with established diagnoses T-ALL which, in at least one case, is clonally related. This raises the possibility of a novel pathologic phenomenon with associated diagnostic and biological implications.

Conflicts of Interest

The authors declare that they have no conflicts of interest.

Acknowledgments

The authors thank the supporting staff at the Moffitt Cancer Center including the departments of Malignant Hematology and Hematopathology.

TABLE 2: Patient 2 pathological findings, by site.

Site (days from original diagnosis)	Diagnosis	Morphology	IHC (T-cell population of interest)	Flow (T-cell population of interest)	Gene rearrangements	Peripheral blood CBC with 100-cell differential count (%)*	Cytogenetics
5/2009 Mediastinal mass	T-cell ALL	Monotonous population of immature lymphoid cells with high N:C ratio, round to oval nuclei, mild nuclear irregularity, and scant cytoplasm	Positive: TdT (90%)	Positive: CD2, CD3, CD5 (d), CD7, CD4, CD8, CD45, CD10 Negative: CD20, EpCAM, Cytokeratin	TβA Germline; TβB Germline; TβC Germline; TγA Germline; TγB 185.23, 193.82	WBC[a] 6.4; Hemoglobin[b] 12.8; MCV[c] 87.2; Platelets[a] 209; Lymphocytes 18.7; Atypical lymphocytes 0; Blasts 0	No mitotic activity
Pleural fluid 17 days	T-cell ALL	Immature lymphoid blasts	Positive: CD3, CD4, CD8, TdT, CD99 Negative: CD79a	np	np	nc	
Right iliac crest 18 days	T-cell ALL	Sheets of lymphoblasts with high N:C ratio, immature chromatin, visible nucleoli, scant cytoplasm with occasional cytoplasmic vacuoles	np	Positive: CD45 (d), cyCD3, CD7, CD4, CD8, TdT (d), CD117, CD10 Negative: CD20, CD34; loss of surface CD3 and CD5	np	WBC[a] 9.94; Hemoglobin[b] 13.9; MCV[c] 86.2; Platelets[a] 262; Lymphocytes Few; Atypical lymphocytes 22; Blasts 0	
9/2009 Left iliac crest 131 days	Normocellular marrow with NEM	nc	nc	nc	Germline	nc	Normal
3/2013 Right iliac crest† 1417 days	Normocellular marrow with NEM	nc	np	nc	TβA 262.3; TβB 261.10, 266.54; TβC 188.74; TγA Germline	WBC[a] 6.39; Hemoglobin[b] 1.7; MCV[c] 90.6; Platelets[a] 165	

TABLE 2: Continued.

Site (days from original diagnosis)	Diagnosis	Morphology	IHC (T-cell population of interest)	Flow (T-cell population of interest)	Gene rearrangements	Peripheral blood CBC with 100-cell differential count (%)*	Cytogenetics
Pleural fluid 1419 days	PTCL, NOS with 75% large T-cells	Abundant large lymphoid cells with condensed chromatin, markedly irregular nuclear contours, frequent horseshoe-shaped nuclei, occasional binucleation, inconspicuous nucleoli, moderate-to-abundant pale blue cytoplasm, and cytoplasmic azurophilic granules	np	Positive: CD3c, CD8, CD45 Negative: CD3, CD7, CD4, TdT, CD117, CD20, CD34, CD56	TγB 174.32; TβA 259.6 (+/−); TβB 252.79, 272.24; TβC 326.3; TγA 208.3, 216.77; TγB Germline	Lymphocytes 19.7; Atypical lymphocytes 0; Blasts 0; WBC[a] 6.12; Hemoglobin[b] 10.4; MCV[c] 91.5; Platelets[a] 190; Lymphocytes 19.6; Atypical lymphocytes 0; Blasts 0	SNP ARRAY
3/2013 Left chest wall mass 1419 days	PTCL, NOS**	Skeletal muscle extensively involved by a diffuse infiltrate of large lymphoid cells with granular chromatin, marked nuclear pleomorphism, markedly irregular nuclear contours, occasional horseshoe-shaped nuclei, and occasional conspicuous nucleoli	Positive: CD2, CD3, CD8 (b), ki67 (80%) Negative: CD5, CD7, CD4, TdT, CD15, CD20, CD30, CD34, CD56, pan-keratin, PAX5, EBV-LMP, EBER	np	np	nc	

TABLE 2: Continued.

Site (days from original diagnosis)	Diagnosis	Morphology	IHC (T-cell population of interest)	Flow (T-cell population of interest)	Gene rearrangements	Peripheral blood CBC with 100-cell differential count (%)*	Cytogenetics
Left flank mass	PTCL, NOS	Large lymphoid cells with granular chromatin, marked nuclear pleomorphism, markedly irregular nuclear contours, occasional horseshoe-shaped nuclei, occasional conspicuous nucleoli, moderate pale eosinophilic cytoplasm, and abundant cytotoxic granules	Positive: CD3 (b), granzyme-B Negative: CD5, TdT, CD20, CD30, CD34, ALK-1, CD1a, myeloperoxidase, EBER ISH	Not representative			

Note: (b) bright; (d) dim; (f) focal; (s) positive in subset; +/− equivocal. NEM, no evidence of malignancy; nc, noncontributory; nd, nondiagnostic due to insufficient specimen; np, not performed. [a]In k/μL; [b]in g/dL; [c]in fL. *Manual differential used when available; otherwise, automated impedance counts were utilized. †The IHC profile is from a chest wall mass biopsy taken on the same day. This biopsy had a dense atypical lymphocytic infiltrate. **Flow photocytometry demonstrated a 5% population of small T-cells. Limited material hindered full evaluation.

References

[1] E. A. Swerdlow, *WHO Classification of Tumours of the Haematopoietic and Lymphoid Tissues*, IARC, Lyon, France, 4th edition, 2008.

[2] C. Terhorst, J. de Vries, K. Georgopoulos et al., "The T cell receptor/T3 complex," *Year in Immunology*, vol. 2, pp. 245–253, 1986.

[3] M. Calvaruso, A. Gulino, S. Buffa et al., "Challenges and new prospects in hepatosplenic γδ T-cell lymphoma," *Leukemia & Lymphoma*, vol. 55, no. 11, pp. 2457–2465, 2014.

[4] P. Gaulard and L. de Leval, "Pathology of peripheral T-cell lymphomas: where do we stand?," *Seminars in Hematology*, vol. 51, no. 1, pp. 5–16, 2014.

[5] P. Gaulard, T. Henni, J. P. Marolleau et al., "Lethal midline granuloma (polymorphic reticulosis) and lymphomatoid granulomatosis. Evidence for a monoclonal T-cell lymphoproliferative disorder," *Cancer*, vol. 62, no. 4, pp. 705–710, 1988.

[6] T. Saito, Y. Matsuno, R. Tanosaki, T. Watanabe, Y. Kobayashi, and K. Tobinai, "γδ T-cell neoplasms: a clinicopathological study of 11 cases," *Annals of Oncology*, vol. 13, no. 11, pp. 1792–1798, 2002.

[7] S. Al Omran, W. A. Mourad, and M. A. Ali, "Gamma/delta peripheral T-cell lymphoma of the breast diagnosed by fine-needle aspiration biopsy," *Diagnostic Cytopathology*, vol. 26, no. 3, pp. 170–173, 2002.

[8] P. Gaulard, K. Belhadj, and F. Reyes, "γδ T-cell lymphomas," *Seminars in Hematology*, vol. 40, no. 3, pp. 233–243, 2003.

[9] A. S. Bourgault-Rouxel, T. P. Loughran Jr., R. Zambello et al., "Clinical spectrum of γδ+ T cell LGL leukemia: analysis of 20 cases," *Leukemia Research*, vol. 32, no. 1, pp. 45–48, 2008.

[10] S. Lepretre, G. Buchonnet, A. Stamatoullas et al., "Chromosome abnormalities in peripheral T-cell lymphoma," *Cancer Genetics and Cytogenetics*, vol. 117, no. 1, pp. 71–79, 2000.

[11] F. Vega, L. J. Medeiros, and P. Gaulard, "Hepatosplenic and other γΔ T-cell lymphomas," *American Journal of Clinical Pathology*, vol. 127, no. 6, pp. 869–880, 2007.

[12] K. Miyazaki, M. Yamaguchi, H. Imai et al., "Gene expression profiling of peripheral T-cell lymphoma including γδ T-cell lymphoma," *Blood*, vol. 113, no. 5, pp. 1071–1074, 2009.

[13] B. T. Tan, K. Seo, R. A. Warnke, and D. A. Arber, "The frequency of immunoglobulin heavy chain gene and T-cell receptor γ-chain gene rearrangements and Epstein-Barr virus in ALK$^+$ and ALK$^-$ anaplastic large cell lymphoma and other peripheral T-cell lymphomas," *Journal of Molecular Diagnostics*, vol. 10, no. 6, pp. 502–512, 2008.

[14] C. Schutzinger, H. Esterbauer, G. Hron et al., "Prognostic value of T-cell receptor gamma rearrangement in peripheral blood or bone marrow of patients with peripheral T-cell lymphomas," *Leukemia & Lymphoma*, vol. 49, no. 2, pp. 237–246, 2008.

[15] J. Iqbal, D. D. Weisenburger, A. Chowdhury et al., "Natural killer cell lymphoma shares strikingly similar molecular features with a group of non-hepatosplenic γδ T-cell lymphoma and is highly sensitive to a novel aurora kinase A inhibitor in vitro," *Leukemia*, vol. 25, no. 2, pp. 348–358, 2011.

[16] L. Zhang, R. Ramchandren, P. Papenhausen, T. P. Loughran, and L. Sokol, "Transformed aggressive γδ-variant T-cell large granular lymphocytic leukemia with acquired copy neutral loss of heterozygosity at 17q11.2q25.3 and additional aberrations," *European Journal of Haematology*, vol. 93, no. 3, pp. 260–264, 2014.

[17] A. Gutierrez, A. Kentsis, T. Sanda et al., "The BCL11B tumor suppressor is mutated across the major molecular subtypes of T-cell acute lymphoblastic leukemia," *Blood*, vol. 118, no. 15, pp. 4169–4173, 2011.

Permissions

List of Contributors

Mihaela Găman, Ana-Maria Vlădăreanu, Camelia Dobrea, Minodora Onisâi, Cristina Marinescu, Irina Voican, Daniela Vasile, Horia Bumbea and Diana Cîşleanu
Carol Davila University of Medicine and Pharmacy, Bucharest, Romania

Mihaela Găman, Ana-Maria Vlădăreanu, Minodora Onisâi, Cristina Marinescu, Irina Voican, Daniela Vasile, Horia Bumbea and Diana Cîşleanu
Department of Hematology, University Emergency Hospital Bucharest, Bucharest, Romania

Aristides Armas, Martha Mims and Gustavo Riveros
Baylor St. Luke's Medical Center, Houston, TX 77030, USA

Chen Chen, Martha Mims and Gustavo Rivero
Baylor College of Medicine, Section of Hematology and Oncology, 1 Baylor Plaza, Houston, TX 77030, USA
Department of Pathology, Baylor College of Medicine, 1 Baylor Plaza, Houston, TX 77030, USA
The Dan L. Duncan Comprehensive Cancer Center at Baylor College of Medicine, 1 Baylor Plaza, Houston, TX 77030, USA

Geoffrey Shouse
Division of Hematology and Oncology, Loma Linda University School of Medicine, Loma Linda, CA, USA

Miemie Thinn
Division of Hematology and Medical Oncology, Loma Linda Veterans Administration Medical Center, Loma Linda, CA, USA

Ensi Voshtina
Department of Medicine, Medical College of Wisconsin, Milwaukee, WI, USA

Huiya Huang
Department of Pathology, Medical College of Wisconsin, Milwaukee, WI, USA

Renju Raj and Ehab Atallah
Department of Hematology and Oncology, Medical College of Wisconsin, Milwaukee, WI, USA

Zurab Azmaiparashvili, Vinicius M. Jorge and Catiele Antunes
Albert Einstein Medical Center, Philadelphia, PA, USA

Abhishek Mangaonkar, Hassan Al Khateeb, Narjust Duma, Mrinal Patnaik, William Hogan, Mark Litzow and Taxiarchis Koureliss
Division of Hematology, Department of Medicine, Mayo Clinic, Rochester, MN, USA

Erik K. St. Louis and Andrew McKeon
Department of Neurology, Mayo Clinic, Rochester, MN, USA

James C. Barton
Department of Medicine, University of Alabama at Birmingham, Birmingham, AL, USA
Southern Iron Disorders Center, Birmingham, AL, USA
Department of Medicine, Brookwood Medical Center, Birmingham, AL, USA

Hayward S. Edmunds Jr.
Cunningham Pathology Associates, Birmingham, AL, USA

Dhauna Karam, Sean Swiatkowski, Mamata Ravipati and Bharat Agrawal
Rosalind Franklin University, 3333 Green Bay Road, North Chicago, IL 60064, USA
Captain James A. Lovell Federal Health Care Center, 3001 Green Bay Road, North Chicago, IL 60064, USA

Suheil Albert Atallah-Yunes and Myat Han Soe
Department of Medicine, Baystate–University of Massachusetts Medical School, Springfield, MA, USA

Alba Colell and Adrià Arboix
Cerebrovascular Division, Department of Neurology, Hospital Universitari del SagratCor, Universitat de Barcelona, Barcelona, Catalonia, Spain

Francesco Caiazzo
Department of Neurosurgery, Hospital Universitari del SagratCor, Universitat de Barcelona, Barcelona, Catalonia, Spain

Elisenda Grivé
Department of Neuroradiology, Hospital Universitari del SagratCor, Universitat de Barcelona, Barcelona, Catalonia, Spain

Yasuhiro Tanaka, Atsushi Tanaka, Akiko Hashimoto and Isaku Shinzato
Department of Hematology and Clinical Immunology, Nishi-Kobe Medical Center, Hyogo, Japan

Kumiko Hayashi
Molecular Genetic Analysis Department, LSI Medience Corporation, Tokyo, Japan

Martina Pennisi, Micol Giulia Cittone, Valentina Mancini and Roberto Cairoli
Division of Hematology, Niguarda Ca' Granda Hospital, Milan, Italy

Clara Cesana, Laura Bandiera, Barbara Scarpati, Silvia Soriani, Silvio Veronese, Mauro Truini and Silvano Rossini
Department of Laboratory Medicine, Niguarda Ca' Granda Hospital, Milan, Italy

Agata M. Bogusz
Department of Pathology and Laboratory Medicine, Hospital of the University of Pennsylvania, Philadelphia, PA 19104-4283, USA

Koken Ameku and Mariko Higa
Department of Respiratory Medicine, Okinawa Prefectural Nanbu Medical Center and Children's Medical Center, Okinawa, Japan

Jessica Corean and K. David Li
Department of Pathology, ARUP Laboratories, University of Utah, Salt Lake City, UT, USA

Khaled Algashaamy, Yaohong Tan, Nicolas Mackrides, Jing-Hong Peng, Joseph Rosenblatt, Juan P Alderuccio, Izidore S. Lossos, Francisco Vega and Jennifer Chapman
Department of Pathology, Division of Hematopathology, University of Miami, Sylvester Comprehensive Cancer Center and Jackson Memorial Hospital, Miami, Florida, USA

Alvaro Alencar, Joseph Rosenblatt, Juan P Alderuccio, Izidore S. Lossos and Francisco Vega
Department of Medicine, Division of Hematology-Oncology, University of Miami, Sylvester Comprehensive Cancer Center and Jackson Memorial Hospital, Miami, Florida, USA

Jasjit Kaur Rooprai
Faculty of Medicine, University of Ottawa, Ottawa, Ontario, Canada

Karima Khamisa
Division of Hematology, Department of Medicine, e Ottawa Hospital, Ottawa, Ontario, Canada

Panayotis Kaloyannidis, Eshrak Al Shaibani, Ioannis Apostolidis, Hani Al Hashmi and Khalid Ahmed Al Anazi
Adults Hematology and Stem Cell Transplantation Department, King Fahad Specialist Hospital, Dammam, Saudi Arabia

Miral Mashhour
Department of Pathology and Laboratory Medicine, King Fahad Specialist Hospital, Dammam, Saudi Arabia

Mohammed Gamil
Dermatology Department, King Fahad Specialist Hospital, Dammam, Saudi Arabia

Vikrant Singh Bhar and Vasudha Gupta
Associate Consultant, Department of Haematopathology, Artemis Hospitals, Gurgaon, India

Mahak Sharma
Senior Resident, Department of Haematopathology, Artemis Hospitals, Gurgaon, India

Rishi Dhawan
Assistant Professor, Department of Hematology, AIIMS, New Delhi, India

Shilpi Modi
Associate Consultant, Department of Histopathology, Artemis Hospitals, Gurgaon, India

Mona Vijyaran
Associate Consultant, Department of Hematooncology, Artemis Hospitals, Gurgaon, India

Nieves Gascón, Héctor Pérez-Montero, Sandra Guardado, Rafael D'Ambrosi, María Ángeles Cabeza and José Fermín Pérez-Regadera
Radiation Oncology Department, Hospital Universitario 12 de Octubre, Madrid, Spain

Dina Sameh Soliman, Ahmad Al-Sabbagh, Feryal Ibrahim, Zafar Nawaz, Abdulrazzaq Haider and Susanna Akiki
Department of Laboratory Medicine and Pathology, National Center for Cancer Care and Research, Hamad Medical Corporation, Doha, Qatar

Dina Sameh Soliman
Department of Clinical Pathology, National Cancer Institute, Cairo University, Cairo, Egypt

Ruba Y. Taha, Sarah Elkourashy and Mohamed Yassin
Department of Hematology and Medical Oncology, National Center for Cancer Care and Research, Hamad Medical Corporation, Doha, Qatar

Sameera A. Alsafwani
Qatif Central Hospital (QCH), Qatif, Saudi Arabia

Abdulwahed Al-Saeed
Dammam Medical Complex (DMC), Dammam, Saudi Arabia

Rehab Bukhamsin
Dammam Regional Laboratory and Blood Bank (DRL),
Dammam, Saudi Arabia

Fares Darawshy, Issam Hendi, Ayman Abu Rmelieh and Tawfik Khoury
Department of Medicine, Hadassah-Hebrew University Medical Center, Jerusalem, Israel

Yosef Kalish
Department of Hematology, Hadassah-Hebrew University Medical Center, Jerusalem, Israel

Thamer Kassim, Lakshmi Chintalacheruvu, Osman Bhatty, Mohammad Selim, Osama Diab, Ali Nayfeh and Maryam Gbadamosi-Akindele
Department of Internal Medicine, Creighton University, Omaha, NE, USA

Jayadev Manikkam Umakanthan
University of Nebraska Medical Center, Omaha, NE, USA

William A. Hammond, Pooja Advani and James M. Foran
Division of Hematology and Oncology, Mayo Clinic, Jacksonville, FL, USA

William A. Hammond
Baptist MD Anderson Cancer Center, Jacksonville, FL, USA

Rhett P. Ketterling and Daniel Van Dyke
Division of Laboratory Medicine and Pathology, Mayo Clinic, Rochester, MN, USA

Liuyan Jiang
Division of Laboratory Medicine and Pathology, Mayo Clinic, Jacksonville, FL, USA

Amy G. Starr, Joeffrey J. Chahine and Bhaskar V. Kallakury
MedStar Georgetown University Hospital, Department of Pathology, 3800 Reservoir Rd NW, Medical Dental Building, SE 200, Washington, DC 20007, USA

Sushma R. Jonna and Chaitra S. Ujjani
Lombardi Comprehensive Cancer Center, Department of Hematology and Oncology, MedStar Georgetown University Hospital, 3800 Reservoir Rd. NW, Washington, DC 20007, USA

Elham Vali Betts, Denis M. Dwyre and Hooman H. Rashidi
Department of Pathology and Laboratory Medicine, University of California, Davis, Davis, CA, USA

Huan-You Wang
Department of Pathology, University of California, San Diego, La Jolla, CA, USA

Stephen E. Langabeer and Lisa Preston
Cancer Molecular Diagnostics, St. James's Hospital, Dublin 8, Ireland

Johanna Kelly
Department of Clinical Genetics, Our Lady's Children Hospital, Dublin 12, Ireland

Matt Goodyer, Ezzat Elhassadi and Amjad Hayat
Department of Haematology, Galway University Hospital, Galway, Ireland

Takanori Fukuta, Takayuki Tanaka, Yoshinori Hashimoto and Hiromi Omura
Department of Hematology, Tottori Prefectural Central Hospital, Tottori, Japan

Vadim R. Gorodetskiy and Vladimir I. Vasilyev
Department of Intensive Methods of Therapy, V.A. Nasonova Research Institute of Rheumatology, Kashirskoye Shosse 34A, Moscow 115522, Russia

Wolfram Klapper
Department of Pathology, Hematopathology Section and Lymph Node Registry, Christian-Albrecht University Kiel and University Hospital Schleswig-Holstein, 24105 Kiel, Germany

Natalya A. Probatova
Department of Pathology, N.N. Blokhin Russian Cancer Research Center, Kashirskoye Shosse 24, Moscow 115478, Russia

Elena V. Rozhnova
Department of Therapeutic Dentistry, I.M. Sechenov First Moscow State Medical University, Trubetskaya, 8, Building 2, Moscow 119991, Russia

Andrew C. Tiu
Department of Medicine, Einstein Medical Center, Philadelphia, PA, USA

Rashmika Potdar and Mark Morginstin
Division of Hematology and Medical Oncology, Einstein Medical Center, Philadelphia, PA, USA

Vivian Arguello-Gerra
Department of Pathology and Laboratory Medicine, Einstein Medical Center, Philadelphia, PA, USA

Eric Granowicz
Scripps Mercy Hospital, Department of Internal Medicine, San Diego, CA, USA

Kiyon Chung
Scripps Mercy Hospital, Department of Cardiology, San Diego, CA, USA

X. A. Andrade, H. E. Fuentes and H. Manns
Department of Medicine, John H. Stroger Jr. Hospital of Cook County, Chicago, IL, USA

D. M. Oramas
Division of Pathology, University of Illinois at Chicago, Chicago, IL, USA

P. Kovarik
Department of Pathology, John H. Stroger Jr. Hospital of Cook County, Chicago, IL, USA

D. Swan and E. Elhassadi
Haematology Department, University Hospital Waterford, Regional Cancer Center South East, University College Cork, Cork, Ireland

M. Murphy
Pathology Department, University HospitalWaterford, Regional Cancer Center South East, University College Cork, Cork, Ireland

Hanyin Wang
Department of Internal Medicine, Tufts Medical Center, 800 Washington St., Boston, MA 02111, USA

Hande Tuncer
Division of Hematology/Oncology, Tufts Medical Center, 800 Washington St, Boston, MA 02111, USA

Kirill A. Lyapichev, Jennifer R. Chapman, Oleksii Iakymenko, Offiong F. Ikpatt, Sandra Patricia Sanchez and Francisco Vega
Division of Hematopathology, Department of Pathology and Laboratory Medicine, University of Miami and Sylvester Comprehensive Cancer Center, Miami, FL, USA

Uygar Teomete
Department of Radiology, University of Miami and Sylvester Comprehensive Cancer Center, Miami, FL, USA

Francisco Vega
Division of Hematology-Oncology, Department of Medicine, University of Miami and Sylvester Comprehensive Cancer Center, Miami, FL, USA

Yekaterina Kim and Daniel C. Choi
Montefiore Medical Center, Albert Einstein College of Medicine, Bronx, NY, USA

Ali N. Zaidi
Montefiore Heart and Vascular Care Center, Albert Einstein College of Medicine, Bronx, NY, USA

H. Coelho, M. Badior and T. Melo
Serviço de Hematologia, Centro Hospitalar de Vila Nova de Gaia/Espinho, Vila Nova Gaia, Portugal

David Ferreira and Royston Ponraj
Conjoint Associate Lecturer, University of New South Wales, Sydney, Australia
Medical Department, Medical Registrar, Liverpool Hospital, Elizabeth St., Liverpool, NSW 2170, Australia

Adrian Yeung
Haematology Department, Haematology Advanced Trainee, Liverpool Hospital, Elizabeth St., Liverpool, NSW 2170, Australia

Jillian de Malmanche
Haematology Department, Haematology Staff Specialist, John Hunter Hospital, Lookout Rd., New Lambton Heights, NSW 2305, Australia

Stephen E. Langabeer and Karl Haslam
Cancer Molecular Diagnostics, St. James's Hospital, Dublin 8, Ireland

Maria Anne Smyth, John Quinn and Philip T. Murphy
Department of Haematology, Beaumont Hospital, Dublin 9, Ireland

Shyam Ravisankar and Maya Shah
Division of Hematology and Oncology, Newark Beth Israel Medical Center, Newark, NJ, USA

Yair Levy
Department of Radiology, Newark Beth Israel Medical Center, Newark, NJ, USA

Naomi Fei and Sarah Sofka
Department of Internal Medicine, West Virginia University Hospital, 1 Medical Center Dr., Morgantown, WV 26505, USA

Andrew Chu, Thu Thu Aung, Mauricio Danckers, Mohi Mitiek and Jonathan Leslie
Internal Medicine Residency Department, Aventura Hospital and Medical Center, 20900 Biscayne Boulevard, Aventura, FL 33190, USA

Minni Shreya Arumugam
Internal Medicine Residency Department, SUNY Upstate Medical University, 750 East Adams Street, Syracuse, NY 13210, USA

Michael Markow
Department of Pathology, Ohio State University, Columbus, OH, USA

Abu-Sayeef Mirza
Department of Internal Medicine, University of South Florida, Tampa, FL, USA

Lia Perez
Bone Marrow Transplant Program, Moffitt Cancer Center, Tampa, FL, USA

Haipeng Shao, Claudio Anasetti, Lubomir Sokol and Mohammad O. Hussaini
Moffitt Cancer Center, Tampa, FL, USA

Index

www.ingramcontent.com/pod-product-compliance
Lightning Source LLC
Chambersburg PA
CBHW080522200326
41458CB00012B/4297